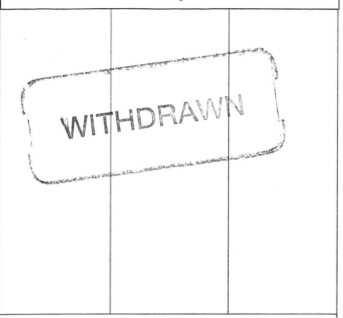

Risks and Challenges in Medical Tourism

Risks and Challenges in Medical Tourism

Understanding the Global Market for Health Services

**Jill R. Hodges, Leigh Turner, and
Ann Marie Kimball, Editors**

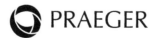 PRAEGER

AN IMPRINT OF ABC-CLIO, LLC
Santa Barbara, California • Denver, Colorado • Oxford, England

Library of Congress Cataloging-in-Publication Data

Risks and challenges in medical tourism: understanding the global market for health services / Jill R. Hodges, Leigh Turner, and Ann Marie Kimball, editors.
   p. ; cm.
  Includes bibliographical references and index.
  ISBN 978-0-313-39935-0 (hardcopy : alk. paper) — ISBN 978-0-313-39936-7 (e-ISBN)
  I. Hodges, Jill R.   II. Turner, Leigh.   III. Kimball, Ann Marie.
  [DNLM: 1. Medical Tourism.   2. Bioethical Issues.   3. Health Expenditures.
4. Health Services Accessibility.   5. Internationality. W 84.1]

   362.1—dc23   2012008764

ISBN: 978-0-313-39935-0
EISBN: 978-0-313-39936-7

16 15 14 13 12   1 2 3 4 5

This book is also available on the World Wide Web as an eBook.
Visit www.abc-clio.com for details.

Praeger
An Imprint of ABC-CLIO, LLC

ABC-CLIO, LLC
130 Cremona Drive, P.O. Box 1911
Santa Barbara, California 93116-1911

This book is printed on acid-free paper ∞

Manufactured in the United States of America

Contents

PART II. BORDER CROSSINGS: RISKS, CONTROVERSIES, AND CONSEQUENCES

PART III. LEGAL AND REGULATORY QUESTIONS

PART IV. ETHICAL CONSIDERATIONS

Chapter 1

Introduction: Health Care Goes Global

Leigh Turner and Jill R. Hodges

Patients now have access to a global marketplace for health services. Even a cursory Internet search reveals a multitude of hospitals, clinics, and medical tourism companies marketing knee surgeries, dental implants, in vitro fertilization, stem cell therapies, kidney transplants, cosmetic treatments, and "wellness" tours, among other services. Many of these offerings include package deals that bundle medical care with air travel, ground transport, hotel accommodations, and guided tours. Some countries, such as Singapore and India, have national medical tourism initiatives to attract foreign investment and revenues, and other nations are building large "medi-cities" to accommodate international patients. There are media reports of botched bariatric procedures[1] and life-saving surgeries abroad;[2] superbugs crossing borders via patients;[3] and illegal and yet readily accessible markets for human organs.[4] We read that Apple founder Steve Jobs went from the United States to Switzerland to receive a special cancer treatment;[5] that Pakistan President Asif Ali Zardari traveled to Dubai to monitor a heart condition;[6] that National Football League quarterback Peyton Manning flew to Europe for a stem cell procedure intended to treat his injured neck;[7] and that ordinary citizens are combining trips for colonoscopies with deep sea fishing and zip lining adventures in Costa Rica.[8] Reports from national ministries, business consulting firms, and industry groups claim that medical tourism is an expanding, multibillion-dollar global industry.

Despite the attention medical tourism receives in both popular media and scholarly literature, much about this phenomenon is poorly documented and superficially analyzed. Researchers disagree about what exactly the term "medical tourism" encompasses, how many people actually engage in it, and how increased medical tourism may affect both "sending" and "receiving" nations. While we know that patients increasingly are crossing national borders and seeking health care at international medical facilities, there are many gaps in our understanding of how the global health care marketplace is developing and what impact it has, or will have, upon public health, health systems, and health human resources in both the countries from which patients depart and the countries to which they travel for medical care. This book tries to fill some of these gaps. The chapters that follow examine various dimensions of medical tourism using a variety of research methods and interpretive lenses drawn from such fields as anthropology, bioethics, economics, geography, legal studies, medicine, and public health.

A MULTIFACETED LOOK AT MEDICAL TOURISM

This volume is organized in four sections that provide a multidisciplinary examination of key facets of the medical tourism industry. The first section, which includes chapters 2–5, examines medical tourism in the context of four significant and very different regions. The second section, chapters 6–8, explores some of the risks and controversies that arise with a global health care market, from cross-border spread of disease to the emergence of organ markets and exploitation of vulnerable people. In the third section, chapters 9–11 explore what legal and regulatory frameworks exist to address these and other concerns. Chapters 12 and 13 investigate various ethical implications of the global market for health care. Finally, we conclude with an examination of what can and should be done to address some of the major risks related to medical tourism and the globalization of health services.

DRIVERS, DEPARTURE POINTS, AND DESTINATIONS

In chapter 2, a team of researchers from Rush University and University HealthSystem Consortium (UHC) examine medical tourism to and from the United States. The United States has for decades been a major destination country for patients traveling to access advanced technologies. While the United States continues to attract medical tourists seeking state-of-the art treatments and medical expertise, it also has become a significant source of outbound medical travelers due to its comparatively high health care costs and the growing number of U.S. residents without health insurance. Rush University economist Tricia J. Johnson and colleagues Andrew

Garman, Samuel F. Hohmann, Steven Meurer, and Molly Allen describe the current dynamics as hospitals, clinics, and commerce and trade organizations in the United States attempt to attract and retain more international patients.

In chapter 3, health economist Richard D. Smith and sociologist Helena Legido-Quigley of the London School of Hygiene and Tropical Medicine, along with Neil Lunt and Daniel Horsfall of the University of York, explore medical tourism in the European Union (EU), another region known for both inbound and outbound flows of patients. In contrast to the United States, in the European Union, universal health care predominates, and patients tend to travel to expedite access to medical services or to obtain access to procedures that are not available in their home countries. Of particular interest in this region is the extent of cross-border travel among neighboring nations and the recently adopted Directive on the Application of Patients' Rights in Cross-Border Health Care. In addition to articulating the rights of medical travelers within EU member states, the Directive establishes common standards for different aspects of care to foster better continuity and collaboration among health care providers.

In chapter 4, Mahidol University sociologist Churnrurtai Kanchanachitra and colleagues examine medical tourism in Southeast Asia, one of the most dynamic and important destinations for medical travelers. The chapter examines four nations with different economies and health systems: Malaysia, the Philippines, Singapore, and Thailand. Despite their differences, all four countries embrace medical tourism on a national level as a revenue-generating strategy intended to promote economic development. These countries invest significant resources in supporting and promoting the industry, partly in response to the 1997 financial crisis that left many private hospital beds unoccupied. Joining Kanchanachitra in this analysis are Manuel M. Dayrit of the World Health Organization (WHO) and Cha-aim Pachanee and Viroj Tangcharoensathien of the International Health Policy Program (IHPP) in Thailand's Ministry of Public Health. The authors highlight how each of these countries struggles to promote economic development through medical tourism without draining resources from their public health systems and undermining health equity.

In chapter 5, University of Colorado, Denver-based anthropologist Courtney A. Lee investigates a similar struggle in the context of Latin America. Lee provides an ethnographic profile of Costa Rica, a country with a highly successful socialized medical system that in recent years has sought to attract medical tourists and expanded its private, for-profit health sector. Drawing upon interviews with providers, government officials, and business representatives as well as patient surveys, this chapter provides a detailed account of the experiences and concerns of Costa Ricans as their nation opens its borders to patients traveling from other countries.

RISKS, CONTROVERSIES, AND CONSEQUENCES

In chapter 6, Seattle-based health policy analyst Jill R. Hodges and epidemiologist and physician Ann Marie Kimball examine medical travel's potential role in the spread of infectious disease. This concern took on increased significance when researchers proposed that medical travel facilitated the migration of the gene that makes the multidrug resistant enzyme NDM-1 from India and Pakistan to various European destinations in 2009–2010.[9] The chapter illustrates how medical travel combines two practices known to contribute to the spread of disease—travel and hospital stays—theoretically elevating the risk of dissemination, particularly when patients with compromised immune systems are involved.

Chapter 7 investigates the global markets for commercial organ transplantation and unproven stem cell treatments, which have experienced significant growth in the last decade. Melbourne-based bioethicist and physician Dominique Martin describes why these markets, in which patients suffering from chronic or life-threatening diseases embark on desperate searches for treatment, represent some of the most dangerous dimensions of medical travel. Similarly, individuals selling organs, who are typically people with few resources, are vulnerable to coercion that may result in choices that can endanger their lives.

Comparable forces are at play in the transnational market for reproductive services, the subject that anthropologist Andrea Whittaker, an Australian Research Council Future Fellow at Monash University, explores in chapter 8. Couples and individuals hoping to conceive a child may travel thousands of miles and undertake multiple trips and stays of several months to access a variety of resources and procedures. These cross-continental quests can have health and ethical implications for the couples themselves, the surrogates and donors enlisted to participate in the process, and the resulting children. At times, these procedures can involve exchanges among three or even four countries, depending on where the procedure takes place and who is involved.

LEGAL AND REGULATORY QUESTIONS

Potentially increasing the risks associated with medical tourism is the fact that it in many respects occurs in a regulatory vacuum. As Southern Methodist University Law Professor Nathan Cortez observes, while the health care industry is highly regulated in the United States, the global market for health services operates for the most part without effective regulatory frameworks. In chapter 9, Cortez considers several of the major legal issues related to medical tourism, including what legal remedies are available to patients who experience problems with treatments abroad, and whether it is legal for insurance companies to ask patients to travel across borders for care.

Chapter 10 addresses legal questions that arise in the case of what Harvard Law Professor I. Glenn Cohen calls "circumvention tourism." This practice, Cohen writes, involves travel to obtain services that are not legal in a patient's home country but are legal in the treating country. He examines this issue in the context of four cases—assisted suicide, female genital cutting, abortion, and surrogacy. In each case, he explores whether countries can or should criminally prosecute citizens who undertake travel for these services.

In chapter 11, Stephen T. Green, an infectious disease specialist and a director of the UK-based QHA Trent Accreditation Scheme, and Hannah King of the Department of Social Policy and Social Work at the University of York, consider accreditation of international clinics and hospitals as one significant tool for establishing global standards. While accreditation is voluntary, many facilities targeting medical travelers consider it a critical credential that signals an international level of quality in their facilities. This chapter examines the relationship between accreditation and quality of care, along with related issues, including whether uniform, one-size-fits-all accreditation standards are appropriate or feasible, and whether the high cost of undergoing accreditation review unfairly disadvantages low-resource facilities that nonetheless provide good quality care.

ETHICAL ISSUES

Our final chapters review the risks, controversies, and ethical issues that emerge when patients shop for care in the global health services marketplace. In chapter 12, Leigh Turner, of the University of Minnesota's Center for Bioethics, identifies the risks medical tourism poses to patients, public health, and health systems. Turner argues that while medical tourism can benefit individual patients and might in some instances generate benefits for health systems, there also are many risks associated with the expansion of medical tourism and globalization of health services. Among the risks he examines are inadequate disclosure to medical tourists of the risks and benefits of particular medical procedures, disruption of the continuum of health care, inadequate quality of care, fraud, and lack of sufficient privacy protections. Turner also argues that sending and receiving health systems face risks, including the costs of treating medical tourists who return with postoperative complications, and the potential for undermining health equity in medical tourism destinations.

In chapter 13, Simon Fraser University bioethicist Jeremy Snyder, health geographer Valorie A. Crooks, and colleagues Alexandra Wright and Rory Johnston review some of the ethical issues surrounding the medical tourism facilitators that market and coordinate medical travel. They examine the many roles that facilitators play, from travel agents to medical advisors, as well as the training and qualifications that facilitators may or may not have to effectively serve their clients. The authors also address the conflicts of interest that can arise when the people who are advising patients and arranging for their care are paid by medical providers who want to sell their services.

In chapter 14, we conclude by examining the composite that results from this multidisciplinary, global exploration by some of the leading researchers investigating medical tourism and the globalization of health care. We discuss what their analyses reveal about the expanding and dynamic industry of medical tourism as well as what remains to be investigated. In addition, we highlight critical issues and potential policy responses that require consideration if this market continues to grow.

It is important to note that while this collection provides a rich and wide-ranging examination of medical tourism, it does not attempt to address every aspect of this continually evolving and complex industry. Critical regions such as India and China are addressed only briefly. In addition, our book does not offer detailed analyses of the dynamics of medical tourism and regional and bilateral trade agreements. Rather than attempting to provide an all-encompassing "final word" on medical tourism—an impossible task given the scope of the subject and the rapidity with which this market is changing—we regard this book as an attempt to enrich, expand, and deepen current debates concerning the ethical, legal, public health, and social dimensions of medical tourism and the globalization of health services.

WHAT DO WE MEAN BY MEDICAL TOURISM?

While the phrase "medical tourism" is commonly used to describe the movement of patients across borders, it is a contested concept used in at least four distinct ways. The phrase serves to describe health care providers who travel to under-resourced settings and provide medical care for a brief period, individuals who travel to other countries to obtain free access to medical interventions provided by publicly funded health care systems, individuals who travel solely to access health care services, and individuals who travel for medical care and engage in side trips or other activities commonly associated with tourism. Acknowledging the multiple ways in which the phrase medical tourism is used, and recognizing that the term is in many respects more a marketing device than a serious analytic category, many researchers have nonetheless adopted it because, whatever its limitations, it remains the most widely recognized term for describing the practice of travel for the purpose of gaining access to various types of health-related care.[10]

We define "medical tourism" as the practice of traveling, primarily across international borders, with the intent to access medical care, including dental services, screenings, and exams. However, depending on the available data and the nature of the topics examined, authors of individual chapters employ a variety of definitions and terms, including "health travel," "medical travel," and "cross-border health care." For example, discussions about patients who travel to nearby countries, as is typical within the European Union, feature the term "cross-border health care." Similarly, some researchers addressing topics such as travel for abortions, suicide, and transplants have understandable concerns that the word "tourism" trivializes the matter at hand and use other terms. In light of these considerations, while we appreciate the value of defining terms and using concepts in a consistent manner, we have not attempted to impose a uniform vocabulary upon our contributors.

OLD PRACTICE, NEW PATTERNS

For centuries, people seeking relief for their ailments have traveled to access healing waters, temples, shrines, and exotic treatments. Crossing borders for cures is not a new concept; what is different today is the size and scope of the market. Spurring the recent surge in the number of patients traveling for medical care are a growing interest in medical tourism as an economic development strategy, mounting challenges confronting national health systems and the individuals that rely upon them, and the emergence of global communication and transportation networks.

Economic crises around the globe and increased commercialization of health care have prompted health care providers and health ministries alike to identify medical tourists, who generally pay higher, out-of-pocket rates, as prime targets for filling private hospital beds and generating revenue. Within specific countries, various enterprises provide financial and organizational support to foster their medical tourism industries, and governments provide tax breaks, incentive payments, and special visas for medical tourists.

Facilitating this exchange are global, regional, and bilateral trade agreements that reduce barriers to trade, including trade in health services. Although international trade historically was principally in goods, trade in services—the fastest-growing sector of the global economy—now constitutes approximately 20 percent of international trade.[11] In 1995, the World Trade Organization (WTO) created the General Agreement on Trade in Services (GATS), which provides a legal framework and deliberative forum for negotiating trade in services and describes different "modes" of trade (Table 1.1). The basic premise of GATS, as with other WTO agreements, is nondiscrimination; that is, countries commit to treat all international trading partners (and domestic providers) equally and refrain from imposing barriers, standards, or restrictions on particular partners. GATS allows countries to determine the particular sectors they want to open to trade in services and to limit the extent to which they open those sectors. To date, only a limited number of countries have elected to open their health sectors.[12] This is unlikely to change in the near future, since progress on the latest round of WTO multilateral trade talks, the Doha Round, remains stalled in early 2012 after more than 10 years of negotiations. Nonetheless, GATS, and increasingly, bilateral and regional trade agreements, provide a potential framework for expanding foreign investment in health care facilities, promoting greater cross-border mobility among health care providers and enabling more medical travel covered by private or public insurance. Bilateral, regional, and multinational trade agreements, when they are negotiated in a manner intended to promote increased trade in health services, make it possible for investors and providers in high-cost countries to establish medical facilities or create partnerships in lower-cost countries. They can also help to establish the terms for reimbursement for care provided to patients who cross borders for care.

Also contributing to the expansion of medical travel is the fact that a number of the world's major economies are confronting aging populations with growing rates of chronic disease, often in tandem with soaring health care costs. As a result, in many settings, individuals increasingly are unable to afford or access the health services that they want or need. At the same time, air travel is faster and more affordable than it was in previous decades, and the Internet, a key marketing tool in medical tourism, makes it possible for hospitals, clinics, and medical tourism companies to promote health services to a global clientele. Consequently, today's medical tourist is not necessarily a member of the economic elite boarding a jet to purchase the best care in the world. To the contrary, she could just as easily be an uninsured real estate agent enduring an economy class trip to India for hip surgery she needs so she can return to work.

Table 1.1
GATS supply modes

Mode	Example
Mode 1: Cross-border supply.	Tele-health services—A physician in India provides postsurgical consultation to a patient in Canada via teleconference.
Mode 2: Consumption abroad, aka movement of consumers.	Medical tourism—An Australian resident seeking inexpensive cosmetic surgery travels to Thailand for her procedure.
Mode 3: Commercial presence.	Foreign-owned hospitals—A Singapore-based health care group establishes a health care facility in China.
Mode 4: Temporary movement of service providers.	Health worker migration—A nurse from the Philippines goes to work in Saudi Arabia.

Note: Medical tourism is considered "Mode 2" trade under the General Agreement on Trade in Services (GATS).

TRAVEL FOR COST, QUALITY, AND ACCESS

Patients' motives for engaging in medical tourism often provide a mirror image of their respective health systems' shortcomings. "Push" factors promoting medical tourism include high costs, long wait times, poor quality care, limited access to technology and expertise, and public health policies that restrict access to certain services.

Regional differences in the cost of medical care are a key driver of intranational and transnational medical travel, particularly within and from the United States. At present there are more than 47 million uninsured U.S. citizens.[13] Many other Americans are classified as "underinsured" because they have health insurance plans with high deductibles or low annual caps for health insurance coverage. Medical debt and health-related bankruptcy are serious problems in the United States.[14,15] As a result, some uninsured and underinsured U.S. citizens seek health care services in regions where medical procedures can cost a fraction of what they would pay at home, even when travel costs are figured into the cost of going abroad for care (Table 1.2). In one widely publicized case, Howard Staab, a carpenter from Durham, North Carolina, traveled to India for a cardiac procedure. There, for less than $10,000, travel costs included, he obtained care for which he was quoted a price of $200,000 in the United States.[16]

Some residents of countries such as Canada and the United Kingdom travel abroad for health care to avoid the long waits they face in their publicly funded health insurance systems. Though medically necessary health services are covered by these plans, wait times for hip replacements, knee replacements, spinal surgery, and other procedures prompt some citizens to travel abroad for expedited access to treatment.[17] In addition, publicly funded health insurance plans do not cover all medical procedures. As a result, some individuals travel for care because the procedures they seek are not insured.

Some patients engage in medical travel because they want to access interventions that have not received regulatory approval in their country of residence. For example, some individuals with multiple sclerosis, Amyotrophic lateral sclerosis, and other diseases travel to medical facilities in such countries as China, India, Mexico, Russia, Thailand, and Ukraine to obtain stem cell interventions that have not undergone testing in clinical trials or received regulatory approval.[18,19] Other individuals travel to undergo medical procedures that are illegal in their home countries.[20] These patients may travel to purchase a kidney or perhaps the services of a surrogate mother.[21,22]

Several additional factors prompt medical tourism. In many social settings, family members living in countries with better-resourced health care systems will help ill relatives from abroad obtain care in these locations.[23] Some of what is routinely described using the catch-all term "medical tourism" is regional medical travel in which individuals from such countries as Bangladesh, Egypt, and Libya travel to nearby countries with far

Table 1.2
Procedure costs for medical tourists (in selected countries)

Procedure	United States	India	Thailand	Singapore	Malaysia	Mexico	Cuba	Poland	Hungary	United Kingdom
Heart bypass (CABG)	113,000	10,000	13,000	20,000	9,000	3,250		7,140		13,921
Heart valve replacement	150,000	9,500	11,000	13,000	9,000	18,000		9,520		
Angioplasty	47,000	11,000	10,000	13,000	11,000	15,000		7,300		8,000
Hip replacement	47,000	9,000	12,000	11,000	10,000	17,300		6,120	7,500	12,000
Knee replacement	48,000	8,500	10,000	13,000	8,000	14,650		6,375		10,162
Gastric bypass	35,000	11,000	15,000	20,000	13,000	8,000		11,069		
Hip resurfacing	47,000	8,250	10,000	12,000	12,500	12,500		7,905		
Spinal fusion	43,000	5,500	7,000	9,000		15,000				
Mastectomy	17,000	7,500	9,000	12,400		7,500				
Rhinoplasty	4,500	2,000	2,500	4,375	2,083	3,200	1,535	1,700	2,858	3,500
Tummy tuck	6,400	2,900	3,500	6,250	3,903	3,000	1,831	3,500	3,136	4,810
Breast reduction	5,200	2,500	3,750	8,000	3,343	3,000	1,668	3,146	3,490	5,075
Breast implants	6,000	2,200	2,600	8,000	3,308	2,500	1,248	5,243	3,871	4,350
Crown	385	180	243	400	250	300		246	322	330
Tooth whitening	289	100	100		400	350		174	350	500
Dental implants	1,188	1,100	1,429	1,500	2,636	950		953	650	1,600

Note: Data for costs of surgeries around the world compiled from medical tourism providers and brokers online in March 2011. The price comparisons for surgery take into account hospital and doctor charges but do not include the costs of flights and hotel bills for the expected length of stay.
Source: Lunt et al. *Medical tourism: Treatments, markets and health system implications: A scoping review*, OECD 2011.

more health care providers, better-equipped hospitals, and more advanced treatment regimens. Other patients travel because of their familiarity with health care providers and medical facilities in their former countries of residence.[24,25] Finally, medical tourism is not always driven by efforts to obtain biomedical interventions. Rather, the prospect of access to alternative medicine leads some individuals to journey in search of healing.[26]

PATIENT FLOWS AND DESTINATIONS

Some medical travelers cross oceans to reach destination health care facilities. Other individuals engage in what is best characterized as regional, cross-border medical travel. In Eastern Europe, leading medical travel destinations include Czech Republic, Hungary, Poland, and Ukraine, and dental services are among the common offerings. In North America, the United States and Mexico are important departure points and destinations for medical travelers. In South America, Argentina, Brazil, and Venezuela all attempt to attract international patients, who typically come for cosmetic and other elective procedures. Within the Caribbean, Barbados, Cuba, Dominican Republic, Jamaica, and Puerto Rico are trying to draw medical travelers. In Asia, India, Indonesia, Malaysia, Singapore, South Korea, Thailand, and the Philippines are leading destinations for medical travelers.

Of these countries, India, Singapore, and Thailand have been particularly effective at crafting identities as "medical tourism" destination nations. India is well known as a country offering inexpensive health services. Singapore positions itself as a regional hub for medical travelers while also attracting clinical trials, building an infrastructure for medical education and translational research, and trying to establish a knowledge-based "bioeconomy." Popular services include orthopedic, neurological, and heart procedures. In Thailand, Bumrungrad International attracts many medical travelers and other hospitals and clinics in Bangkok, Phuket, and elsewhere have had success drawing international patients for a range of services, including orthopedic, heart, and cosmetic procedures. While Asian nations are among the most popular destinations in the global health services marketplace, many different regions compete for medical travelers, and the number of countries trying to attract medical tourists is increasing. At present, various nations in both the Caribbean and the Middle East are attempting to establish themselves as destinations for medical tourists.

THE DATA CHALLENGE

Although medical travel is increasingly studied and discussed in a variety of forums, it has proven remarkably difficult to document. There are little reliable quantitative data concerning how many patients engage in medical tourism. In the United States, many newspaper articles and academic analyses mention a report by the business consulting firm Deloitte LLP estimating that in 2007, approximately 750,000 U.S. patients went abroad for health care.[27] When tracked to what appears to be its original source, it becomes apparent that this number is an unsubstantiated claim contained in an editorial posted to an online newspaper.[28] It appears to have no basis in survey research or other credible attempts to estimate how many people leave the United States for the purpose of obtaining access to health care. In chapter 2, Johnson et al. estimate that the number of people traveling from the United States for inpatient services is probably somewhere between 50,000 and 121,500.[29] They acknowledge that these data, too, need to be supplemented by additional efforts to quantify medical tourism in a systematic, rigorous manner.

One major problem in attempting to quantify medical tourism is the lack of a common definition concerning what practices should be considered medical tourism. Some reports classify as medical tourism all care received away from an individual's country of residence, whether or not that care was the result of an accident or illness during holidays, or a trip planned explicitly for the purpose of accessing medical services. Similarly, while some datasets include only inpatient medical services, other records also count trips to dentists, spas, and acupuncturists. Finally, providers may count patients by episodes, visits, or procedures. Depending upon who is counting, and what classification scheme is used, a patient who travels to another country and has an initial hospital visit for radiological services, then returns the next week for a consultation and lab procedures, then comes back a third time for surgery and rehabilitation may be counted as one, three, or five instances of medical tourism.

In an effort to develop consistent definitions and reporting methodologies, the Organization for Economic Co-operation and Development (OECD) published guidelines in June 2011 for "Improving Estimates of Exports and Imports of Health Services and Goods Under the SHA Framework."[30] The report uses as its basis the System of Health Accounts Framework, a standard accounting framework that countries employ to measure health care consumption by residents. The guidelines do not distinguish between incidental health services (such as falling ill while traveling) from travel explicitly for the purpose of accessing health care services. But it does address some common concerns, such as whether to include health care consumption by retirees living abroad (for the most part, the guidelines suggest it should not be included) or wellness services (only in cases in which a "clear curative, rehabilitative or preventive nature can be identified"[30(p29)]). While the guidelines provide a useful starting point for better tracking imports and exports of health goods and services, the authors note that they will require time to fully implement, as well as some flexibility in methodologies to accommodate differences among countries.

Consistent use of terms and concepts has potential to improve our understanding of the magnitude of medical tourism. However, other complicating factors are likely to persist. A second factor that inhibits our grasp of the extent to which people travel to access care is the fact that much of this care occurs within private health care facilities, where providers are neither required nor necessarily inclined to divulge their data on visits from medical tourists. Even in instances in which government entities are involved in supporting or providing services to medical tourists, the data are not always readily available or reliable. There might, for instance, be reasons to exaggerate counts for marketing or public relations purposes. Finally, to the extent that figures are derived from patient self-reporting, either through health providers or travel and tourism surveys, not all patients are comfortable being forthcoming about their travel for medical care. The desire for privacy is sometimes a motivation for traveling for care. Also, some patients may feel that their home providers will not approve of their decision to go elsewhere for care or to pursue a procedure that the provider may have recommended against. Consequently, self-reporting of involvement in medical tourism may result in undercounting.

The lack of accurate data about how many people are traveling and what procedures they are traveling for makes it equally difficult to estimate the value of the industry to the global and individual economies. Some estimates place the value of the global market in the tens of billions. A 2006 report by the Tourism Research and Marketing group estimated that medical travelers took more than 19 million trips in 2005, accounting for a global market valued at $20 billion.[31] In 2008, Deloitte estimated the value of the global medical tourism market was around US $60 billion.[32] As with volume estimates, estimates of value vary based on what is included in the calculations. Some estimates include tourism dollars (travel and hotel stays, for instance), while other calculations include only medical expenditures.

OPPORTUNITIES AND RISKS

Though accurate estimates of the volume and value of medical tourism are elusive, it appears that the industry enriches some providers and hospitals and boosts foreign revenues in leading destination countries. Medical travel can benefit individuals as well, enabling them to access medical services that are unaffordable or otherwise out of reach. But the expansion of medical tourism is not without costs or controversy. Medical tourism can disrupt domestic health systems and worsen inequities by draining resources from public sector services.[33,34] It also can promote exploitation of vulnerable individuals living in countries where organ trafficking or commercial surrogacy occurs. And while the possibility of traveling for care might empower some patients by enabling them to select what procedures they want, it can also endanger them by exposing them to numerous risks.[35,36] Moreover, given the extent to which most medical travel is self-funded and relies on the patient's ability to pay, the practice also prompts questions about whether health care should be understood as a human right to which all individuals are entitled or as a service to be sold and purchased in the marketplace.[37] Using a variety of interpretive lenses, this volume explores this complex mix of risks and possibilities. We hope that the following chapters provoke debate, encourage further critical analysis of medical tourism, and help inform future discussions of these important issues.

REFERENCES

1. Carpenter B. Medical tourism: Dangers of medical procedures abroad. 2010. http://www.the33tv.com/news/kdaf-medical-tourism-dangers-story,0,440773.story. Accessed December 14, 2011.

2. Grace M. *State of the heart: A medical tourist's true story of lifesaving surgery in India.* 1st ed. Oakland, CA: New Harbinger Publications; 2007.

3. Associated Press. NDM-1, Superbug gene, could spread worldwide, doctors warn. *Huffington Post.* 2010. http://www.huffingtonpost.com/2010/08/11/ndm-1-new-superbug-gene-c_n_678427.html. Accessed December 14, 2011.

4. Ritter P. Legalizing the organ trade? *Time.* 2008. http://www.time.com/time/world/article/0,8599,1833858,00.html. Accessed December 14, 2011.

5. Levin D. Steve Jobs went to Switzerland in search of cancer treatment. *Fortune Tech.* January 18, 2011. http://tech.fortune.cnn.com/2011/01/18/steve-jobs-went-to-switzerland-in-search-of-cancer-treatment/. Accessed December 14, 2011.

6. Denyer S. Pakistan's Zardari to leave Dubai hospital, rest at home. *Washington Post.* 2011. http://www.washingtonpost.com/world/pakistans-president-to-be-discharged-from-dubai-hospital-rest-at-home/2011/12/14/gIQAQVowtO_story.html. Accessed December 14, 2011.

7. Khan A. Peyton Manning: Can stem cell therapy get Colts QB back in game? *Los Angeles Times.* 2011. http://articles.latimes.com/2011/sep/19/news/la-heb-peyton-manning-stem-cell-treatment-colts-quarterback-20110919. Accessed January 12, 2012.

8. Martin A. Entrepreneur delves into medical tourism. *Brookfield Now.* October 11, 2011. http://www.brookfieldnow.com/news/131564068.html. Accessed December 14, 2011.

9. Pitout JDD. The latest threat in the war on antimicrobial resistance. *Lancet Infect Dis.* 2010;10(9):578–579.

10. Crooks VA, Kingsbury P, Snyder J, Johnston R. What is known about the patient's experience of medical tourism? A scoping review. *BMC Health Serv Res.* 2010;10:266.

11. World Trade Organization. Understanding the WTO: The Agreements—Services: Rules for growth and investment. *WTO.* http://www.wto.org/english/thewto_e/whatis_e/tif_e/agrm6_e.htm. Accessed December 13, 2011.

12. World Trade Organization. Services: Sector by Sector—Health and social services. http://www.wto.org/english/tratop_e/serv_e/health_social_e/health_social_e.htm. Accessed December 13, 2011.

13. Milstein A, Smith M. America's new refugees—seeking affordable surgery offshore. *N Engl J Med.* 2006;355(16):1637–1640.

14. Doty MM, Collins SR, Rustgi SD, Kriss JL. Seeing red: The growing burden of medical bills and debt faced by U.S. families. *Issue Brief (Commonw Fund).* 2008;42:1–12.

15. Seifert RW, Rukavina M. Bankruptcy is the tip of a medical-debt iceberg. *Health Aff.* 2006;25(2):w89–92.

16. Milstein A, Smith M. America's new refugees—seeking affordable surgery offshore. *N Engl J Med.* 2006;355(16):1637–1640.

17. Eggertson L. Wait-list weary Canadians seek treatment abroad. *Canadian Medical Association Journal.* 2006;174(9):1247.

18. Kiatpongsan S, Sipp D. Medicine. Monitoring and regulating offshore stem cell clinics. *Science.* 2009;323(5921):1564–1565.

19. Enserink M. Selling the stem cell dream. *Science.* 2006;313:160–63.

20. Cohen IG. Medical tourism: The view from ten thousand feet. *Hastings Cent Rep.* 2010;40(2):11–12.

21. Budiani-Saberi DA, Delmonico FL. Organ trafficking and transplant tourism: A commentary on the global realities. *Am J Transplant.* 2008;8(5):925–929.

22. Naqvi SA, Ali B, Mazhar F, Zafar MN, Rizvi SA. A socioeconomic survey of kidney vendors in Pakistan. *Transpl Int.* 2007;20(11):934–939.

23. Kangas B. Therapeutic itineraries in a global world: Yemenis and their search for biomedical treatment abroad. *Med Anthropol.* 2002;21(1):35–78.

24. Lee JY, Kearns R, Friesen W. Seeking affective health care: Korean immigrants' use of homeland medical services. *Health & Place.* 2010;16:108–115.

25. Bergmark R, Barr D, Garcia R. Mexican immigrants in the U.S. living far from the border may return to Mexico for health services. *J Immigr Minor Health.* 2010;12(4):610–614.

26. Hoyez AC. The "world of yoga": The production and reproduction of therapeutic landscapes. *Soc Sci Med.* 2007;65(1):112–124.

27. Keckley P, Underwood H. Medical tourism: Consumers in search of value. Deloitte Center for Health Solutions. 2008:1–30.

28. Baliga H. Medical tourism is the new wave of outsourcing from India. *India Daily.* December 23, 2006.

29. Johnson T, Garman A. Impact of medical travel on imports and exports of medical services. *Health Policy.* 2010;98(2–3):171–177.

30. OECD. *Improving estimates of exports and imports of health services and goods under the SHA framework.* OECD; 2011. www.oecd.org/dataoecd/4/18/49011758.pdf.

31. Tourism Research and Marketing. *Medical tourism: A global analysis.* Arnhem, The Netherlands: ATLAS, 2006.

32. Keckley P, Underwood H. *Medical Tourism: Consumers in Search of Value.* Deloitte Center for Health Solutions; 2008.

33. Thomas G, Krishnan S. Effective public-private partnership in healthcare: Apollo as a cautionary tale. *Indian J Med Ethics.* 2010;7(1):2–4.

34. Pachanee CA, Wibulpolprasert S. Incoherent policies on universal coverage of health insurance and promotion of international trade in health services in Thailand. *Health Policy Plan.* 2006;21(4):310–318.

35. Furuya EY, Paez A, Srinivasan A, et al. Outbreak of Mycobacterium abscessus wound infections among "lipotourists" from the United States who underwent abdominoplasty in the Dominican Republic. *CID.* 2008;46:1181–1188.

36. Birch DW, Vu L, Karmali S, Stoklossa CJ, Sharma AM. Medical tourism in bariatric surgery. *Am J Surg.* 2010;199(5):604–608.

37. Connell J. A new inequality? Privatisation, urban bias, migration and medical tourism. *Asia Pacific Viewpoint.* 2011;52 (3):260–271.

Part I

Drivers, Departure Points, and Destinations: Situated Studies of Medical Tourism

Chapter 2

The United States: Destination and Departure Point

Tricia J. Johnson, Andrew Garman, Samuel F. Hohmann, Steven Meurer, and Molly Allen

International medical travel to the United States began the 1960s, when open heart surgery became available, and patients traveled from abroad to access this sophisticated procedure.[1] In the decades that have followed, wealthy patients have continued to travel from overseas to access U.S. medical technology and expertise, and certain U.S. providers have marketed to international patients, particularly during economic downturns. But in more recent years, U.S. patients have begun to flow out of the country in what may be almost equal numbers, principally in search of more affordable medical services. This chapter focuses on international medical travel from the perspective of the United States, examining both inbound

This chapter reflects some of the initial research and work completed for the U.S. Cooperative for International Patient Programs (USCIPP), a three-year project funded by the U.S. Department of Commerce to improve measurement and increase the volume of inbound international medical travel to the United States.

travel of international patients into the country and outbound travel of U.S. patients to other countries.

Medical travel is an important issue at both the national level and for individual hospitals and communities. From a national balance of trade standpoint, international medical travel represents both potential gains when patients come into the United States for care (and U.S. providers are in essence exporting care) and potential losses when U.S. patients turn to other countries for care (and U.S. patients are importing care). In 2010, President Barack Obama announced his National Export Initiative, which calls for doubling exports by 2015 to increase U.S. jobs and boost the economy overall. The National Export Initiative focuses on further developing existing markets, opening new markets abroad, and developing public-private partnerships to strengthen the U.S. brand. Service industries, including health care, are an important component for new business growth. Health care is an important contribution to the U.S. economy overall, accounting for 17.6 percent of the gross domestic product in 2009[2]; and attracting international patients for medical care is one opportunity for growth in this sector. Relative to other service industries, health care has relatively high revenue per encounter, particularly for inpatient care. Patients leaving the country for medical care abroad, meanwhile, represent U.S. dollars spent in other countries rather than domestically. Despite the potential importance of patient flows in and out of the United States, historically there have been no coordinated efforts at the national level to facilitate medical travel to the United States—or to stem the flow of patients from the United States.

Similarly, for individual hospitals, inbound international patients represent an additional source of revenue, while outbound patients are lost revenue that potentially would have been earned had patients sought care at home. International medical travelers represent a small proportion of total patient discharges in U.S. hospitals, even in those that cater to this population. But international patients may become a more prominent source of revenue as hospitals aggressively compete for contracts with health insurers and medical care continues to shift to the outpatient setting, leaving hospitals with more unoccupied beds. The growth of international medical travel is both an opportunity for U.S. hospitals, since there are potentially more international patients seeking care outside of their home countries to attract—and also a risk, since growing numbers of hospitals abroad are offering similar high quality, Western-style medicine that may, in the future, divert patients away from the United States.

Inbound medical travelers are a unique patient population for U.S. hospitals. As we will discuss, while it has been claimed that these inbound travelers are a proverbial cash cow for these hospitals, this group of patients is not without costs. Additionally, the sources of revenue, both direct foreign dollars and foreign payments made through a domestic insurer, vary widely. Understanding this patient population and the associated funding sources will help health care providers to plan strategically for growing or bypassing this book of business.

In this chapter, we describe trends in medical travel into, out of, and within the United States. We restrict this discussion to imports and exports for final use; that is, health care services provided to individuals.[3] We also specifically limit our focus to medical travel, meaning travel to another region with the main purpose of obtaining medical care.[4] This includes both international medical travel (travel to another country) and domestic medical travel (travel to another area within the United States).

BALANCE OF HEALTH CARE MOBILITY FOR THE UNITED STATES

While there has been considerable attention devoted to both outbound and inbound medical travel from and to the United States, there is a nontrivial gap in knowledge about the actual numbers of patients traveling into and out of the country and their reasons for travel. From a methodological perspective, collecting data on inbound and outbound medical travelers is particularly challenging in the United States. There are no centralized data repositories that track patient origin at the national level and no national reporting requirements for the volume or value of inbound medical travel into or outbound travel from the country. Surveying individual hospitals about the number of international patients would be tremendously costly and time consuming. There were 5,795 hospitals in the country in 2010,[5] and although only a small subset of hospitals with reputations for world class care have historically been the primary destinations for international medical travelers into the United States, the number of U.S. hospitals marketing to international patients has expanded in recent years. As the following discussion illustrates, quantifying the extent of medical travel into and out of the United States is further complicated by varying definitions of what, exactly, constitutes medical travel.

Estimating Inbound Medical Travel

Establishing valid data for the number of inbound medical travelers into the United States, the reasons for travel, and the value of care provided to these travelers is critical for understanding the current impact of medical travel on the country and on U.S. providers specifically. This information is essential for developing strategies on a national, regional, and hospital level to attract medical travelers. And if quality of care is a major determinant of medical travel, understanding who travels to the United States for care and why can help inform efforts to improve patient value. These data are also important for forecasting the impact of global events that could influence inbound medical travel in the future.

Table 2.1 examines two sources for the number of international patients traveling to the United States for medical care. The first source is a study by Tricia J. Johnson and Andrew Garman,[6] which estimates a lower and upper bound for inbound medical travel into the United States using data collected through (1) interviews with 18 U.S. providers with established international patient programs, and (2) the U.S.

Table 2.1
Estimates of international patients traveling to the United States for medical care

Authors	Johnson and Garman (2010) Estimates for 2007	UHC (2011) Estimates for 2010
Source	Provider interviews and Survey of International Air Travelers (SIAT)	UHC Clinical Database
Inclusion criteria	Interviews: 18 U.S. hospitals with international patient programs SIAT: health treatments as primary purpose of travel	91 member hospitals of UHC with patient records that included an international payer or zip code YYYYY
Number of patients		
Inpatient	42,469	12,680
Outpatient hospital	–	21,172
Total	102,869 (inpatient, outpatient, other health treatments)	33,852 (inpatient and outpatient hospital only)
Total charges (in 2010 dollars)		
Inpatient	$2.0 B[a]	$539 M
Outpatient hospital	–	$119 M
Total	–	$658 M (inpatient and outpatient hospital only)

B = billion USD; M = million USD.
[a] Number of inpatients multiplied by total charges per inpatient from UHC.
Note: Differences between estimates of medical tourism volumes and revenues reflect varying inclusion criteria and data sources.

Department of Commerce Survey of International Air Travelers (SIAT), which surveys between 65,000 and 95,000 inbound and outbound travelers each year about reasons for air travel into and out of the country. The lower bound is an estimate of inpatient medical care based only on data from provider interviews, and the upper bound is an estimate of both inpatient and outpatient medical care and other nonmedical spa treatments based on data from the SIAT. The study estimated that there were between 42,000 and 103,000 international medical travelers seen in the United States in 2007, depending on the inclusion criteria and comprehensiveness of the definition.

The second source is UHC, an alliance of nonprofit academic medical centers and their affiliated hospitals. UHC collects patient-level data from approximately 200 member hospitals through its Clinical Data Base, which includes information about the primary and secondary payer and the zip code of the patient's home residence. In 2010, UHC reported 12,680 inpatient discharges and 21,172 outpatient, nonemergency department encounters for international patients across 91 hospitals.[7] (International patients were identified based on hospital patient records noting an international payer or the zip code "YYYYY" to indicate non-U.S. zip codes.) In addition, there were 22,126 emergency department visits, presumably for medical care that was incidental to the primary purpose of travel. While UHC is not a census of all hospitals that provide care to international patients in the United States, it is the most detailed source of information for counting international patients for the 200 hospitals that are members of UHC's Clinical Data Base. Furthermore, the Data Base represents the vast majority of the U.S. academic medical center market and majority of those that are likely to cater to large numbers of international patients.

The discrepancy between the two estimates may be attributed to different inclusion criteria—for inpatient discharges, Johnson and Garman's estimate was based on interviews with programs known to serve international patients while UHC's estimate was based on data collected directly from its hospital members, so although the two samples were similar, they were not identical. Both estimates included many of the largest U.S. hospitals catering to international patients, with considerable overlap in the hospitals included; however, there were differences. In addition, UHC's number was based on administrative data collected from the hospitals' billing systems, while Johnson and Garman's number was based on self-reported information that was likely to be an approximation. Because UHC collects administrative data on an ongoing basis for hospital quality improvement and benchmarking purposes, data collection is routine—requiring no ad hoc surveying of hospitals—and, therefore, has the ability to provide estimates for the number of medical travelers over time.

Estimating Outbound Medical Travel

Despite anecdotal evidence that international trade in health services has grown, there are few sources of data-driven estimates of the volume of medical travelers leaving the United States for health care services. The lack of credible, substantiated data has resulted in a wide range of estimates for outbound medical travel from the United States, from tens of thousands to hundreds of thousands of people a year.

Table 2.2 describes data-driven estimates of outbound medical travel from two sources. In 2008, Tilman Ehrbeck, Ceani Guevara, and Paul D. Mango[8] estimated between 60,000 and 85,000 medical travelers worldwide (including travel to and from the United States); however, they limited their count to patients traveling for inpatient medical care only and excluded travel between contiguous geographic areas where cross-border care is the closest available (e.g., travel from Tijuana, Mexico, to San Diego, California). In an analysis using data collected from the SIAT, Johnson and Garman[6] estimated that between 50,000 and 121,000 Americans traveled abroad for inpatient medical care in 2007.

The methodological approaches and inclusion criteria used might explain the discrepancies between estimates. The estimate that Ehrbeck et al. published in 2008 used the most restrictive definition of medical travel—purposeful travel to another country for inpatient medical care, excluding treatments provided in contiguous geographic regions where that care was the closest available. They used primary data and interviews with an unknown number of providers, patients, and intermediaries to estimate the number of international travelers worldwide. Like Ehrbeck et al., Johnson and Garman[6] reported estimates of international travelers

Table 2.2
Estimates of U.S. patients traveling abroad for medical care

Authors	Data Source(s)	Year	Types of Medical Care Included	Number of Medical Travelers
Ehrbeck, et al. (2008)	Interviews and other data	2008 or earlier	Inpatient medical travel only, excluding travel in contiguous areas	60,000–85,000 worldwide (not limited to Americans)
Johnson and Garman (2010)	Interviews and Survey of International Air Travel	2007	Inpatient medical travel only	50,329–121,392

Note: As with inbound medical travel to the United States, estimates for outbound medical travel from the United States vary widely as a result of diverse data sources and definitions.

for whom medical care was the primary reason for travel. They used data from the SIAT, and because the SIAT classifies medical travel very broadly and includes nonmedical spa treatments in addition to medical care, they estimated an upper and lower bound for the number of medical travelers, with the upper bound representing all inpatient and outpatient travel for the primary purpose of health treatments (including both medical and spa treatments) and the lower bound representing the number traveling specifically for inpatient medical care.

Both estimates above are considerably smaller than the widely quoted but unsubstantiated estimate that some 750,000 U.S. patients went abroad for care in 2007.[9] This number first appeared as a projection for 2007 in an article in the *India Daily* in 2006[10] and was subsequently reported as actual experience for the United States in 2007 by the Deloitte Center for Health Solutions.[9,11] Despite the fact that this number has been cited broadly, our research suggests that it is a considerable overestimate of the actual number of outbound medical travelers from the United States.

Remaining Data Challenges

The diversity of methods to count the number of international medical travelers and the range of estimates themselves demonstrate the difficulty in tracking inbound and outbound travel. In addition to the challenge of determining what patients and procedures to count is the challenge of identifying all the potential providers marketing to medical travelers. Decreasing profit margins for domestic patients and the ease of marketing medical care across the world via the Internet has encouraged even some small hospitals to attempt to attract potentially lucrative international patients as a means to diversify patient portfolios and increase revenue. One example is Galichia Heart Hospital, an 82-bed acute care hospital in Wichita, Kansas. Galichia's medical travel website, galichiamedicaltourism.com, markets "Fixed Prices, American Quality Healthcare." The website compares its prices with other medical travel destinations across the world, including its special offer for a low-dose CT scan for $299. While domestic cosmetic and LASIK surgery providers have posted prices for years, to date few U.S. providers have posted prices for nonelective surgeries or other major treatments that are generally covered by health insurance.

COMING FOR QUALITY: MEDICAL TRAVEL TO THE UNITED STATES

Although there is a lack of definitive data about the volume of medical travelers arriving and leaving the United States, more is known about who is coming and going and why. Wealthy patients first began coming in significant numbers to the United States in search of state-of-the art health technologies and world-renowned medical expertise in the 1960s. Since that time, international patients arriving in the United States have primarily come from four geographic regions: Latin America, the Middle East, Europe, and Asia.[6,8] McKinsey & Company estimated that 87 percent of Latin American medical travelers go to the United States or Canada, while 58 percent of those from the Middle East, 33 percent of those from Europe, and 6 percent of those from Asia go to the United States or Canada for medical care.[8] The high numbers of Latin Americans and small numbers from Asia reflect the United States' proximity to these respective geographic regions. Additionally, Latin American patients do not need to cross multiple time zones when traveling to the United States, which may reduce the barriers to travel. While anecdotal evidence suggests that there is substantial cross-border travel between Canada and Mexico and the United States, more work is needed to quantify the number of cross-border travelers. The largest competitors for international patients coming from other regions are other countries that are closer to the patients' home countries. One of the largest barriers for potential patients considering travel to the United States for medical care is the U.S. visa requirement. Patients must apply for and be granted a visitor visa (generally the B2 visa for pleasure, tourism, and medical treatment) unless they are residents of one of the 35 countries that participate in the U.S. Visa Waiver Program. Because of the time required to obtain a visa for travel to the United States, anecdotal evidence suggests that potential patients bypass the United States for care provided in another country that has a quicker visa application process or where a visa is not required.

The Value Proposition of U.S. Health Care

The long-standing attraction for patients traveling from other countries to the United States has been the perception that U.S. providers offer some of the highest quality care in the world. Anecdotal evidence suggests that international patients traveling to U.S. academic medical centers and other hospitals do so in search of care that is either not available locally or for which the quality of care locally is below the desired quality. Accounts from U.S. providers suggest that international patients often use publicly available hospital rankings, such as *U.S. News & World Report*'s ranking of U.S. hospitals and Thomson Reuter's top 100 hospitals survey as a resource for seeking out the highest quality care in the United States.

Interviews with administrators and directors of the international patient programs of nationally ranked academic medical centers in the United States suggest that growth in international patient revenues has been due to an increased demand for the most sophisticated, technologically complex medical care, also referred to as quaternary care.[12] Using data from UHC, Samuel F. Hohmann and colleagues[13] reported that the common service lines for international patients included cardiology, cardiothoracic surgery, and vascular surgery (23%); spinal surgery, neurosurgery, and neurology (14%); urology (8%); and orthopedics (7%).

Benefits of Inbound Medical Travel to the United States

Although international patient revenue may be as small as 1 percent or less of gross revenue, even for hospitals that proactively cater to international patients, the per-patient revenue is disproportionately high because international patients tend to have more complex medical conditions, require more intensive care, and stay longer than domestic patients.[14] International patients are also far less likely to benefit from prices negotiated by third party payers.

Hohmann and colleagues showed that while international patient volumes for U.S. academic medical center members of UHC were decreasing between 2001 and 2004, lengths of stay and charges were increasing.[13] Furthermore, Siriporn Satjapot, Tricia J. Johnson, and Andrew Garman[14] found that the most critically ill international patients stayed 25 percent longer than domestic patients with similar conditions.

UHC estimated that in 2010, total charges for international patients in its member hospitals that identify international patients by either payer source or zip code were $539 million for inpatient care and $119 million for nonemergency outpatient care for a total of $658 million. This translates into approximately $47,000 per inpatient discharge, and $5,620 per outpatient encounter. The average total charge per inpatient discharge for all patients discharged from U.S. hospitals in 2009 was $33,359 (in 2010 dollars), supporting the notion that international patients generate substantially more revenue than other patients for U.S. hospitals.

Unlike employer-sponsored health plans in the United States, which can often negotiate discounted payment rates with domestic providers in exchange for access to a large number of health plan enrollees, international payers and self-pay patients generally do not have negotiating leverage, because the potential volume and associated revenue is substantially smaller. International patients, therefore, have historically represented a disproportionate share of revenue since payment rates have been higher than those for similar care provided to domestic patients.[15] Recently, international payers have started to negotiate rates that are somewhat comparable to those negotiated by domestic insurers, which has reduced profit margins on services to some international patients.

Care provided to an international patient that is reimbursed at a domestic payer rate may, in fact, be less profitable to a U.S. hospital than care for a domestic patient, due to the cost of additional services that are often provided to international patients, such as interpretation services.

In additional to individual providers, local communities also benefit from international patients traveling to the United States for medical care. As with U.S. patients traveling abroad, international patients coming to the United States often travel with family members or friends who stay in the local communities while the patient receives care. The patient's travel companions spend money on lodging, transportation, food, and potentially on tourist activities while the patient receives medical care. While the collateral benefit of international patients for the local communities has not been studied systematically, it is clear that the revenues that medical tourists generate extend beyond money spent directly on medical care itself.

In response to the potential for growth in health care exports to the United States and their resulting contribution to the U.S. economy, the U.S. Department of Commerce in 2010 funded a three-year project to improve measurement and increase the volume of inbound international medical travel through its Market Development Cooperator Program. The project, the U.S. Cooperative for International Patient Programs (USCIPP), is a partnership between UHC, Rush University, the International Trade Administration of the U.S. Department of Commerce, and U.S. hospitals. The specific goals are to increase the global competitiveness of U.S. health care providers, improve access to U.S. health care for international patients, and improve the ongoing measurement of the number of inbound patients traveling to the United States and the ensuing revenue for U.S. providers. These national efforts to create an industry for international patient programs are intended to strengthen U.S. providers' position in the global market.

LEAVING FOR COST: MEDICAL TRAVEL FROM THE UNITED STATES

Long-haul international medical travel from the United States to countries such as Thailand and Singapore gained attention around 2005 when national news programs such as *60 Minutes* published stories about U.S. patients seeking care abroad. As hospitals in Mexico, Costa Rica, and other Central American countries have become Joint Commission International accredited, indicating they have met certain quality standards, more U.S. patients searching for lower cost and higher value care also have begun considering the option of so-called short-haul international medical travel.

Today, the destinations for U.S. patients traveling abroad for medical care are concentrated in three geographic regions: Asia; Latin America; and within region, or Mexico and Canada. Ehrbeck et al.[8] estimate that 45 percent of North American medical travelers seek care in Asia and 26 percent in Latin America. In addition, there is also a substantial amount of within-region medical travel among the United States, Mexico, and Canada, with 27 percent of North American travel occurring among these three countries.[8]

Cost as a Primary Driver

One of the primary reasons that U.S. patients travel abroad for care is cost. Surveys have suggested that a substantial number of U.S. patients would be willing to travel abroad for care in exchange for a considerable reduction in out-of-pocket costs. The Deloitte Center for Health Solutions reported reported that 39 percent of Americans would consider traveling abroad for an elective procedure if the quality was at least equivalent to care in the United States, and they could save at least 50 percent in out-of-pocket costs.[9] In a survey of U.S. households with a sick family member, a substantial portion indicated that they would be willing to travel abroad for major surgery if it saved them money.[16] Of people who were uninsured or stressed by spending, 25 percent said that they would be willing to travel abroad for surgery if it saved $1,000 to $2,000, and nearly 40 percent said they would be willing to travel abroad for surgery if it saved at least $10,000; more surprising, approximately 25 percent of those who were insured and not stressed by spending (based on self-reports from the respondent) said that they would be willing to travel abroad if they could save at least $10,000.

While uninsured people are more likely to be unemployed or in low wage jobs, 10 percent are in households with incomes of 400 percent or more of the federal poverty level (FPL) ($88,200 or more for a family of four in 2009), which means they would not be eligible for Medicaid or subsidized coverage under the Patient Protection and Affordable Care Act.[7] This segment of uninsured people is strongly motivated to find more affordable health care. In the Kaiser Family Foundation's Health Tracking Poll,[17] which surveyed American adults ages 18 to 64 with and without health insurance, 27 percent of the uninsured responded that they had used up all of their savings on medical bills in the prior 12 months, demonstrating the financial distress created by the cost of medical care in the United States.

In 2009, there were approximately five million uninsured people with incomes of 400 percent of the FPL or greater.[17] While not all uninsured people with higher incomes could actually afford to pay out of pocket for medical and travel expenses for care received abroad, a portion of them are already paying out of pocket for care received in the United States, and could potentially reduce their expenses by traveling abroad for care.

Another group of uninsured who could potentially benefit from lower-cost care abroad are those who are delaying care in the United States because they cannot afford it, but could afford the lower costs of care from providers abroad. In a national representative, random survey of American adults conducted in 2008, 12 percent of individuals with incomes $75,000 or greater reported problems in paying for health care or health insurance, 11 percent of these individuals reported that they had skipped a medical test or treatment that was needed, and 15 percent reported that they had postponed necessary health care because of cost.[18] It is clear that even for individuals with insurance or with relatively high incomes, the high costs of health care in the United States have severe economic consequences, which could further encourage some individuals to seek care abroad.

Table 1.2 in the Introduction shows the average prices for a variety of procedures that are common treatments sought abroad in nine international travel destinations, compared to estimated prices in the United States. Estimated costs for nearly all of the nine major procedures (i.e., procedures with charges of US$10,000 or more), were less than 50 percent of U.S. prices for all but one of these procedures, and two-thirds had an estimated cost of 25 percent or less of U.S. prices. The medical care prices in other countries do not take into account nonmedical travel costs, which could add an extra $11,000 or more ($2,000 per person for the patient and one companion for air travel; $4,000 for lodging and $3,000 for meals for a three-week stay) and opportunity costs for the patient and travel companion. After accounting for nonmedical travel costs, more than half of the procedures and country destinations would still reduce out-of-pocket costs by 50 percent. More data are needed that reflect actual payments made out of pocket by consumers, rather than estimated prices.

Patient Experiences with Medical Travel

There are few data-driven studies that examine patients' experiences with international medical travel. A recent review of the literature reported only five empirically based studies of patients' experience with international medical travel, but none specifically examined either U.S. patients' experiences with medical travel abroad or the experience of foreign patients traveling into the United States for care.[19] Quantitative and qualitative research are needed to understand the experiences of international medical travelers into and out of the United States. This information could help to shed light on strategies to increase medical travel into the country and to reduce the number of Americans traveling abroad for care.

MEDICAL TRAVEL WITHIN THE UNITED STATES

In addition to international travel, another option for U.S. patients searching for high-value care is domestic medical travel, also known as intra-country travel. There is anecdotal evidence that Americans have long traveled across the country in search of the highest quality of care available, but the number of people who have traveled domestically for care has not been quantified. In a market research survey conducted by Deloitte, 39 percent of Americans reported that they would be willing to travel outside of their home region, but within the United States, for necessary care; and 32 percent would be willing to travel domestically for elective medical care that offers either better quality or faster access.[20]

Health insurers and employers historically have contracted locally with health care providers, and regionally if services were not available locally. But there is a large body of research that supports the notion that "practice makes perfect," that is, that health care outcomes are better when using high-volume hospitals and surgeons.[21,22] A small number of stakeholders have strategically attempted to steer patients to these high-volume providers or "centers of excellence" as a way to improve quality. The Leapfrog Group,[23] a national consortium of employers and health care purchasers focused on improving patient safety, quality, and value in the U.S. health care system, awards an "Evidence-Based Hospital Referral" Safety Standard to hospitals that meet volume recommendations for certain procedures to help payers and consumers identify high-quality providers.

Self-funded employers in particular have begun strategically contracting with providers across the United States for high value care.[24–26] In 2010, Lowe's Companies, Inc. embarked on a three-year agreement with Cleveland Clinic, the top-ranked hospital for heart surgery by *U.S. News & World Report,* to provide heart procedures for its 228,000 employees and dependents across the United States.[27] This arrangement covered transportation and lodging for the patient and one companion as a way to reduce out-of-pocket payments for the consumer, thereby incentivizing travel. Early evidence showed that one-third of employees needing serious heart surgery elected to travel to the Cleveland Clinic for care; however, there is no information to date about the outcomes for these patients.

Patients who travel for care in the United States rather than internationally will experience less dramatic cost savings. But domestic medical travel presents fewer barriers than international medical travel; it generally requires less time away from home and work due to shorter travel distances, and patients benefit from more information about the quality of care, easier post-discharge care coordination, and providers who share the same native language.

Domestic medical travel to centers of excellence within the United States has the potential to improve quality and long-term health outcomes and decrease long-term health care spending. Health insurers and employers may follow the lead of Lowe's Companies by proactively contracting with the highest-quality providers. However, more work is needed to fully understand the tangible and intangible costs of domestic medical travel, including out-of-pocket costs and the psychological stress of being away from one's own social and community support when receiving major treatments.

FUTURE WORK

The field of international and domestic medical travel to, from, and within the United States is ripe for study. With few exceptions, most of the published work to date has been either conceptual or reports of individual case studies. Basic empirical work is needed to quantify the volume of patients traveling into and out of the country on an annual basis and to identify the geographic regions from which and to where patients are traveling. An evaluation of payment sources for inbound medical travelers is needed, starting with the distribution of international patients by source of payment (e.g., self-pay out of pocket, Ministry of Health, private international health insurer, private domestic health insurer) and type of financial arrangement (e.g., fee-for-service, case based, per diem based). Trends in volumes, payment sources, and types of financial arrangements by geographic region would provide important information for providers and the government to understand whether the international medical travel market is growing or contracting, and in what areas.

While objective, data-driven research to quantify the financial contributions of foreign patients to U.S. health care providers and the tourism economy is in the early stages, it is clear that inpatient, rather than outpatient, medical care has the largest impact. Not only do inpatient hospital stays generate the largest health care revenue, but they also tend to translate into longer stays in the local community and consequently more significant contributions to local economies. It is therefore critical that systematic efforts to collect data on the number of inbound and outbound travelers be stratified by the type of health treatment to further understand the potential implications of medical travelers for the U.S. economy. Revisions to the SIAT, for example, to include questions about the types of health treatment received in the United States could be used to estimate spending in the local economies by type of treatment. Expansion of UHC's Clinical Data Base to include information about international patients from both member and nonmember hospitals would enhance estimates of international patient volumes and the value of international patients' contributions to the U.S. economy.

An additional challenge lies in getting hospitals to report information about international patients. Historically not all hospitals have tracked the number of international patients for whom they provide care; and even those that track the number of international patients do so in different ways. These data are not only important for individual hospitals, but also at the national level to systematically measure on an ongoing basis the growth in global competition for medical care exports.

Future estimates of international medical travelers should carefully track cross-border care (e.g., Mexicans traveling to Texas, Arizona, or California; U.S. patients traveling to Mexico or Canada; Canadians traveling to Washington, Minnesota, and other border states), because short-haul cross-border travel may be one of the largest opportunities for increasing inbound and stemming outbound travel for medical care to and from the United States. For example, if it is determined that a substantial number of U.S. patients are going to Toronto or Vancouver for less costly medical care, it's possible to evaluate the financial benefit of providing lower-cost services within the country, particularly in these border areas.

Cross-border travel is becoming increasingly common in other regions of the world, such as the European Union (see chapter 3). The European Union's new Directive on the Application of Patients' Rights in Cross Border Health Care, slated to take effect in 2013, encourages cooperation in health care for cross-border patients among member countries. These illustrations suggest that the United States has an opportunity to develop infrastructure at the national level to facilitate inbound medical travel from neighboring regions for patients who are seeking access to high quality tertiary and quaternary care.

Assessing the Impact of Health Reform

One frequently debated question is the extent to which the Patient Protection and Affordable Care Act (PPACA) or other changes to the U.S. health care system might increase or decrease U.S. residents' demand for medical care abroad. At the time of this writing, the U.S. Supreme Court was considering the constitutionality of certain aspects of the PPACA. But if the law stands, by 2014, the PPACA is slated to expand health insurance coverage to most Americans who were previously uninsured. If these health insurance plans have large coinsurance rates or deductibles, there may be an increase in the number of underinsured Americans who have a continued incentive to travel abroad for more affordable care. High-deductible health plans (HDHPs) that are coupled with health savings accounts encourage consumers to shop for high value care—care that is either higher quality for the same cost, lower cost for the same quality, or both higher quality and lower cost. Money invested in a health savings account can only be used for qualifying medical expenses (without paying a penalty), and the account earns interest over time. Because consumers pay out of pocket for all medical care until health care spending exceeds the deductible, there is a direct financial incentive to search out high value care. An increase in the number of Americans enrolled in a HDHP in the coming years is likely to increase the number of consumers who turn to providers abroad as an affordable solution to medical care unless there are radical changes in the pricing of medical care domestically.

CONCLUSION

While outbound travel by Americans searching for lower-cost care has been in the spotlight since the mid-2000s, American hospitals have been catering to international patients for a much longer time. The cottage industry of international medical travel has largely been fragmented in the United States, with no coordination or tracking at the national level. Competition for international patients searching for high quality care has increased with hospitals across the world entering the market and aggressively marketing quality with credentials such as Joint Commission International accreditation, while offering lower prices than those in the United States. This increased competition from abroad has precipitated greater collaboration across U.S. hospitals and at the national level to grow inbound medical travel. At the same time, U.S. patients have been traveling in increasing numbers in search of affordable health care. This trend may continue as health reform measures leave more patients with health plans that require them to cover a larger portion of their health care costs. While evidence suggests that there are slightly more patients leaving the United States for care abroad than coming into the country to receive care, the balance of trade from international medical travel currently favors the United States. If the trend toward travel into the United States for highly specialized quaternary care continues, revenue per international patient will continue to increase for U.S. hospitals as well. This may be tempered, however, as international payers become more sophisticated in their contract negotiations, which would put downward pressure on payment rates. The balance of these two forces will ultimately determine the contribution of international patients to the U.S. economy overall.

REFERENCES

1. Schroth L, Khawaja R. Globalization of healthcare. *Front Health Serv Manage.* 2007;24(2):19–30.

2. Centers for Medicare and Medicaid Services. National health expenditure data: NHE factsheet. https://www.cms.gov/NationalHealthExpendData/25_NHE_Fact_sheet.asp. Accessed October 15, 2011.

3. OECD. Improving estimates of exports and imports of health services and goods under the SHA framework. Final report. June 2011.

4. Garman AG, Milstein A, Anderson M. Medical travel. In: Mullner R, ed. *Encyclopedia of Health Services Research*. Thousand Oaks, CA: Sage; 2009.

5. American Hospital Association. Fast facts on U.S. hospitals. http://www.aha.org/aha/resource-center/Statistics-and-Studies/fast-facts.html. Accessed October 15, 2011.

6. Johnson TJ, Garman AG. Impact of medical travel on imports and exports of medical services. *Health Policy*. 2010;98:171–177.

7. UHC. International patient encounters for calendar year 2010 based on payer or zip code YYYYY. [data file]. Chicago: UHC; Retrieved from UHC Clinical Data Base.

8. Ehrbeck T, Guevara C, Mango PD. Mapping the market for medical travel. *McKinsey Quarterly*. May 2008.

9. Deloitte Center for Health Solutions. Medical tourism: 2008 survey of health care consumers. http://www.deloitte.com/assets/Dcom-UnitedStates/Local%20Assets/Documents/us_chs_ConsumerSurveyExecutiveSummary_200208.pdf. Accessed March 9, 2008.

10. Baliga H. Medical tourism is the new wave of outsourcing from India. *India Daily*. December 26, 2006.

11. Deloite Center for Health Solutions. Medical tourism: Update and implications—2009 report. Washington, DC: Deloitte Development LLC; 2009; Publication #9112.

12. Garman AG, Johnson TJ, Clapp JR. The future of medical tourism: Niche market or disruptive innovation? Chicago: Oral presentation, American College of Healthcare Executives Congress on Healthcare Leadership; 2008.

13. Hohmann S, Garman AN, Johnson TJ, Anderson M. Medical tourism: Characteristics of international patients & the care they receive at U.S. academic medical centers. Washington, DC: Oral presentation, AcademyHealth 25th Annual Research Meeting; 2008.

14. Satjapot SP, Johnson TJ, Garman AN. International medical travelers, length of stay, and the continuum of care: Inquiry and comparison. *Qual Manage Health Care*. 2011;20(1):76–83.

15. Agency for Healthcare Research and Quality. HCUPnet: 2009 national statistics, outcomes for all discharges: Weighted national estimates from HCUP nationwide inpatient sample. hcupnet.ahrq.gov. Accessed December 8, 2011.

16. Milstein A, Smith M. Will the surgical world become flat? *Health Affairs*. 2007;26(1):137–141.

17. Kaiser Commission on Medicaid and the Uninsured. The uninsured and the difference health insurance makes. Washington, DC: Henry J. Kaiser Family Foundation; 2011;Publication #1420–1413.

18. Kaiser Family Foundation. Kaiser public opinion: Economic problems facing families. Menlo Park, CA: Henry J. Kaiser Family Foundation; 2008;Publication #7773.

19. Crooks VA, Kingsbury P, Snyder J, Johnston R. What is known about the patient's experience of medical tourism? A scoping review. *BMC Health Services Research*. 2010;10.

20. Keckley P, Couglin S. 2011 survey of health care consumers global report key findings, strategic implications. Washington, DC: Deloitte Center for Health Solutions; 2011.

21. Birkmeyer JD, Dimick JB. Understanding and reducing variation in surgical mortality. *Annu Rev Med*. 2009;60:405–415.

22. Luft HS, Hunt SS, Maerki SC. The volume-outcome relationship: Practice-makes-perfect or selective-referral patterns? *Health Serv Res*. 1987;22(2):157–182.

23. The Leapfrog Group. Factsheet: Evidence-based hospital referral (EBHR). http://www.leapfroggroup.org/media/file/FactSheet_EBHR.pdf

24. Wojcik J. Employers consider short-haul medical tourism. *Business Insurance*. 2009;43(29). http://www.businessinsurance.com/article/20090823/ISSUE01/308 239988#. Accessed April 11, 2012.

25. Chordas L. Heading for home. *Best's Review*. 2009;110(5):40–44.

26. Lapowsky I. Doctors within borders: The allure of domestic medical tourism. *Inc*. 2011;June:25–26.

27. Cleveland Clinic. Lowe's expands heart healthcare benefits with Cleveland Clinic. www.my.clevelandclinic.org/news/2010/lowes_expands_heart_healthcare_benefits.aspx. Accessed May 7, 2010.

Chapter 3

Medical Tourism the European Way

Richard D. Smith, Helena Legido-Quigley,
Neil Lunt, and Daniel Horsfall

Within the European context, a medical tourist—a patient who elects to travel across international borders with the intention of receiving some form of medical treatment—may be categorized in one of two ways. The first is an EU citizen who seeks medical care outside of the European Union, or a non-EU citizen who seeks care in the European Union. This is the archetypal medical tourist, who pays out of pocket for care in another country. However, for European citizens and governments, there is a second form, and it is travel within the European Union by EU citizens who have the rights to access publicly and privately provided medical care in other EU member states. Some of these patients will soon be covered by the Directive on the Application of Patients' Rights in Cross-Border Healthcare. The Directive, adopted by the European Parliament and the Council of the European Union in 2011, was introduced in response to ongoing confusion among patients, commissioners, and providers alike around patient rights to reimbursement for cross-border treatment. A number of high-profile cases taken to the European Court of Justice fueled the need to codify existing rights. The Directive aims to facilitate patients' decisions about cross-border health care by providing patients with information about what treatments they are entitled to;

what reimbursement they will be eligible for; and what costs they will have to meet themselves, along with other issues that will be discussed in detail later in the chapter.[1] The Directive, which has been expanded by successive rulings of the European Court of Justice on private cases regarding consumption of health care in other EU member states and reimbursement by the (national) purchasing body in the home country,[2] establishes the legal framework for all patients traveling abroad to receive treatment in another member state who are not covered by current social security legislation.[3]

The Directive builds on a 1971 regulation, 1408/71 (updated in 2004 with regulation EC 883/2004), which covers people in need of treatment while temporarily abroad, EU citizens living abroad, and those with advance authorization from their own health payers to receive treatment in another member state. The differences in practice between the two routes are not yet clear, and only when the Directive is implemented by October 2013 will we have a clearer idea of how the Directive and regulation EC 883/2004 will work concurrently.

This chapter focuses on those patients who make a personal decision to travel within the European Union to receive health care under the Directive; those paying out-of-pocket payments for services within the European Union not available in their own systems and not covered under the Directive; and patients traveling outside the European Union (see Table 3.1 for a typology of cross-border and international health care travel according to the regulations under which they operate).

The movement of patients within and without Europe for health-related reasons is not a new phenomenon; individuals have traveled for health benefits since ancient times. During the 19th century in Europe,

Table 3.1
Typology of patient mobility

Patients covered by Regulation EC 883/2004
Temporary visitors abroad
Retirees living abroad
People sent abroad by their home system
Patients covered by the new Directive*
Patients taking their own initiative to travel abroad
Patients paying out of pocket for services not available in their own publicly funded systems in the European Union* (often underpinned by legal considerations or because it is cheaper elsewhere) Note: this group is not covered by the Directive.
Patients traveling outside the EU*

Note: Patients traveling for medical care can be categorized by the type of regulations and reimbursement models that apply.
*= The categories marked with an asterisk are the focus of this chapter.

for example, there was a fashion for the growing middle classes to travel to spa towns to "take the waters," which were believed to have health-enhancing qualities. During the 20th century, wealthy people from less-developed areas of the world traveled to European nations to access better facilities and highly trained medics. But this flow is now complemented by outbound travel, and the shifts that are currently underway are quantitatively and qualitatively different from earlier forms of health-related travel. The main difference is that in the past, only the privileged few could travel, whereas nowadays travel is more accessible to the general population. Fundamentally, such developments point toward a paradigm shift in the understanding and delivery of health services. The medical tourism market is growing, with far-reaching implications for the publicly funded health care that predominates in Europe, including a new role for patients as "consumers" of health care rather than "citizens" with rights to health care services. This will, of course, bring a range of attendant risks and opportunities for patients.

Predictions for this emerging global market are difficult to make, since most of the available evidence about medical tourism is anecdotal. Accurate statistics on patients moving across borders are almost nonexistent. Research by the Europe for Patients project found that national health systems did not systematically record provision of health care to foreign patients, and that even when visits from foreign patients were documented, the information was sometimes lost or details were missing, and the data were rarely analyzed. The Europe for Patients report also noted that there is a particular lack of information about foreign patient visits to the commercial sector, as for-profit providers are less willing to share data and collaborate in research programs.[4]

This chapter examines medical tourism from the perspective of the European Union, where universal health care systems predominate, some funded with general taxation and others through social insurance. Our focus is principally on aspects related to the increasing level of out-of-pocket medical tourism within the European Union and between the European Union and the rest of the world. However, this development needs to be set within the context of all patient mobility across EU member states. We will discuss inward and outward flows of patients; industry trends; medicolegal and ethical issues facing the European Union (quality of care, redress, rights and responsibilities, liability, litigation); and health system implications for EU members as source and destination countries.

EUROPE AND THE MARKET FOR MEDICAL TOURISTS

We know that European residents go to other European countries and outside of the European Union for medical care; and residents from other regions, including the Middle East and Asia, come to the European Union to seek medical care, generally paying directly out of pocket. While EU member states are meant to record visits from foreign patients, in reality we know very little about the numbers and flows of medical tourists among nations and continents—partly because this information is rarely reported. Although there is a general consensus that the out-of-pocket medical tourism industry has burgeoned over the past decade and that there is scope for even further expansion, there remains disagreement as to the current size of the industry and even as to how that should be measured. (For example, do we count patients or treatment episodes, day treatments or only in-stay treatments, expatriates and those funded by their multinational employers, all visits or only those to large and accredited providers?) Without robust, routine, and widespread collection of such information, it is not possible to quantify health and economic impacts, or assess opportunities and risks presented to health systems. What follows needs to be understood within this broad and pervasive caveat.

Travel Patterns

In terms of intra-regional trade, or movements of patients within the European Union, the patterns (if not absolute figures) are fairly well established. For example, individuals accessing medical treatment in Hungary tend to be from Western Europe, and some patient flows reflect historical ties: for example, between Hungary and Austria, or between the United Kingdom and Malta or Cyprus. The opening of Eastern Europe and the former USSR has led some Western Europeans to become familiar with and consider health care facilities in these destinations (for example, patients may travel between the United Kingdom and Poland). Nonetheless, the scale of patient mobility within European boundaries is small compared to overall health care expenditure. The European Commission in several of its official documents has estimated the scale at around 1 percent of public health care expenditure, although this figure has not been validated.

Although medical tourism may not currently account for a significant portion of health expenditures in the European Union, there is some evidence to suggest that European citizens are showing a greater interest in traveling to other member states to receive treatment. The Flash Eurobarometer (2007),[5–6] which surveyed European citizens of all member states, reported that 53 percent of those surveyed expressed willingness to search for treatment in another member state. In addition, the results of one of the few studies exploring patient mobility illustrated a marked increase over the years. The study, which surveyed German patients enrolled with a nationwide health insurance fund, found that while in 2003 only 7 percent of patients had obtained nonurgent treatment in another EU country, by 2008, this figure had increased to 40 percent.[5] The Techniker Kranken-kasse (TK) insurance fund contacted patients at 88 clinics in the Nether-lands, Belgium, Austria, and Italy, as well as 28 health and spa institutions in Austria, Italy, the Czech Republic, Hungary, Poland, and Slovakia.

Beyond European boundaries, destinations for EU patients include Asia (India, Malaysia, Singapore, Thailand, and South Korea); South Af-rica; South and Central America (including Brazil, Costa Rica, Cuba, and Mexico); and the Middle East (particularly Dubai). It would appear that proximity is an important, but not a decisive, factor in shaping individual decisions to travel to specific destinations for treatment.[7] For patients in some European countries, the colonial connections, such as the ties be-tween the United Kingdom and India, are important.[8-9] Again, there re-mains substantial disagreement concerning the current size of the industry regionally and globally, with estimates ranging from tens of thousands to millions traveling the globe for care each year.

Reasons for Travel

The key reasons that patients surveyed in the TK Europe study re-ported for opting for treatment in another European country were to save money and to combine treatment with a holiday, illustrating the growing trend toward health care tourism. Although this may not be our archetypi-cal group of patients, since most of the patients in the study were over the age of 60, their practices may be indicative of larger trends. The study also suggested that even though it is widely agreed that most patients prefer to be treated as close to their home as possible, it also appears that patients are willing to seek health care abroad in order to receive treatment with-out delay. As a result, in those member states where there is an increase in waiting times, it could be the case that larger numbers of patients will decide to travel abroad to receive treatment.

Irene Glinos et al.[10] identify four drivers behind the increases in de-mand for foreign medical care: familiarity, affordability, perceived qual-ity, and availability (including international travel for abortion services, fertility treatment, and euthanasia services). Familiarity is often a factor for expatriates, who access medical services on their visits back to their "home" countries—for example, members of the large Indian diaspora in the United Kingdom who return to India for care.[11]

The Flash Barometer survey (2007),[6] focused on the EU market, lists lack of availability of treatment at home, superior quality of treatment abroad, provision of services by specialists, faster treatment, and afford-ability of care among the key drivers that motivate citizens of EU member states to seek treatment outside their home countries. There is, however, little firm evidence on the *relative* importance of these different factors in influencing decisions to seek treatment abroad.

Overall, there is a need for a greater understanding of how decisions are made and how these choices differ for different treatments and consumer groups.[7] We know relatively little about the sociodemographic profiles, age, gender, and existing health conditions of those who cross borders for medical care. Similarly, it remains to be determined whether out-of-pocket medical tourism is a luxury good or not: for example, whether consumers spend proportionately more on medical tourism treatments as incomes rise, how the use of services varies with price (whether there's price elasticity), and whether a worsening of wider economic conditions impacts deleteriously or favorably on medical tourism. Demand for services may be volatile, with travel determined by both wider economic and external factors, as well as shifting consumer preferences and exchange rates.

INDUSTRY TRENDS WITHIN EUROPE

Medical tourism is an emerging global industry with a range of key stakeholders, including providers, brokers, and national governments. At stake are potentially significant revenues from both health services and tourism activities. For the most part, medical tourists from the European Union currently pay out of pocket when they travel abroad for health services. To date, medical tourist providers have had relatively little success tapping the potentially more lucrative income sources of private and workplace insurance systems, apparently due to lack of insurance portability from European countries and the legal uncertainties around cross-border health care. The adoption of the new Directive may potentially benefit health care providers within the European Union by enabling them to attract patients who will be reimbursed for care in member states, or even to be paid directly through the patients' home systems. In addition, the Directive provides clearer information on how decisions around prior authorization will work and how the cost of cross-border health care will be calculated.[1]

A diverse selection of providers participates in the medical tourism industry in the European Union, from solo practices and dual partnerships to extremely large medical tourism facilities. Many emergent medical tourism destinations model their strategies on those of established UK and U.S. private and not-for-profit hospitals, emphasizing quality and customer service. Some hospitals are part of large corporations, such as the Barcelona Medical Centre in Spain, which encompasses 20 health centers, including general clinics, specialty, and diagnostic centers. Providers are primarily from the private sector but are also drawn from the public sector. Some institutions within the UK National Health Service (NHS), for instance, have private facilities for treating foreign patients who pay out of pocket. In addition, within Europe, the new Directive establishes a system of European Reference Networks for highly specialized care for patients with rare diseases. These networks will concentrate knowledge in medical domains and promote progress in the treatment of rare conditions by enabling information sharing and learning through collaborations. Ultimately, since most providers serving medical tourists come from the commercial sector, where companies tend to be reluctant to disclose competitive information, we know relatively little about the development of European and international industries and markets trading in medical tourism.

Less obvious, but perhaps more important, there has been a steady rise in the number of companies and consultancies within Europe offering brokerage arrangements for services and providing web-based information for prospective patients about available services and choices for movement to and from Europe. Typically brokers and their websites tailor packages to meet individuals' requirements, including arrangements for flights, treatment, hotel, and recuperation.[12–15] Brokers may specialize in particular target markets or procedures: for instance, treatments such as dentistry or cosmetic surgery, or in certain destination countries. A series of interrelated issues exist around the precise role of these intermediaries in arranging overseas care, such as how they determine their market, get their information, choose providers, and subsequently determine the most appropriate advice for patients. It is noteworthy that these website facilitation businesses may disappear as quickly as they enter the market.[14] Of future interest will be how such European-based brokers adapt marketing strategies to maximize opportunities from the Directive for patient mobility.

In Europe as elsewhere, the Internet plays a key role in enabling consumers to access health care information and advertising from anywhere in the world—and in enabling providers to target nondomestic markets, often through brokers. While websites might provide reassurance about the quality of care, they remain largely unregulated, and their content may run counter to legal requirements to uphold advertising standards.[16] This online, direct-to-consumer marketing, which helps drive out-of-pocket medical tourism,[17] raises issues of patient safety and informed choice since many medical tourism websites are primarily adverts and infomercials. While there is some wider evidence that the presence of advertising reduces a website's credibility,[18] there is no specific evidence on this topic with relation to medical tourism websites, where it can be difficult for consumers to discern advertising from non-biased information. (For further discussion about brokers, also known as facilitators, and related issues, see chapter 13.)

In addition to individual providers and brokers, national governments seek to stimulate and promote medical tourism in their countries through a range of agencies and policy initiatives. Some countries see significant economic development potential in the emergent field of medical tourism.

Thai, Indian, Singaporean Malaysian, Hungarian, Polish, and Maltese governments have all sought to promote their comparative advantage as medical tourism destinations at large international trade fairs, via advertising within the overseas press, and by providing official support for activities as part of their economic development and tourism policies.[12,19–21] For example, the Polish government is actively attempting to harness the potential of its recent EU ascension to compete with more far-flung destinations for European medical tourists. Poland has established itself as a popular destination for dental and cosmetic care, and many of the state-owned clinics serve Polish citizens alongside medical tourists, reflecting the Polish government's desire to capture the potential of medical tourism. Also supporting the industry are the Polish Medical Tourism Chamber of Commerce[20] and Polish Association of Medical Tourism. Hungary has also sought to utilize the opportunities presented by EU ascension to help develop its medical tourism industry. While many of the clinics offering treatment are private, the Hungarian government has promoted free spa days to tourists and designated 2003 as the Year of Health Tourism. Nicolas Terry refers to Hungary as the "dental capital of the world"[22(p419)] and Hungarian clinics actively market a wide range of dental procedures to tourists on the Internet.

MEDICOLEGAL ISSUES FACING EUROPE

The most significant limitation to the expansion of medical tourism is reservations related to a variety of issues that may be summarized as *medicolegal*. Principle among these concerns is what happens in the event of an adverse outcome arising from failings in clinical and professional practice. This problem is particularly acute where destination countries are not regulated according to source country standards and regulations. This tends to be a greater issue with care sought by EU citizens outside of the European Union than within Europe, since the new Directive reaffirms that member states retain responsibility for care provided in their territory and that cross-border health care should be provided according to the treating country's standards.[3] There are also likely to be stronger consumer safeguards within the European context—although the precise scope of such protections has not been fully tested.

There are a range of dimensions related to the quality and safety of medical treatment abroad. Many of these are not necessarily unique to medical tourism; health care in most any context is replete with information asymmetries and potential threats to quality and safety. But in the case of medical tourism, if patients experience poor quality treatment that results in adverse outcomes; and, as a result, they or their health system wish to bring a civil or criminal case, they face potential confusion with a number of issues not fully clarified by case law and legislation.[23]

Presently, there is a lack of internationally comparative outcome, quality, and safety data. Importantly, bodies such as the World Health Organization have yet to publish guidance on this, and there does not appear to be any immediate intention to develop standards and protocols. For some, a lack of transparency on quality is an impediment to a fully developed market in medical tourism.[24] Availability of reliable evidence about the quality of a particular surgeon or clinical team could encourage more people to pursue medical tourism. What can be gleaned from the literature concerning risk and safety-related incidents for medical tourism is limited. While there is evidence regarding, for example, the occurrence of adverse events in UK hospitals,[25] there are no similar international data.

In addition, medical tourism potentially adds new risks to health care, due to the potentially lengthy overseas travel involved and the nature of treatments and decision-making processes. The journey home can be difficult and painful, especially following surgery. A study of Norwegian patients found that this factor was perceived as the most negative aspect of visiting overseas providers.[26] Traveling when unwell can lead to further health complications, including the possibility of deep vein thrombosis, or blood clots, that can result from the pressure changes entailed in long-haul air travel.

Patient follow-up by providers in cases involving medical travel is rare; a study of 20 patients presenting at a German university hospital after overseas refractive surgery concluded that there was insufficient management of complications and a lack of postoperative care.[27] Even patients traveling within the European Union for medical procedures experience problems with continuity of care. Interviews with 24 English patients treated in Germany revealed a mixed picture of the quality of follow-up care in England. A total of 10 patients rated aftercare as not satisfactory, and some did not receive any aftercare at all.[28] A survey of subscribers of two Dutch health insurers who had received hospital treatment in Belgium showed the aspects of care that patients rated most negatively were related to their experiences once discharged from the hospital.[29]

Many patients travel without a clear understanding of the risks to which they are exposed.[30] Organ transplantation overseas raises particular risks, including infection and graft rejection (for a full discussion of the risks of travel for transplants, see chapter 7). With regard to cosmetic surgery, a survey by the British Association of Plastic, Reconstructive and Aesthetic Surgeons indicated that 37 percent of respondents had seen patients in the NHS with complications arising from overseas cosmetic surgery,[31] and in an audit of the pan-Thames region, 60 percent of consultants replying to a survey indicated that they had seen complications, with the majority (66%) requiring inpatient admission.[32]

In the event that problems occur, there are complexities regarding who could be subject to legal proceedings, where these proceedings would be held, and which country's law would govern.[23] (For a full discussion of these issues, see chapter 9.) The Directive potentially provides some protections for patients. Under the Directive, national authorities can refuse patients permission to go abroad if the treatment would expose the patient to risk or if the treatment raises quality or safety concerns.[3] In those cases where specialized clinical investigations and procedures are involved, member states can create a system of prior authorization to manage the flow of patients.[3] Furthermore, the Directive confirms that the legislation and requirements that apply to safety and liability are those of the member state where the health care is being provided. However, until the Directive is implemented into national law, the existing rules on cross-border health care as established in several court rulings still prevail.[1]

The current legal uncertainly with regard to medical tourism also raises key issues for those providing medical tourism treatments and services. As Laurence Vick[23] observed, providers who promote their services abroad run the risk of becoming subject to other countries' laws if problems arise. New insurance products are increasingly becoming available to provide legal and financial protection for the patient if medical malpractice arises while they are overseas undergoing treatment, but clearly "the devil is in the detail," and medical tourists need to check carefully any exemptions the policy may carry. It may also be advisable for medical tourist brokers to consider insurance coverage since they potentially could become subject to claims for damages via commercial or even criminal routes.

IMPLICATIONS FOR EUROPEAN HEALTH SYSTEMS

Most European countries simultaneously act as countries of origin and destination in the medical tourism marketplace. In both these roles, there are a range of financial, social, political, ethical, and legal issues, as well as implications for local industry.

Impacts on Sending Countries

Important for many European countries are the financial impacts that may arise for their publicly funded health care systems as a result of residents crossing borders for care. Costs may result from elective, overseas cosmetic surgery, or dental work that requires emergency or remedial treatment within home countries upon the patient's return.[31,33-35] Infection outbreaks resulting from travel will also bring their own costs. Similarly, there may be health and social care costs that arise from multiple births associated with overseas fertility treatments.[36] There also may be impacts on domestic private health providers, who potentially lose business to overseas providers. In addition, there are costs associated with residents seeking care overseas—the necessity to monitor or regulate advertising, or provide detailed information and advice to support potential or actual medical tourists, for instance. However, there has been little systematic collection of evidence or attempts to estimate overall system costs.

In addition to the potential extra costs, there is the likelihood that large numbers of medical tourists traveling from the European Union to other countries could have other impacts on the sending country's own health system. Outflows of high-income patients, for example, may reduce revenue and dilute political support for developing local services. Such flows could also reduce the pressure for investment in certain kinds of facilities or technologies. Indeed, there is an argument that some types of outflows of medical tourists for treatments that could be provided locally signals a failure of policy and delivery in the sender country. Within higher-income countries, medical tourism may also exacerbate the emergence of a two-tier system. If, for example, eligibility for services such as fertility or dental work is tightened, then those with private resources may choose to travel overseas to maintain access (thus exercising choice and exit). Those lacking the resources to travel may retain only the option of voicing their discontent with domestic provision or lack thereof. Patients who are able to circumvent waiting times point to familiar concerns of access and equity. In those countries where third party insurers are exploring medical tourism as a provider option, those who are insured under these plans—perhaps unable to get alternative cover—may find themselves disadvantaged by the expectation that they travel overseas for particular procedures.

Clearly, however, source country payers may benefit from outflows of patients–employers and employees contributing to health plans and the public insurance system itself could benefit financially if medical tourism is an option. For instance, individual flows may become consolidated into bilateral relationships with wider benefit. For example, the UK NHS reduced waiting times by outsourcing certain cases to France and Germany during 2001–2002.[37] A total of 190 patients (153 orthopedic and 37 ophthalmology) were treated on an inpatient basis. This arrangement, which included a focus on "long waiters," enabled NHS providers to meet targets and reduce waiting lists. More than 80 percent of patients who participated reported that they were very satisfied with their experiences. Similarly, a recent study looking at possible bilateral medical tourism trade between the United Kingdom and India suggested that by funding patients who wished to go to India for select services, the UK NHS could realize substantial benefits, both financially and by alleviating waiting lists.[8,11,38] The study, which looked at patients on waiting lists for certain procedures suitable for medical tourism such as hip and knee replacements, compared the costs of getting treatment in the United Kingdom with the cost of sending patients to India with an accompanying adult and found the savings would be approximately £120 million (US$187 million). This figure becomes £200 million (US$312 million) if expenses associated with sending accompanying adults are not covered. Some subsets of the population, such as first- and second-generation Indian nationals, may prefer to go back "home" for treatment and may be happy to cross-subsidize some of the costs, or may not need an accompanying adult, further increasing the amount saved. Plausibly the health systems within source countries could develop relations with off-shore medical tourism facilities to leverage costs savings, providing individuals with a choice of overseas destinations. In addition to reducing costs, this form of outsourcing or more "collective" medical travel could also reduce waiting lists.[8]

One of the drivers for medical tourism is price; patients may travel for treatments that are available locally within the private sector but at greater cost. There are arguments that some medical systems are inefficient and face restrictive barriers to entry. A development such as medical tourism can potentially exert competitive pressure on these systems and help drive down the costs and prices offered in domestic systems. This was the case when the NHS outsourced some services to France and Germany during 2001–2002. Some commentators argued that this was a short-term move designed to challenge domestic monopolies and thus bring about change in the home health care system.[1] And, in fact, medical tourism encourages economies to maximize their comparative advantages in labor costs, technology, or capacity. However, there are criticisms that numbers treated in such initiatives as the above are relatively small, and therefore any capacity created is small relative to the large organizational effort required to arrange such outsourcing schemes. These arrangements also have an impact on local health systems that is more political and ethical; the possibility that patients may access overseas treatments that are not provided, or are illegal, within the source country may generate public debate about the importance of providing them locally (for example, latest fertility treatments, gender reassignment, organ transplantation, or even euthanasia services).

Thus, source counties (those importing health services) may benefit from medical tourism through alleviating waiting lists and lowering health care costs but may risk quality of care and legal liability.

Impacts on Receiving Countries

Many European countries, especially those in Eastern Europe, are also destination countries that export health services. Most countries that engage in delivering care to medical tourists do so to increase the level of direct foreign exchange earnings coming into their country to improve their balance of payments position. To some extent, this might be thought of as income accruing directly to the health system. For instance, foreign patients purchase health care services and hence provide an income that can be used within hospitals to cross-subsidize care for domestic patients or to help fund capital investments that benefit all patients who use the hospital. It is therefore possible that some countries may seek foreign patients in order to develop facilities to better serve local patients. However, these arguments are more likely to be "window dressing," while the core motive is to increase foreign exchange earnings. One must remember that foreign patients may represent a significant or insignificant addition to the number of domestic patients—the addition of medical tourists might amount to more than 50 percent of the private market in some instances but in others may only top up a thriving domestic private market by 10 to 20 percent. There may also be different economic implications depending upon whether these patients are simply using spare capacity in the private sector, or competing with domestic patients.

Although medical tourism may bring some income to the health sector, it is typically not health care income that concerns destination countries, but instead general increases in tourist income and hence foreign exchange. A 2006 report by the Tourism Research and Marketing Group estimated that worldwide, there are 37 million health-related trips for patients and their companions each year, generating €33 billion ($US39 billion) in revenues from health care and tourism.[39] Indeed, it is the promise of these earnings that often drives governments to invest directly or indirectly (e.g., through tax incentives) in private hospitals and actively promote medical tourism.[40–42] Thus, sectors other than medical care—especially those associated with hospitality and travel—may benefit to some degree from increased medical tourism, as will the government more centrally through increased taxation revenue.

Nonetheless, the net income from medical tourism may not be as significant as it appears. For instance, in many cases medical tourists are either diaspora or patients who have previously visited the country and are likely to return again. Thus, they are regular visitors who on one trip happen to add in an element of medical care, so it is highly likely that the non–health care revenue would have been raised irrespective of their visit for medical reasons. In this situation, clearly the additional income generated by the "medical" element of medical tourism is far more limited, and the overall addition to the economy consequently less, which may put a different perspective on the balance of benefits and risks. Further, there are also financial costs associated with drawing medical tourists to a country. As mentioned above, often there are requirements for upgraded infrastructure, either specifically within the health sector—for example, enhanced hospital facilities; or outside of that sector—for instance, roads and telecommunications. There are also likely to be costs associated with providing appropriate staffing of facilities, possible accreditation schemes, and other requirements to attract medial tourists.

CONCLUSION

Where does this analysis take us in considering what a European perspective contributes to the study of medical tourism? Explorations of medical tourism commonly address implications and actions of low- and middle-income countries, principally as destination countries; the movement of patients from high-income countries, especially the United States and some European nations, to low- and middle-income countries; the role of multilateral trade agreements, especially under the World Trade Organization's General Agreement on Trade in Services (GATS); and the potential damages, costs, and risks presented.[43-44] The European perspective emphasizes, in addition, the implications for social health systems and the role of regional cross-border trade (applicable to other regions such as Asia, with ASEAN—the Association of Southeast Asian Nations; and North America, with NAFTA—the North American Free Trade Agreement).

The key issues facing European health systems principally relate to the finance and regulation of medical tourism. Despite concerns generated by the current financial crisis, there is no sign that economic liberalization is slowing down. As trading opportunities in other sectors become exhausted, as experience within the services trade generally expands, and as the financial climate stabilizes into (and out of) recession, European countries will increasingly look to the opportunities that international trade has to offer. For importing services, this will center on cost, quality, and timeliness. For exporting services, this will center on technology transfer, skill enhancements, and foreign income.

A limit to international health care trade in Europe is that, at present, medical tourism is driven by commercial interests lying outside of organized and state-run health policy making and delivery. There are possibilities to bring it more within the remit of domestic policy competency, involving, for example, third party (state) payers sending patients abroad. Given the heavily politicized nature of health care (even in countries with substantial private health care sectors), there will be concerns about the threats this poses, but increasing levels of regional cross-border movement is certainly more amenable than wider movement beyond EU borders. For instance, there are some specific opportunities presented by intra-EU movement of patients across borders; smaller countries, or regions with low population densities, may benefit from treatments being available that would otherwise be unavailable, for example, and border regions could make more rational use of scarce capacities.[4]

On a global level, medical tourism raises questions for transnational and global structures and processes. There is currently a lack of agreed-upon international standards for assessing and ensuring the quality and safety of medical tourism providers and health professionals, and consequently no obligation for them to ensure quality and safety other than an ethical one. There is a range of possible solutions (both national and transnational), from interventions that provide more information (although by whom and at what points is not clear); to those that restrict potential consumers' choices (either directly or through discouragement); to attempts to restrict supply (whether approving or licensing providers or intermediaries). There are also interventions that may aim to offer consumer protection around poor quality treatments, such as encouraging independent holistic accreditation by recognized schemes, advising clinicians responsible for delivering services to take out personal medical indemnity that would compensate their patients in the event of problems, or requiring medical tourists themselves to purchase insurance coverage.[45] It is important for European countries to engage in such debate, and perhaps lead developments, as they share common concerns when their citizens increasingly go outside of the European Union for care.

The Directive has introduced new provisions that will benefit all types of patients. National contact points will be established to provide patients with information on rights and procedures. These national contact points will have to provide information on health care providers, including assessments, procedures for reimbursement, and complaint and redress mechanisms.[3] Each health care provider must supply patients with information on availability, quality, and safety of care. This new mechanism will make the process more transparent, and all patients (including out-of-pocket travelers and even those who do not travel abroad) will benefit by having more information about their health care options. The Directive also may encourage more direct marketing by providers aimed at both reimbursable patients eligible under cross-border payments and those paying out of pocket. This *may* lead to better improved information on provider outcomes data being available for prospective travelers. Alternatively, such marketing may eschew an evidence-based approach.

The Directive represents a first step in setting some common standards for cross-border care within the European Union. However, the divergent health policies and public health practices across Europe require further coordination. Knowledge exchange in this field is already taking place both informally and formally in the form of collaborating networks. There is considerable experience in the realm of best practice with collaborating platforms endorsed on a European level, such as the European network for Health Technology Assessment (EUnetHTA) program, which has been quite successful in promoting the optimization of HTA methodology and knowledge transfer. Another possibility would be to introduce the "open method of coordination" for particular initiatives (such as clinical guideline development) in which member states share best practices and increase policy convergence in areas that remain a primary responsibility of national governments. More specific strategies can be facilitated by exchange of information on best practices as suggested in the health strategy and in the work of the health information unit for the European Union's Directorate General for Health and Consumers (DGSANCO).

The new Directive is the first example of EU legislation in the area of health care services; this responsibility has been traditionally the sole preserve of member states. Once it is transposed into national law, the Directive will establish common standards for how the process of prior authorization will work, how patients can access information about entitlements, how many and who will be responsible for establishing a national contact point(s), what data providers will have to collect, and how the cost for cross-border health care will be calculated.[1] The Directive encourages cooperation between member states in a number of areas related to cross-border health care and has great potential to clarify patients' rights and to establish clearer rules.

Our analysis in this chapter has to be set in the context of a significant absence of systematic data concerning health services trade, both overall and at a disaggregated level, in terms of individual modes of delivery and activities in specific countries. Data are lacking in both the terms and extent of the trade itself, as well as its implications. While the numbers of patients traveling with costs reimbursed under the Directive will be clear, the size of out-of-pocket patient flows and spending will continue to remain opaque. For instance, there is little robust evidence that medical tourism adds especially to the economies of destination countries, as figures tend to be quoted in aggregate, not at the marginal level of the additional tourist-related income specifically resulting from *medical* tourism. Prior to any state intervention or regulation, we need more information and understanding.

The lack of data must be addressed if European countries are to keep fully informed about the significance (potential or actual) of medical tourism for their health systems. Quantitative data are needed about patient flows, further information is needed on risks to cross-border health care and possible impacts on national health care systems, and more research is needed on patients' and health care professionals' experiences and preferences.

REFERENCES

1. NHS. *Patient choice beyond borders: Implications of the EU Directive on cross-border healthcare for NHS commissioners and providers.* Brussels: NHS European Office; May 2011.

2. Bertinato L, Busse R, Fahy N, et al. *Cross-border health care in Europe.* Denmark: WHO; 2005.

3. Legido-Quigley H, Passarani I, Knai C, et al. Cross-border healthcare in the European Union: Clarifying patients' rights. *BMJ.* 2011; 342.

4. Rosenmöller M, McKee M, Baeten R, eds. *Patient mobility in the European Union: Learning from experience.* Denmark: European Observatory on Health Systems and Policies; 2006.

5. Wahner C, Verheyen F. *TK in Europe: TK Europe Survey, 2009—German patients en route to Europe.* Hamburg: Techniker Krankenhause; 2009.

6. The Gallup Organization. *Cross-border health services in the EU: Analytical report.* Budapest: The Gallup Organization with the European Commission; 2007.

7. Exworthy M, Peckham S. Access, Choice and travel: Implications for health policy. *Social Policy & Administration.* 2006; 40:267–287.

8. Smith RD, Martinez-Alvarez M, Chanda R. Medical tourism: A review of the literature and analysis of a role for bi-lateral trade. *Health Policy.* 2011; 103:276–282.

9. Bergmark R, Barr D, Garcia R. Mexican immigrants in the U.S. living far from the border may return to Mexico for health services. *Journal of Immigrant and Minority Health.* 2008; 12(4):610–614.

10. Glinos IA, Baeten R, Boffin N. Cross-border contracted care in Belgian hospitals. In: Rosenmöller M, Baeten R, McKee M, eds. *Patient mobility in the European Union: Learning from experience.* Denmark: European Observatory on Health Systems and Policies; 2006.

11. Martinez Alvarez, M., Chanda, R. & Smith, R. D. The potential for bi-lateral agreements in medical tourism: A qualitative study of stakeholder perspectives from the UK and India. *Globalization and Health.* 2011; (7)11.

12. Whittaker A. Pleasure and pain: Medical travel in Asia. *Global Public Health: An International Journal for Research, Policy and Practice.* 2008; 3(3):271–290.

13. Reddy S, Qadeer I. Medical tourism in India: Progress or predicament? *Economic and Political Weekly.* 2010; 45(10). http://epw.in/epw/uploads/articles/14762.pdf.

14. Cormany D, Baloglu S. Medical travel facilitator websites: An exploratory study of web page contents and services offered to the prospective medical tourist. *Tourism Management.* 2010; 32(4):709–716.

15. Lunt N, Carrera P. Advice for prospective medical tourists: Systematic review of consumer sites. *Tourism Review.* 2011; 66(1/2):57–67.

16. Legido-Quigley H, McKee M, Nolte E, Glinos IA. *Assuring the quality of health care in the European Union. A case for action.* Vol 12. Copenhagen 2008.

17. Lunt N, Hardey M, Mannion R. Nip, tuck and click: Medical tourism and the emergence of web-based health information. *The Open Medical Informatics Journal.* 2010; 4:1–11.

18. Walther BJ, Wang Z, Loh T. The effect of top-level domains and advertisements on health web site credibility. *J Med Internet Res.* September 3, 2004; 6(3):e24.

19. Mudur G. Hospitals in India woo foreign patients. *BMJ.* June 5, 2004; 328 (7452):1338.

20. Reisman D. *Health tourism: Social welfare through international trade.* Cheltenham, UK: Edward Elgar; 2010.

21. Chee HL. Medical tourism in Malaysia: International movement of healthcare consumers and the commodification of healthcare. *ARI Working Paper* 2007; 83. http://www.ari.nus.edu.sg/docs/wps/wps07_083.pdf.

22. Terry NP. Under-regulated health care phenomena in a flat world: Medical tourism and outsourcing. *Western New England Law Review.* 2007; 29:421.

23. Vick L. Medical tourism: Legal issues. *Destination Health Medical Tourism Conference.* Olympia, London: Michelmores Solicitors; 2010.

24. Ehrbeck T, Guevara C, Mango PD. Mapping the market for medical travel. *The McKinsey Quarterly.* 2008. https://www.mckinseyquarterly.com/Mapping_the_market_for_travel_2134.

25. Sari AB-A, Sheldon TA, Cracknell A, Turnbull A. Sensitivity of routine system for reporting patient safety incidents in an NHS hospital: Retrospective patient case note review. *BMJ.* January 13, 2007; 334(7584):79.

26. HELTEF. *Evaluering: Pasienterfaringer I kjøp av helsetjenester i utlandet [Evaluation: patient experiences from purchasing healthcare abroad.* Oslo: Norwegian Knowledge Centre for Health Services; 2003.

27. Terzi E, Kern T, Kohnen T. Complications after refractive surgery abroad. *Ophthalmologe.* May 2008; 105(5):474–479.

28. Birch I, v. Boxberg M. *The international market for medical services: The UK-Germany experience.* London: Anglo-German Foundation for the Study of Industrial Society; 2004.

29. Boffin N, Baeten, R. *Dutch patients evaluate contracted care in Belgian hospitals: Results of a patient survey.* Brussels: European Social Observatory; 2005.

30. Krishnan N, Cockwell P, Devulapally P, et al. Organ trafficking for live donor kidney transplantation in Indoasians resident in the West Midlands: High activity and poor outcomes. *Transplantation.* 2010; 89(12):1456–1461.

31. Jeevan R, Armstrong A. Cosmetic tourism and the burden on the NHS. *Journal of Plastic, Reconstructive & Aesthetic Surgery.* 2008; 61(12):1423–1424.

32. Birch J, Caulfield R, Ramakrishnan V. The complications of "cosmetic tourism"—an avoidable burden on the NHS. *Journal of Plastic, Reconstructive & Aesthetic Surgery.* 2007; 60(9):1075–1077.

33. Healy C. Surgical tourism and the globalisation of healthcare. *Irish Journal of Medical Science.* 2009; 178(2):125–127.

34. Cheung IK, Wilson A. Arthroplasty tourism. *Med J Aust.* Dec 3–17, 2007; 187(11–12):666–667.

35. Miyagi K, Auberson D, Patel AJ, Malata CM. The unwritten price of cosmetic tourism: An observational study and cost analysis. *Journal of Plastic, Reconstructive and Aesthetic Surgery.* Jan 2012; 65(1):22–8.

36. Ledger WL, Anumba D, Marlow N, Thomas CM, Wilson ECF, Group TCoMBS. Fertility and assisted reproduction: The costs to the NHS of multiple births after IVF treatment in the UK. *BJOG: An International Journal of Obstetrics & Gynaecology.* 2006; 113(1):21–25.

37. Lowson K, West P, Chaplin S, O'Reilly J. *Evaluation of Patients Travelling Overseas: Final Report.* York: York Health Economics Consortium; 2002.

38. Martinez Alvarez, M., Chanda, R. & Smith, R. How is Telemedicine perceived? A qualitative study of perspectives from the UK and India. *Globalization and Health.* 2011; (7)17.

39. TRAM. *Medical Tourism: A Global Analysis.* Bruxelles: Tourism Research and Marketing. 2006.

40. Ramírez de Arellano AB. Patients without borders: The emergence of medical tourism. *International Journal of Health Services.* 2007; 37(1):193–198.

41. Reed CM. Medical tourism. *Medical Clinics of North America.* 2008; 92(6):1433–1446.

42. Lee CG. Health care and tourism: Evidence from Singapore. *Tourism Management.* 2010; 31(4):486–488.

43. Smith RD, Rupa C, Viroj T. Trade in health-related services. *The Lancet.* 2009; 373(9663):593–601.

44. Blouin C, Drager N, Smith R, eds. *International trade in health services and the GATS: Current issues and debates.* Washington, DC: World Bank; 2006.

45. Cohen IG. Protecting patients with passports: Medical tourism and the patient protective-argument. *Iowa Law Review.* 2010; 95(5):1467–1567.

Chapter 4

Medical Tourism in Southeast Asia: Opportunities and Challenges

Churnrurtai Kanchanachitra, Cha-aim Pachanee, Manuel M. Dayrit, and Viroj Tangcharoensathien

Over the last decade, Southeast Asia has witnessed a significant growth in medical tourism, with foreign patients coming to the region for a variety of health services that are either unaffordable, unavailable, or of lower quality in their home countries. This chapter examines four Southeast Asian countries where the medical tourism industry plays a significant role—Malaysia, the Philippines, Singapore, and Thailand—and seeks to contribute to national policy discussions about the potential benefits and challenges that arise in providing medical services to foreign patients. In this comparative perspective, we review the evolution of medical tourism in relation to each country's domestic health system development, discuss their respective policy environments and comparative advantages as medical tourism destinations, and examine the impacts of medical tourism on their economies and on medical service provision for local citizens.

Figure 4.1 presents our framework for considering the many factors that governments must weigh in developing their medical tourism industries to promote economic development without compromising the health of their populations. Achieving both goals requires coherent policies and social consensus. This chapter explores the four selected countries' polices around trade in health services—and medical tourism in particular—and

Figure 4.1
Balancing Trade and Health

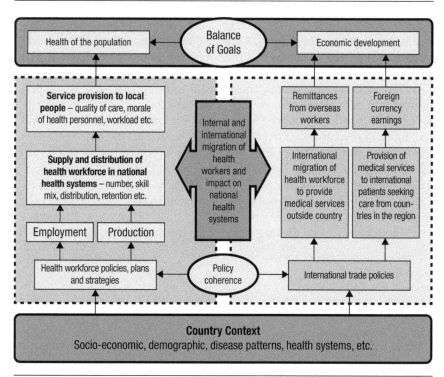

In developing their medical tourism industry, each country must weigh potential foreign currency earnings and other benefits against possible repercussions such as workforce shortages in the public health system.

Source: This article was published in *The Lancet,* Vol. 377 No. 9767. Churnrurtai Kanchanachitra, Magnus Lindelow, Timothy Johnston, Piya Hanvoravongchai, Fely Marilyn Lorenzo, Nguyen Lan Huong, Siswanto Agus Wilopo, Jennifer Frances dela Rosa. Human resources for health in southeast Asia: Shortages, distributional challenges, and international trade in health services, 769–781. © Elsevier (2011).

analyzes whether and how these countries balance these potentially competing goals.

THE RISE OF MEDICAL TOURISM IN SOUTHEAST ASIA

It is difficult to quantify the growth of medical tourism in Southeast Asia with precision because there is no generally accepted definition of medical tourism or methodology for counting medical tourists. Some countries include outpatients in their counts, for example, while others may only count inpatients. The Organisation for Economic Co-operation and Development (OECD) and World Health Organization (WHO) are currently developing common definitions and metrics,[1] and if these are widely adopted, comparisons across countries will improve. In the meantime, this chapter defines medical tourism broadly as those who seek health care abroad regardless of the purpose of their travel—in other words, whether they traveled specifically for medical care or sought medical care because they fell ill while traveling or working—because this definition will encompass all of the data that are collected and provided by the countries included in this analysis.

As Figure 4.2 demonstrates, the medical tourism industry developed differently in each of the four countries that are the subjects of our analysis. Estimates for the number of foreign patients traveling to Malaysia and Thailand for services increased substantially from 2002 to 2008. However, in Singapore and the Philippines, the number of foreign patients has remained rather stable in the past three to five years. Data show that most international patients come from within the intra-Asia region. In 2005, most of Singapore's international patients came from Indonesia and Malaysia, for example.[2] Similarly, during the period of 2006–2008, some 77 percent of international patients visiting Malaysia came from Indonesia.[2]

Figure 4.2
International Patient Visits*

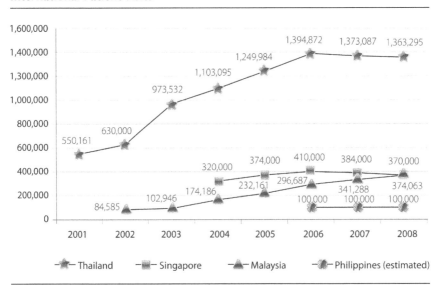

*Estimates for Malaysia and Thailand reflect all international patients; estimates for Singapore and the Philippines are for patients who traveled specifically for health care.

Reports of visits from international patients, including medical tourists, to Thailand, Malaysia, Singapore, and the Philippines reflect the general growth of medical tourism in the region, particularly in Thailand. *Sources:* Chee HL. Medical tourism and the state in Malaysia and Singapore. *Glob. Soc. Policy.* December 1, 2010;10(3):336–357; Thailand Department of Export Promotion, Ministry of Commerce annual survey, 2001–2008; Joint Foreign Chambers AP. *A business perspective.* Arangkada, Philippines 2010. http://www.investphilippines.info/arangkada/tourism-medical-travel-retirement/.

HEALTH SERVICE AND FINANCING SYSTEMS

The varying complexions of the medical tourism industries in Malaysia, the Philippines, Singapore, and Thailand reflect the countries' different levels of economic development and diverse approaches to health service provision and financing as detailed in Table 4.1. The Philippines is a lower- to middle-income country with more than 20 percent of the population living in poverty, while Malaysia and Thailand are middle-income countries with relatively small portions of the population living in poverty, and Singapore is a high-income country. Their health financing

Table 4.1
Health and economic indicators

	Malaysia	Philippines	Singapore	Thailand
Gross national income per capita (PPP* international $), 2009	$13,710	$4,060	$49,780	$7,640
Population living on <$1 (PPP international $) a day (%), 2000–2008	<0.2%	22.6%	N/A	<2.0%
National Health Account parameters (2008)				
Total Health Expenditure (THE), % Gross Domestic Product	4.3%	3.7%	3.3%	4.1%
THE, per capita, US$	$353	$68	$1,404	$164
THE, per capita PPP int. $	$621	$129	$1,833	$328
General Government Health Expenditure (GGHE), %THE	44.1%	34.7%	34.1%	74.3%
Private health expenditure (Prvt HE), % THE	55.9%	65.3%	65.9%	25.7%
Social Health Insurance, % GGHE	0.8%	21.7%	13.2%	9.0%
Out-of-pocket payment, % Private HE	73.2%	82.5%	94.3%	68.1%
Out-of-pocket payment, % THE (2007)	40.7%	54.7%	63.3%	19.2%
Hospital beds (2000–2009)				
% Public	73.3%	51.0%	72.0%	80.0%
% Private	26.7%	49.0%	28.0%	20.0%

*Purchasing power parity (i.e., factors in cost of living and inflation).
Note: The varying economic and health indicators in Malaysia, the Philippines, Singapore, and Thailand have influenced how medical tourism has developed in each country.
Source: WHO World Health Statistics 2011.

systems also differ; while most health spending is privately funded in Malaysia (55.9%), the Philippines (65.3%), and Singapore (65.9%); the reverse is true in Thailand, where private health expenditure accounts for just over a quarter of health costs (25.7%). In all four countries, most private health expenditure comes from individuals paying out of pocket, especially in Singapore (94.3%). This section describes the health service and financing systems in these four countries and explores the relation with the countries' policies on medical tourism.

Malaysia

Prior to the early 1980s, the health care system of Malaysia was primarily the National Health Service. It was financed mostly from taxation and provided health services for the population either for free or, in some cases, a nominal charge.[3] Since the early 1980s, the private sector has played an increasingly significant role, especially at the higher end of the health care spectrum. The proportion of private hospital beds has increased from 5 percent of total acute care beds in 1980 to 25 percent today, with slight dips along the way due to the economic recession in the mid-1980s and the Asian financial crisis in 1997.[3] Large, corporate hospitals owned by private Malaysian investors has helped drive recent growth. Initially, the private sector consisted of general practitioners operating as small businesses and some small private hospitals. Subsequently, large corporations bought up the small hospitals and built additional facilities. These large hospitals have attracted a substantial flow of medical specialists, physicians, nurses, and other allied health experts from the public sector, resulting in a rapid growth of private specialists. Data from 1999 to 2001 indicate that more than 70 percent of the specialist services in radiotherapy, magnetic resonance imaging, CT scanning, mammography, and cardiothoracic treatment were delivered in the private sector.[3]

Interestingly, while the Malaysian health system originated as a publicly financed system providing free or low cost services to all citizens, the government has strongly backed the corporatization of public hospitals and the burgeoning enterprise of large private hospitals, reflecting a pro-private ideology in public policies. In 1991, the government introduced the Caring Society social policy to make the government health sector more self-supporting and less like a social welfare program. As a result, patients' fees increased in government hospitals, and patients were allowed to tap their Employees' Provident Fund (EPF, a compulsory savings plan for workers), to cover medical treatments.[2] At the same time, the government embarked on a privatization policy that involved corporatizing the National Heart Institute in 1993 and the University of Malaya Medical Centre in 1998, and there are plans to privatize all other government hospitals.

Despite the fact that all citizens are entitled to publicly funded health services, out-of-pocket payments for health services account for 40.7 percent of the country's total health expenditures. This apparent contradiction reflects the comparatively modest public spending on health—44.1 percent of the total health expenditure—that results in limited public services, prompting citizens who can afford to do so to pay out of pocket for more and better services. Overall, in the last two decades, Malaysian health care has become more corporate in nature, and this corporatization has led to the increasing commodification of health care and set the stage for medical tourism.

The Philippines

Over the last 60 years, the Philippines has developed an extensive infrastructure of public hospitals, health centers, and *barangay* (village) health stations that provide services to its population. This public infrastructure exists in parallel with a private sector infrastructure of primary, secondary, and tertiary care hospitals located primarily in urban centers throughout the country.[4] In 2004, there were 1,723 licensed public and private hospitals with a combined bed capacity of 85,040. The government owned and operated 654 (38%) of these hospitals, which accounted for 53 percent of the total bed capacity. By 2009, the total number of licensed public and private hospitals had increased to 1,822, including 729 (40%) public hospitals. While the total bed capacity in the Philippines increased 15 percent between 2004 and 2009 to 97,664, the share of government hospital beds dropped slightly to 51 percent as a result of increased bed capacity in private sector facilities. During this period, the average bed capacity per hospital in the private sector rose from 38 to 44, while the average bed capacity in public facilities remained stable at 68.[5]

At the pinnacle of the government system are the specialty hospitals that include the Philippine Heart Center for Asia, the Lung Center of the Philippines, the National Kidney and Transplant Institute, and the Philippine Children's Medical Center. These specialty centers, located in metropolitan Manila, were established in the 1970s and are among the finest tertiary care facilities in the country. In addition, each of the 16 administrative regions of the country has a government regional tertiary hospital. These specialty and regional hospitals are under the jurisdiction of the national government's Department of Health. There are also provincial and city hospitals under the jurisdiction of their respective provincial and city governments with capacities ranging from 50 to 150 beds.

The government also operates health centers and *barangay* health stations that provide free preventive and primary care services, including maternal and child care, communicable disease control, and family planning to low-income families in both rural and urban areas. There are about

1,000 municipal health centers throughout the country staffed by teams of doctors, nurses, and midwives and 10,000 *barangay* health stations that are visited by midwives and supported by community health workers. In 1992, the Local Government Code moved the management of these health centers and *barangay* health stations from the national Department of Health to local governments.[6]

In 2010, total expenditure on health as a percentage of Gross Domestic Product (GDP) was 3.7 percent.[7] Overall, health care for Filipinos is financed by taxes, social health insurance, and out-of-pocket expenditures. In 2004, total per capita spending for health was US$35.30, which represented roughly 2–3 percent of the total annual expenditure of an average Filipino family.[4] Government expenditure on health has increasingly fallen short of meeting the health needs of the population. In 2010, general government expenditures on health accounted for only 34.7 percent of total health care expenditure, compared with 47.6 percent in 2000.[7] While most of the population is covered by public insurance (77% in 2007), the depth of coverage has remained shallow; expenditures attributable to public insurance comprise only 10 percent of total health expenditures.[8] The private sector, which operates on a fee-for-service basis, provides fair to excellent health services to those who can pay the required fees. In 2010, private sector expenditure accounted for 65.3 percent of total health expenditure, and of that, 82.5 percent was out-of pocket-payments,[9] 12.2 percent from private insurance, and the rest from employers' contributions.[7]

President Benigno Aquino Jr., who was elected into office in 2010 for a six-year term, has launched an ambitious health agenda aimed at providing universal access to affordable, quality care for necessary services. To move toward this goal, the administration recommended the following indicators:

1. Out-of-pocket spending should not exceed 30 percent–40 percent of total health expenditures. (This figure ranged from 40–50% in the early 2000s.[4])
2. Total health expenditure should be at least 4 percent–5 percent of GDP. (In 2009, this figure was 3.8%.[7])
3. More than 90 percent of the population should be covered by prepayment and risk-pooling schemes. (In 2007, this figure was 77%.[6,7,10])
4. Close to 100 percent coverage of vulnerable populations should be provided with social assistance and safety-net programs.[8]

In parallel to the policy on universal coverage, the Philippine government is promoting medical tourism to tap into the global market and earn foreign currency.[11] Issues around the simultaneous implementation of these two policies will be reviewed in a later section.

Singapore

Singapore, with a population of 5.8 million in 2010,[12] has seven public hospitals comprised of five acute general hospitals, a women's and children's hospital, and a psychiatry hospital. The general hospitals provide multidisciplinary acute inpatient and specialist outpatient services and a 24-hour emergency department. In addition, there are six national specialty centers for cancer, cardiac, eye, skin, neuroscience, and dental care. There were 16 private hospitals in 2006 with capacities ranging from 20 to 505 beds.[13] There were 11,509 total hospital beds in 2010, or 3.2 beds for every 1,000 people. About 77 percent of the beds were in public hospitals.[14]

During the 1990s, the government restructured all 13 public hospitals and specialty centers as private companies wholly owned by the government to enable more management autonomy and flexibility and to introduce commercial accounting systems. These restructured hospitals receive an annual government subsidy to provide subsidized medical services to patients. They are managed like not-for-profit organizations and are subject to broad policy guidance by the government through the Ministry of Health. In addition, the government introduced community hospitals to provide intermediate health care to sick and aged people who do not require more intensive care.[13]

Singaporeans co-pay their health care costs under the Medisave, Medishield, Eldershield, and Medifund schemes. These schemes were introduced to reform the health care financing system from one that was primarily tax based to a system that is more patient funded. Patients pay differential subsidies for different hospital bed types; there is no subsidy for class A; a 20–65 percent subsidy for class B; and a 70–80 percent subsidy for class C beds.[13] As in Malaysia and the Philippines, out-of-pocket payments are still high, making up 63.3 percent of total health expenditure in 2007.[15]

Thailand

In Thailand, the Ministry of Public Health owns and operates the majority of health facilities. The Ministry also supervises and licenses private clinics and hospitals. Existing public health facilities provide extensive coverage throughout the country at all levels of care. In 2009, in Bangkok alone, there were five medical schools affiliated with universities, 26 general hospitals, 13 specialty hospitals, and a number of health centers under the Ministry of Public Health. In addition, in the regions outside of Bangkok there were six medical schools, 25 regional hospitals, 48 specialty hospitals, 69 general hospitals, 734 district hospitals and 9,768 health centers covering 100 percent of the country.[16]

In the private sector, the number of hospitals expanded rapidly, from about 10 percent of total beds in the entire health system in 1985 to

23 percent in 1997. This expansion was largely influenced by the rapid economic growth and increased demand for private hospital care by the middle classes in the early 1990s. After the 1997 economic crisis, a number of private hospitals closed down, and many reduced their capacity.[17] In 2009, there were 322 private hospitals with a total of 33,405 beds, or about 20 percent of total beds. Some 30 percent of these private hospitals were in Bangkok.[16] In addition, other government organizations such as defense and local bodies run hospitals that serve the general public, accounting for about 12 percent of beds.[16]

Thailand achieved universal coverage for the population in 2002. Medical service costs are financed through one of the three health insurance schemes: the (1) Universal Coverage of health insurance scheme (UC), (2) Civil Servant Medical Benefit Scheme (CSMBS), or the (3) Social Security Scheme (SSS). Less than 0.9 percent of the total population has private health insurance.[16] Compared to the other three countries included in this analysis, Thailand's government health expenditure is significantly higher (74.3% of total health expenditures or THE), and its per household out-of-pocket payment lower (19.2% of THE), on par with the OECD average in 2007.[15]

THE EVOLUTION OF MEDICAL TOURISM

The growth of medical tourism in Southeast Asia came on the heels of the 1997 Asian economic crisis, which raised new challenges for the private health care industry along with other sectors of the economy. As Figure 4.3 illustrates, the impact of the crisis varied from one country to the next—Singapore, Malaysia, and Thailand experienced huge tolls, while the Philippines was less hard hit. Similarly, the economic turmoil played different roles in the development of medical tourism in each country. Singapore continued to cultivate its status as a regional destination for quality medical services as part of its long-standing national economic and trade strategies. In Malaysia and Thailand, the financial crisis resulted in a significant reduction in demand for private hospital services, and ultimately a substantial decline in the size of the private hospital industry. The surviving hospitals, still left with excess capacity and medical services designed for high-end markets, began to target international patients. Meanwhile, the Philippines eventually turned to medical tourism as a way to boost foreign exchange revenues through tourism.

Malaysia

The 1997 economic crisis severely affected Malaysia, particularly the private sector. Many businesses, including those in health care, scaled down or eventually closed their operations. Managed care companies

Figure 4.3
Gross National Income (GNI) Per Capita (1962–2009)

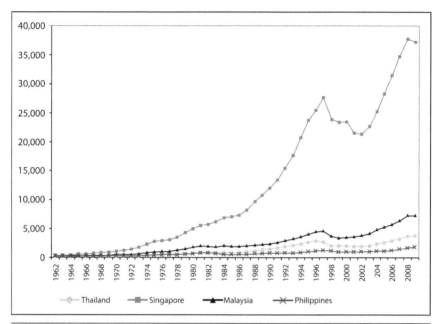

While the 1997 Asian economic crisis affected all four countries, the impact in Singapore, Malaysia, and Thailand was more severe than in the Philippines.
Source: World Bank Atlas.

also cut benefits or introduced more restrictions on per-person spending and choice of providers. The crisis led to the devaluation of the Malaysian Ringgit, which in turn decreased household purchasing power, and families dropped their private medical insurance.[3,18] As a result, many Malaysian patients reverted from private medical services covered by out-of-pocket spending or private insurance to publicly funded health care.[19] The devaluation of the Ringgit not only caused a slump in private hospital utilization rates, but also resulted in soaring prices for imported pharmaceuticals, medical supplies, and medical equipment, ultimately diminishing operating margins and profits for hospitals.[2,3]

To help restore Malaysia's economy, the Ministry of Health formed the National Committee for the Promotion of Medical and Health Tourism in January 1998.[3,18,20] The committee was given three important functions: formulating a strategic plan; promoting a so-called smart partnership among the government, health care facilities, travel organizations, and medical insurance groups; and forging strategic alliances with centers of excellence in other countries, such as the Mayo Clinic, Johns Hopkins

University Medical Center, and Great Ormond Street Children's Hospital. Subsequently, five subcommittees were appointed to indentify suitable target countries for patients; develop tax incentives; and establish fees, accreditation, and advertising guidelines.[3] The government also established the Malaysia Healthcare Travel Council to spearhead promotional activities. Private hospitals established the Association of Private Hospitals Malaysia to complement the government's efforts.[20]

The government further encouraged development of the health care industry by providing a variety of tax incentives for building hospitals, using medical equipment and information technology, and promoting medical services. The national committee on medical and health tourism has proposed additional incentives, including tax exemptions on revenue from foreign patients and additional deductions for money spent on accreditation. In addition, the Malaysia External Trade Development Association (MATRADE) and Tourism Malaysia, both government bodies, have organized and carried out road shows and marketing promotions in target countries. At present, a large number of private hospitals actively participate in medical tourism.[2,20] Two factors contributing to the hospitals' success are linking with hotels and tourist agencies to offer holiday packages that include health screenings and check-ups, and appointing local agents to handle inquiries and other tasks.[3]

Malaysia targets countries with inadequate medical facilities, such as Indonesia, Myanmar, Vietnam, and Laos; countries with high costs for medical services, including Singapore, Japan, and Taiwan; and countries with long waiting lists for public health care and expensive private health care, essentially the United Kingdom. Malaysia also targets the middle classes from the Middle East (United Arab Emirates, Bahrain, Saudi Arabia) and China. Malaysia's image as a Muslim country provides an advantage in promoting medical tourism among Muslim countries such as Brunei, Bangladesh, and those in the Middle East.[3,18] According to figures from the Association of Private Hospitals Malaysia, nearly 375,000 foreign patients sought health services in Malaysia in 2008 (estimates include all foreign patients, not just those who came for medical care).[2] Popular services include cosmetic and reproductive services and health screenings (see Table 4.2).

The Philippines

While the Philippines is known for its faith healers, who attracted foreign patients as far back as the 1960s, the seeds of its current medical tourism market took root in 1970s with the establishment of several high-caliber medical centers in Manila, including the Philippine Heart Center for Asia, which, as its name suggests, was conceived with a vision to cater to patients throughout the Asian region. However, the impetus

Table 4.2
Country-by-country medical tourism industry at a glance

	Malaysia	Philippines	Singapore	Thailand
Annual medical tourism revenue, 2006–2008 (million USD)	$90.5[a] (2008)	$350[b] (2006)	$725.8[a] (2008)	$1,366[c] (2007)
Popular health services				
Cosmetic and reconstructive surgery	✓	✓		✓
Health screening package	✓			✓
Orthopedics			✓	✓
Cardiology			✓	✓
Neurosurgery			✓	
Coronary artery bypass		✓	✓	✓
Coronary angioplasty				✓
Oncology and cancer			✓	
Hip replacement				✓
Ophthalmology	✓	✓		
Dentistry		✓		✓
Dermatology		✓		✓
Stem cell transplant			✓	
Endocrinology	✓			
Internal medicine	✓			
Health rejuvenation packages	✓			
Obstetrics and gynecology	✓			

Note: Popular services vary by location; patients tend to travel to Singapore and Thailand for cardiology treatment and coronary artery bypass surgery, for instance; and to Malaysia, the Philippines, and Thailand for cosmetic and reconstructive surgery.
Sources: [a] Chee HL. Medical tourism and the state in Malaysia and Singapore. *Glob. Soc. Policy.* December 1, 2010;10(3):336–357.
[b] Porter ME, DeVera M, Huang B, Khan O, Qin Z, Tan A. *Medical tourism in the Philippines: Microeconomics of competitiveness: Firms, clusters and economic development.* 2008. http://www.isc.hbs.edu/pdf/Student_Projects/Philippine_Medical_Tourism_2008.pdf. Accessed April 13, 2012.
[c] Na Ranong A, Na Ranong V, Jindarak S. Thailand as a medical hub. Thailand Development Research Institute; 2009.

for medical tourism in recent years has come not from the Department of Health, which has been focused on health care delivery for the local population, but from other branches of the government, particularly the presidency and the Department of Tourism. These government bodies, along with the business sector, have noted the growing market of medical tourism and the potential foreign exchange revenues it might generate.

In October 2004, President Gloria Macapagal-Arroyo created the Public-Private Partnership Task Force on Export Competitiveness to pursue strategies for enhancing exports in three sectors—health and wellness, IT enabled services, and logistics. This partnership was designed to foster interagency collaboration and government support for programs in these areas. As part of this initiative, the Department of Health and the Department of Tourism were tasked to implement policies to support medical tourism through the Philippines Medical Tourism Program (PMTP).[4,18] Following these efforts, the Republic Act 9593, otherwise known as the Tourism Act of 2009, created the Philippine Tourism Promotions Board to develop and promote the Philippines as a center for international medical tourism.[21] Upon his election into office in 2010, President Benigno Aquino Jr. continued the policies initiated by his predecessor.

The Medical Tourism Act, a bill proposing the creation of a Medical Tourism Bureau under the Department of Tourism, was under consideration by Congress at the time of this writing. Critics of the bill argued that the proposed bureau should fall under the Department of Health (DOH), which is responsible for establishing policies on health facility licensing and patient safety guidelines.[22] The DOH has also advocated for a policy to designate select hospitals and clinics as Medical Tourism Economic Zones to enable these DOH-endorsed facilities to benefit from tax incentives and duty-free importation of capital goods and consummables.[22]

Private medical centers in metropolitan Manila are central to the country's medical tourism efforts. Foremost among them are St. Luke's Medical Center, Medical City, Makati Medical Center, and the Asian Hospital (an affiliate of Thailand-based Bumrungrad International), all of which are internationally accredited. While these four private hospitals are well known as a result of their promotions efforts,[10,18] there are other hospitals in Metro Manila and other parts of the country that offer services to medical tourists, including in Cebu, the country's second largest city.

Roughly 3.1 million tourists visited the Philippines in 2009. In 2010, this number increased to 3.5 million.[23] According to a report developed by the Joint Foreign Chambers of Commerce in the Philippines, the Department of Tourism estimates that 100,000 of those visitors can be classified as medical tourists, but at present, the government is unable to determine exact counts of medical tourists.[11] A large proportion of these medical tourists are understood to be Filipinos residing abroad, particularly in the United States, which is home to close to 4 million Filipinos. It is estimated that worldwide, the Filipino diaspora numbers about 10 million. In 2007, 180,739 Filipinos living overseas visited the Philippines; by 2010, the number had almost doubled to 228,445.[24] The most common services medical tourists seek in the Philippines include plastic and cosmetic surgery, dental prosthesis and implants, cataract surgery, kidney transplantation, and coronary artery bypass surgery.[22]

Singapore

The Singaporean government has encouraged private health services since 1965,[2] and as a result, private hospital services have continued to grow to meet the demand of both local and international patients from neighboring countries, especially Indonesia and Malaysia. In addition, the government has promoted specialized medical services targeting foreign patients, helping to establish Singapore as one of the major medical hubs in Asia.

In response to increased demand from international patients, private hospitals in Singapore have established international departments to assist with everything from making appointments with top specialists to hospital transportation, accommodations, and services such as interpretation, visa assistance, and currency exchange. Both private and government hospitals in Singapore regularly collaborate with well-regarded Western hospitals and incorporate the latest medical innovations and procedures. In addition to providing world-class medical care in many branches of medicine, Singapore has developed expertise in procedures such as organ transplantations, infertility services, and joint replacement.[25]

Singapore's medical tourism industry receives strong government support. The government tasked its Healthcare Services Working Group (HSWG) to recommend strategies and provide marketing, research, and development support.[26] In 2003, Singapore Medicine, a multiagency government-industry body supported by the Ministry of Health, Singapore's Economic Development Board, International Enterprise Singapore, and the Singapore Tourism Board, was launched to strengthen Singapore's position as a leading destination for high-quality, affordable, and safe health care.[2,27]

In marketing to international patients, Singapore has emphasized access to highly skilled practitioners and state-of-the-art technology over competitive prices, in part because the high value of its currency makes medical services more expensive there than other medical tourism destinations such as Malaysia, Thailand, and India.[2] According to the Singapore Tourism Board, Singapore attracted some 370,000 medical tourists in 2008.[2]

Thailand

Over the past three decades, Thailand has established itself as a popular travel destination and built upon that reputation to become an international hub for medical services. Thailand's government has helped foster its thriving medical tourism industry as an antidote to the 1997 financial crisis that left an oversupply of private health services. Rapid economic growth during the 1990s and eight years of tax exemptions for private health care facilities resulted in huge investments in large and sophisticated private hospitals and hospital chains.[17] However, during the economic crisis, demands for private health services declined.

The Department of Export Promotion in the Ministry of Commerce recognized that Thailand's health sector, which was well regarded in the region, had the potential to generate foreign currencies and boost economic growth. Accordingly, the Department joined with other agencies and organizations, including the Ministry of Foreign Affairs, Tourism Authority of Thailand, Institute for Small and Medium Enterprises Development, Thai Chamber of Commerce, and Private Hospital Association, to initiate a medical tourism industry. At the same time, big private hospitals adapted their business strategies to attract international patients.

The government continues to support the development of Thailand as a medical hub through the Prime Minister's Special Committee and through the Ministry of Public Health, which has drafted a second strategic plan to enhance and promote Thailand's health services for international patients. The plan outlines four main products: medical services, health promotion services, Thai traditional and alternative medicines, and herbal and health products. The government also continues to support private hospitals; those with 50 beds or more are eligible to apply for three to eight years of corporate income tax exemptions as well as exemptions from or reduction of import duties on machinery to be used in the hospital.

Thailand's medical tourism industry targets two populations—international patients with high purchasing power or insurance coverage, and retired citizens seeking temporary or permanent residency in Thailand. Currently, Thailand is a market leader in Asia for medical services to international patients; according to Anchana NaRanong and Viroj Na Ranong the medical tourism industry generated about US$1.4 billion in 2007.[35]

STRATEGIES FOR DEVELOPING AND SUSTAINING MEDICAL TOURISM

As the foregoing discussion has illustrated, in response to economic pressures, both the private and public health care sectors in these Southeast Asian countries have experienced a general movement away from a not-for-profit orientation toward a for-profit orientation in which health care is essentially a commodity. This has resulted in an emphasis on product standardization, market expansion, and direct marketing to health care to consumers[3]—all elements of a successful medical tourism industry. Each country has developed and employed these features in different ways. This section compares their respective approaches and advantages as they develop their medical tourism industries.

Policy Environment and Actors

The level of state and private sector involvement in the medical tourism industry varies by country (see Table 4.3). State supports are at a much higher magnitude in Singapore and Malaysia, while the private sector

Table 4.3
Principal actors in the medical tourism industry

Country	Government or government-appointed bodies	Private body
Malaysia	• National Committee for the Promotion of Medical and Health Tourism (Medical Tourism Section, Corporate and Health Industry Practice Division, Ministry of Health) • Malaysia Tourism Promotion Board (MTPB) • Malaysia External Trade Development Corporation (MATRADE)	• Association of Private Hospitals Malaysia
Philippines	• Philippine Medical Tourism Program (Department of Health and Department of Tourism, with participation of private hospitals and support from national government)	
Singapore	• Singapore Medicine • Singapore Health Services (SingHealth)	• Individual private hospitals
Thailand	• Office of International Healthcare Center	• Private Hospitals Association and individual hospitals

Note: The role of the government and private sectors in developing and promoting medical tourism varies by country.

plays a leading role in Thailand. The Philippines Medical Tourism Program features more of a public–private partnership. The relative level of involvement of the different sectors is among the factors that influence how the industry has taken shape in each country.

Quality Assurance

Many countries and providers promoting medical tourism pursue accreditation as a quality assurance system and as a marketing tool. In addition to receiving accreditation from international accrediting organizations, such as the Joint Commission International (JCI) and the International Organization for Standardization (ISO) providers can seek accreditation from national bodies that oversee hospital quality, such as the Ministry of Health and the Malaysian Society for Quality in Health in Malaysia; the Healthcare Accreditation Institute in Thailand; and the Philippine Health Insurance Corporation, which not only purchases medical services from public and private providers, but also accredits providers. As Table 4.4 indicates, different markets emphasize different credentials. In Malaysia, the state has selected 35 private hospitals out of more than 220 for official health tourism promotion based on the quality of their services.[29] The Philippines Department of Tourism's website lists 38 health care facilities that the Department has accredited, located in various parts of the country, including Metro Manila and Cebu.[26] Hospitals in Singapore and Thailand have focused on obtaining international accreditation. (For a full discussion of the effectiveness of various accreditation schemes as both quality control and marketing tools, see chapter 11.)

Table 4.4
Quality assurance

	Malaysia	Philippines	Singapore	Thailand
National accreditation	✓	✓		✓
International accreditation—ISO	✓	✓		✓
International accreditation—JCI	✓		✓	✓
JCI accredited hospitals*	7	4	14	15

Note: Hospitals seek both national and international accreditation to distinguish their institutions in the medical tourism market.
*Source: Joint Commission International, December 2011.

Affordability

One of the primary motivations driving medical tourists is the sense that they can receive quality care at lower costs by going abroad for medical services. Lower health provider wages, less expensive medicines, and the absence of significant medical malpractice costs enable each of these Southeast Asian countries to offer health services at substantially lower costs than those in sending countries such as the United States (see Table 4.5). While most patients pay out of pocket, increasingly, insurers are also willing to

Table 4.5
Average costs (USD) for health services

	United States	United Kingdom	Malaysia	Philippines	Singapore	Thailand
Heart bypass	$113,000	$13,921	$9,000	$14,607	$20,000	$13,000
Heart valve replacement	$150,000	–	$9,000	$11,236–12,356	$13,000	$11,000
Hip replacement	$47,000	$12,000	$10,000	$7,865–8,989	$11,000	$12,000
Knee replacement	$48,000	$10,162	$8,000	$7,865–8,989	$13,000	$10,000

Note: Singapore, which has comparatively high costs for the region, emphasizes access to sophisticated technology and high-quality health care in its marketing efforts, while the Philippines attracts medical tourists with its competitive costs.
Sources: Lunt N, Smith R, Exworthy M, Green ST, Horsfall D, Mannion R. Medical tourism: Treatments, markets and health system implications: A scoping review, OECD 2011; del Mundo J, Republic of Philippines Department of Health, personal conversation, Manila, December 2011.

pay for health care abroad if the quality is comparable to that in the patient's home country and the cost is lower,[30] even going so far as to provide full reimbursement and other incentives. If this trend continues, the volume of medical tourists may increase and prompt more investment in and development of popular destination countries' medical tourism industries.

However, research suggests that low prices alone are not likely to attract patients. A study of 200 international patients receiving care in Penang, Malaysia, showed that quality factors such as clinical performance, provision of information, and staff empathy were among the most important factors contributing to patient satisfaction.[32]

Trade Liberalization

Since signing the ASEAN (Association of Southeast Asian Nations) Framework Agreement on Services (AFAS) in 1995, ASEAN countries have been negotiating reduced barriers to trade in services, including health services. Liberalizing regional trade in health services theoretically allows for more foreign investment in health care facilities and enables health care professionals and patients to move more readily across borders in ASEAN nations. It is not clear how much the liberalization of trade in health services ultimately would affect patient flows in this region since Malaysia, the Philippines, Singapore, and Thailand currently allow foreign patients to enter their countries for medical services without significant barriers. The most likely change would be a lifting of certain visa or immigration requirements, but since they are currently minimal, it is unclear whether any change would result in more medical tourism in the region.

On the other hand, countries with higher socioeconomic status such as Singapore, Thailand, and Malaysia could benefit from fewer barriers to investment and health professional migration, since they might be able to attract more health professionals and investment to further develop their medical tourism industries. However, these impacts are at present speculative. While the Mutual Recognition Arrangements (MRAs) among ASEAN countries signed from 2006 to 2008 are expected to facilitate freer flows of health professionals, they have yet to make much difference since local legal structures have not been amended to allow these flows. The necessary amendments may not be quick in coming, since groups representing domestic health professionals are generally not in favor of the inflow of foreign health professionals.

Comparative Advantages and Key Success Factors

Each of the countries discussed has particular advantages and challenges in advancing their medical tourism industries. While Singapore boasts sophisticated technologies and a comparatively large number of

JCI-accredited hospitals, for instance, Thailand is known for not only its high-quality medical services but also its hospitality and comparatively low prices. Table 4.6 highlights some of the primary strategies and advantages that each of these countries offers.

IMPACTS OF MEDICAL TOURISM

The growth of the medical tourism industry in Southeast Asia has played out differently in Malaysia, the Philippines, Singapore, and Thailand as a result of the varying dynamics of their respective economies and health care systems. These changes, in turn, have created new challenges with regard to balancing the goals of promoting population health and

Table 4.6
Strategies and comparative advantages

Malaysia
- Destination for Muslim patients
- Competitive costs
- Strategic alliances with foreign partners
- Easy entry for foreign patients through special visa
- Strong government support, including partnerships with hospitality sector, tax incentives

Philippines
- Destination for Filipinos working overseas
- Competitive costs
- Strong business-government partnership, including tax incentives and infrastructure support
- Liberal policies allowing foreign health professionals to practice in the Philippines
- National specialty hospitals

Singapore
- Well-established medical tourism destination
- Strong government support, including tax incentives and investment
- High technology equipment
- Highly skilled medical professionals
- Large number of hospitals accredited by JCI

Thailand
- National strategic plan to promote as Asian Regional Medical Hub with specialty centers for market segments such as trans-sexual surgery
- Large number of hospitals accredited by JCI
- Highly skilled medical professionals
- Strong private sector participation
- Competitive costs

Note: Malaysia, Singapore, the Philippines, and Thailand leverage their respective strengths to compete in the global medical tourism market.

fostering economic development (Figure 4.1). In theory, medical tourism can benefit health system development by bringing in increased tax revenues that can be used to improve local health care, or by providing jobs that will keep medical professionals from seeking employment abroad. Countries with relatively large numbers of health workers, such as the Philippines, could seek to attract international patients to create a demand for their excess health worker supply. Importing patients may also allow small countries like Singapore, with a population of 4.6 million, to more easily leverage economies of scale when they invest in medical services.[2] On the other hand, there is the danger that governments may focus on the potential benefits of medical tourism at the expense of the domestic health systems, which may suffer from repercussions such as escalating prices for medical services, or the flight of health providers from the public sector. Ultimately, claims that medical tourism benefits the public health sector have yet to be proven.

Even though foreign patients constitute a very small percentage of the total number of patients in any one country's health system,[33] they consume some of the scarcest health resources, namely, medical specialists. Consequently, determining whether to invest the resources to expand medical tourism merits careful consideration. Making an informed policy decision requires weighing evidence on the positive impacts, such as generating foreign currencies, against the negative impacts on local health systems. There is little published data on the impact of medical tourism or well-designed, objective analyses; most studies to date have been primarily descriptive. The following section synthesizes the impacts of medical tourism in these four countries based on available data and literature.

Impact on the Economy

It is estimated that medical tourism in Thailand generated US$1,366 million in 2007[34] and grew an average of 19 percent between 2004 and 2007.[35] In 2008, medical tourism generated an estimated US$90.5 million in Malaysia and US$725.8 million in Singapore, growing at average rates of 30 percent and 28.7 percent per year respectively between 2004 and 2008.[2] In the Philippines, the industry had estimated gross revenues from medical tourism of US$350 million in 2006.[10] As noted earlier in this chapter, there is a lack of reliable data on medical tourism volumes and revenues due in part to different approaches to categorizing international patients, and it is therefore important to recognize that all of these figures are estimates, based on a variety of government and hospital reports.

Although Thailand brings in the highest estimated revenues from medical tourism overall, our calculations based on the volumes and revenues reported above suggest that Singapore realizes the highest average revenue per international patient at US$1,925, followed by Thailand at US$902 and Malaysia at US$225. A reliable comparable figure for the Philippines is not available. The range of per-patient revenues reflects variations in the countries' diagnostic and treatment protocols, personnel costs, and medical service charges. The high-technology medical services and highly qualified medical professionals that draw medical tourists to Singapore, for instance, also contribute to its comparatively high costs. The cost of a knee replacement in these four countries ranges from $US7,800 in the Philippines to US$13,000 in Singapore (Table 4.5) and the per-night cost of a single private hospital room ranges from $US45 in the Philippines to $US229 in Singapore.[22,31] It should be noted that the disparities in these per-patient revenue calculations may also reflect differences in how patients are counted; while Thailand includes both outpatient visits and inpatients admissions in its counts, it is unclear whether Malaysia and Singapore consistently do the same.

It is estimated that around 34 percent to 45 percent of income in big private hospitals in Thailand comes from foreign patients, providing strong incentives for further investment to scale up offerings for medical tourists.[35] It is clear that revenue generated from medical tourism is an important source of income not only for health care professionals but also for others employed in the sizable private health sector. In addition to direct revenues from medical services, medical tourism generates income from associated services and tourism. NaRanong and NaRanong[34] estimated that Thailand brought in an additional US$400–433 million from these related industries in 2008, making for a total added value that amounted to 0.4 percent of the country's GDP. Similarly, in the Philippines, it's estimated that every peso spent by a tourist generates 2.25 pesos in direct and indirect revenues.[4] It is not known whether medical tourists have an even greater multiplier effect.

Having witnessed medical tourism's revenue-generating potential, these countries plan to continue fostering this industry as a way to bring in foreign dollars. Singapore set a target of attracting one million patients by 2012, which it projected would result in S$3 billion (US$2.36 billion and 0.95% of its GDP) in revenue from health care services, and S$400 million (US$315 million and 0.15% of its GDP) from related industries, and create 13,000 new jobs.[35] Thailand set target revenues from medical tourism at US$3.2 billion for 2014, and the Philippines aimed to increase foreign patients from 100,000 in 2006 to 700,000 by 2010 and bring in US$3 billion in gross revenues from medical tourism by 2015.[11] Again, it remains unclear how the respective governments and ministries are measuring progress toward these goals and whether they have met their interim goals.

In pursuit of these aims, Malaysia, the Philippines, Singapore, and Thailand continue to encourage development of their medical tourism industries and consumption of their health services through a variety of tax incentives, subsidies, accommodations, and promotional efforts. Malaysia, for instance, offers tax incentives for building hospitals, provides tax deductions for expenses occurred promoting exports (such as health services provided to foreigners), and offers tax exemptions for revenues from foreign patients.[2] A full accounting of the overall value of medical tourism to these individual economies would take the costs of these incentives and initiatives into account and calculate the return on these investments; however, those figures are not currently available.

Likewise, there are little definitive data on the extent to which the benefits of medical tourism, which at least initially accrue to private hospitals, eventually extend to the public sector. Since tax exemptions help subsidize the private health care sector's services for international patients, reciprocally, it is expected that these private hospitals will provide some health services to local people for free or reduced rates. But whether and how this will happen remains subject to debate. For instance, Thailand's 2010 National Health Assembly, a forum designed to foster public discussion about national health priorities, adopted a resolution that urged the Board of Investment not to provide special tax or investment privileges to health services that are business oriented (i.e., private). At the same time, the Board of Investment adopted a policy that allowed tax exemptions for private hospitals with 30 beds or more. A panel established to address these conflicting policies recommended a compromise solution that calls for private hospitals that receive tax exemptions to provide treatment for patients enrolled in the National Health Security or Social Security plan for at least three years. Not everyone was pleased with the proposed compromise; the private sector argued that providing treatment to patients under these two schemes should be on a voluntary, not compulsory basis. In one such voluntary arrangement, Thailand's two biggest private hospitals that cater to foreign patients have agreed to provide heart surgery for up to 100 patients a year under the Universal Coverage of health insurance scheme for the same price that public hospitals charge.

Given private hospitals' for-profit orientation and the lack of any formal enforcement of obligations to the public sector, medical tourism's benefits beyond the private sector tend to be more theoretical than real. Actualizing these benefits requires adopting formal policies. One such example is an administrative order that the Philippines's Department of Health issued in 2007 in response to concerns that medical tourism would disadvantage local patients. The order requires all private hospitals to allocate at least 10 percent of their authorized bed capacity for charity beds as a condition for licensure.[36] This administrative order was meant to complement an old law passed in 1957 that required all government hospitals to operate with not less than 90 percent of its bed capacity reserved for free or charity care.[37]

So while there have been some efforts to disseminate medical tourism profits more widely, ultimately, available evidence suggests that government subsidies designed to bolster medical tourism tend to benefit the owners, investors, and shareholders of private hospitals at the expense of the majority poor.

Impact on Health Systems

The positive economic impacts of medical tourism must be weighed against the negative consequences on destination countries' health systems, especially those with limited medical services capacity. Among the major concerns are the so-called brain drain of skilled and experienced specialists from the public to the private sector, increasing health care costs for the local population, and ethical concerns that can arise when health services become a commodity.

Internal Brain Drain of Medical Professionals

Many countries suffer from health worker shortages, either in absolute numbers, or in terms of distribution, with adequate numbers overall but shortages in particular areas (often rural) or facilities (typically public). WHO set a threshold of critical shortage at 22.8 health workers (doctors, nurses, midwives) per 10,000 people. By those standards, Thailand and Malaysia are at the margin, with 27 and 25 per 10,000 people respectively. Singapore and the Philippines, with densities of 59 and 73 health workers per 10,000 population respectively, do not have health worker shortages at the national level but do report shortages in the public sector.[33] In the Philippines, for instance, many poor areas lack qualified health personnel, and hospitals in urban centers report high turnover of experienced nurses.

The effects of medical tourism on these long-established problems remain to be seen and may vary from one country to the next given the different forces and historical factors at play. While Malaysia, Singapore, the Philippines, and Thailand have all experienced an outflow of doctors from the public sector, the dynamics of these movements have been different. For example, Thailand's internal migration originated with the 1987–1997 economic boom that led to a rapid expansion of private hospitals spurred on by tax incentives. Some 190 private hospitals were established during this period,[18] and the number of doctors in private hospitals tripled, due in part to doctors migrating from the public sector. The outflow from the public sector reversed during the economic crisis in 1997, which led to a drop in demand for private services. However the drain of health workers from the public sector resumed when the private hospitals began attracting international patients.

Malaysia, Singapore, and the Philippines have experienced similar health worker flows from public to private hospitals. But in addition to internal migration, these countries have had substantial numbers of health workers leave for opportunities abroad. Data from Frederic Docquier and Alok Bhargava[38] showed that in 2006, 12.8 percent of doctors trained in Malaysia, 9.7 percent of those trained in the Philippines, and 10.2 percent trained in Singapore were working in OECD countries, compared with 3.3 percent of doctors who were trained in Thailand.

The Philippines has long been an exporting country for health workers, especially nurses. It is estimated that 163,756 Filipino nurses were working abroad in 2000,[33] accounting for 85 percent of all employed Filipino nurses.[18] Some 68 percent of Filipino doctors were working abroad during the same period.[18] The ongoing out-migration of experienced nurses from the Philippines's tertiary private hospitals to work in Middle Eastern and OECD countries poses a challenge not only for its domestic health system but also for its medical tourism industry, which relies on retaining well-trained and experienced nurses to provide quality care. These countries have adopted a variety of strategies to address these shortages, such as offering incentives for working in public hospitals and allowing doctors to practice simultaneously in the public and private sectors. Malaysia and Singapore have turned to foreign doctors. In 2005, 387 general practitioners (or 5.3% of all general practitioners) and 238 specialists (or 18% of all specialists) working in Malaysia were from other countries.[2] In Singapore, some 59.2 percent of doctors newly registered in 2008 were foreigners.[2] Thailand has not pursued this strategy, focusing instead on building the domestic health workforce, and the Philippines only allows foreign doctors and health managers from countries with which it has reciprocal relations. Some opponents of medical tourism argue that from an ethical standpoint, a country should not import medical professionals from other shortage countries to bolster their workforces to serve medical tourists.

In Thailand, proponents of the medical tourism industry argue that it will help alleviate shortages by providing attractive jobs that will keep health workers from moving abroad, and even attract Thai professionals back from the United States and Europe to practice in medical hubs in Bangkok. Opponents contend that this argument overlooks unmet needs of the population who receive their care not at these private hospitals but in public facilities. In response to these concerns, a resolution at Thailand's 2010 National Health Assembly urged the development of a plan to monitor and address health work resource issues arising from medical tourism and established a public–private partnership to train health workers, especially in fields with shortages.

Rising Costs in Public Sector Care

There is no clear evidence on the impact of medical tourism on the domestic cost of health services. However, it stands to reason that medical tourism will drive up costs in both the private and public sectors. To compete for scarce human resources, the private hospitals that cater to medical tourists offer comparatively high salaries and benefits to medical professionals, resulting in larger income gaps between the public and private sectors. Governments, in turn, have to provide additional incentives to retain doctors in the public sector. This gradually drives up the cost of health services and the annual health budget.

It is clear that patients will bear at least some of the burden of these rising costs. Singapore has responded to rising health care costs by introducing cost containment measures in its public health insurance programs, including deductibles, co-payments, and maximum benefit limits. In 2008, the portion of health care costs that the most subsidized patients in Singapore (C Class) pay increased from 20 percent to 30 percent, leaving some patients with chronic conditions unable to afford their medications.[2] Similarly, in the Philippines and Malaysia, where private health expenditure is high—65.3 percent and 55.9 percent respectively—patients will feel the toll of rising health costs acutely. Thailand still provides publicly financed and administered health services for the general population, continuing the policy of universal health coverage that was established in 2001. However, medical tourism in Thailand has exacerbated the movement of health professionals from the public to the private sector, resulting in shortages of specialists in public hospitals. As a result, access to some specialists requires paying for private medical services, something that only affluent Thai people and international patients are able to afford.

Ethical Concerns

Medical tourism raises a number of ethical concerns for destination countries. As the previous discussion suggests, one potential issue is the creation of a two-tiered medical care system. In this scenario, rich or well-insured foreign patients can access higher quality care in private hospitals, while local people with limited resources are relegated to public facilities grappling with limited resources and shortages of medical specialists. This scenario is based on the assumption that medical tourism will promote the movement of health workers, especially specialists and experienced nurses, from rural to urban areas and from the public to the private sector.[33]

Another concern is the growing for-profit orientation of health care services in the public sector. In Malaysia, Singapore, and the Philippines, for instance, public hospitals and centers of excellence that have historically focused on providing low- or no-cost medical services to the local population have become privatized, for-profit entities. As a result, these hospitals have implemented strategies to generate additional income, including strategies designed to attract foreign patients. As Heng Leng Chee[2] points out, this business orientation can conflict with the public mandate of providing services for local patients. If the government is focusing on gaining revenue from international patients, there is the risk that they will not act in favor of and protect local patients.[39]

Another aspect of commercializing health services that raises ethical issues is organ sales. While the magnitude of this practice is small, the accompanying problems are significant. Of particular concern is the potential exploitation of poor people selling their kidneys for transplantation, a problem that led the Philippines, one of the countries that allowed organ sales, to eventually ban the practice. Between 2002 and 2008, the Department of Health allowed organ sales under a program called the Philippine Organ Donation Program, in which prospective kidney providers could sign up, be connected with prospective recipients, and receive some form of payment for their kidneys. Transplant tourism flourished during this period. By 2007, 528 of the 1,046 kidney transplants in the Philippines were transplants from living, unrelated Filipino donors to foreigners.[40] By 2007, the Philippines had been named by the WHO as one of the five "organ trafficking hotspots" in the world.[40] As the potential for coercion and exploitation became evident, even in the case of "voluntary" donations, the Philippine government intervened. In 2003, the legislature passed the antihuman trafficking law (Republic Act 9208) that made it illegal for organ seekers "to recruit, hire, adopt, transport or abduct a person by means of threat or use of force, fraud, deceit, coercion or intimidation for purpose of removal or sale of organs of said person." The law was not fully implemented until 2011. For a more detailed discussion of travel for transplants and the accompanying issues, see chapter 7.

CONCLUSION AND RECOMMENDATIONS

Medical tourism, one of the promising, growing service trades in Asia, surged in response to the 1997 Asian economic crisis in these four countries. Malaysia, Singapore, and Thailand saw the opportunity to revitalize their economies by capitalizing on their extensive medical service infrastructures. In the Philippines, the current medical tourism market emerged in 2004 when the government launched the Philippines Medical Tourism Program (PMTP) to promote services for international patients as a way of bolstering tourism.

Medical tourism in the region has gradually transformed from a market serving primarily affluent patients in nearby developing countries to one that also includes patients from developed countries who pay both out of pocket and with insurance. Patients' reasons for traveling for medical services have also evolved, from seeking services or quality not available in their home countries to seeking more affordable or timely services. At the same time, the ideology around health services has changed. Health care, traditionally perceived in large part as a public good for patients in need, has turned into a international commodity that can be traded, marketed, and used to generate revenues for the government and private health sector. This has resulted in aggressive marketing with a focus on increasing market size, maximizing profit margins, and designing health systems that are attractive to foreign patients. This market ideology has extended to both the private and government health sectors.

These transitions come at a cost to the public in these destination countries. These costs come in the form of government expenditures to promote and support medical tourism, lost revenues due to tax breaks, and lost import duties for medical equipment. They also come in the form of heightened competition for scarce health workers, especially specialists. The uncontrolled influx of international patients is one of the key drivers of domestic migration of highly qualified super-specialists from teaching hospitals and tertiary care public hospitals to private facilities, a movement that can disrupt services for patients at public hospitals.[33] These shortages may be mitigated to some extent by importing health workers from other countries, a strategy that Malaysia and Singapore have embraced. Other strategies include allowing professionals to split their time between public and private facilities. Field observations suggest that this dual practice option requires careful regulation to ensure quality care and responsiveness to public sector patients. One potential solution is to introduce a levy on private hospitals that benefit from medical tourism to fund more educational opportunities for health workers in these destination countries,[34] but this proposal is not popular with private hospitals.

On the other side of the scale are the potential benefits of medical tourism, including new opportunities to retain health professionals who might otherwise go abroad, and considerable revenue in both the health and hospitality sectors. The Philippine Department of Tourism takes the view that medical tourism will have an overall effect of boosting the health care industry and driving the improvement of health facilities and services. This general upgrade is envisioned to pave the way for hospitals to improve their capacity to serve local patients. Critics of the program are pessimistic that revenues from medical tourism will, in fact, be used to improve health facilities or even increase the salaries of health workers.[41] Still, there are anecdotal reports of benefits from medical tourism. For example, in the Philippines, St. Luke's Medical Center is said to have increased its income from two billion to three billion pesos ($US46 million–$US70 million) from 2007 to 2008 due to revenues from medical tourism patients, and in turn, it has spent about 30 million pesos ($US693,000) on services for charity patients. St. Luke's also has donated its three-year old furniture and equipment to the local government and some Department of Health hospitals. Another private firm, the Belo Medical Group, which specializes in cosmetic surgery, is said to have earned US$12 million from medical tourism.[26] And there are reports that government medical centers like the Philippine Heart Center and the National Kidney and Transplant Institute are using revenues from medical tourism patients to improve services for the local population.[22]

However, there are few such anecdotal reports from the other three countries examined here, much less any systematic analysis of the balance between how much revenue medical tourism generates in these countries and how much their governments spend on promotions and subsidies and forego in tax revenues. In the end, the impact of medical tourism on both sides of the balance sheet has yet to be rigorously evaluated. A series of well-designed studies is required to systematically evaluate the overall effects of medical tourism in these countries. Such studies will need to address:

1. How governments can accurately track the number of medical tourists and their expenditures. Today, different countries use different definitions and methodologies to count medical tourists, making it difficult to draw any meaningful conclusions or comparisons. Furthermore, getting private facilities to provide information on the services provided to medical tourists has been difficult.
2. How and where medical tourism will have the greatest impacts. The present pattern of growth and accreditation of health facilities involved in medical tourism is determined by the supply and distribution of health facilities in the country. One can expect that medical tourism will largely be an urban phenomenon, concentrated in medical centers in the urban areas. The smaller accredited health facilities in the provinces will by and large cater to expatriates whose homes are located in those provinces, and, particularly in the Philippines, to returning overseas workers.
3. How government policies around developing medical tourism can work in synergy with policies to achieve universal health care coverage, and how revenues from medical tourism can be used to address inequities in health care.

This analysis documents the scarcity of data and the need for more conclusive evidence about the costs and benefits of medical tourism. Developing common definitions and methodologies for counting medical tourists is an important step toward a better understanding. In addition, in response to a WHO resolution adopted in 2010, the Global Code of Practice on International Recruitment of Health Personnel,[50] the OECD and WHO are working together to improve the Human Resources for Health (HRH) information system, which captures international migration among health workers. These and other data can help inform governments about the overall value of medical tourism so they can develop coherent policies on trade in health services that balance the societal goals of fostering the health of their populations with the economic goal of generating additional wealth by attracting and serving foreign patients.

ACKNOWLEDGMENTS

The authors would like to thank Ms. Kay Flores, researcher at the University of Asia and the Pacific, School of Economics and Dr. Ramon Quesada, Chairman and CEO of Small Business Corporation for their invaluable support by providing ideas, materials, and references on medical tourism in the Philippines; and former DOH Undersecretary Jade del Mundo, who has been involved with the Philippine medical tourism program since it started, for providing updates and reviewing the article. We would also like to thank Dr. Suwit Wibulpolprasert for his most valuable comments and suggestions to strengthen the chapter.

REFERENCES

1. Helble M. The movement of patients across borders: Challenges and opportunities for public health. *Bull World Health Org.* 2011;89:68–72.

2. Chee HL. Medical tourism and the state in Malaysia and Singapore. *Glob Soc Policy.* December 1, 2010;10(3):336–357.

3. Chee HL. Medical Tourism in Malaysia: International Movement of Healthcare Consumers and the Commodification of Healthcare: A Working Paper Series No. 83. 2007, Asia Research Institute, National University of Singapore.

4. Dacanay J, Rodolfo M. Challenges in Health Services Trade: Philippine Case, Discussion Paper Series No. 2005–30. Manila: Philippine Institute for Development Studies; 2005.

5. Lavado R. How are DOH hospitals funded? *PIDS Policy Notes.* No. 2010-15. Philippine Institute for Deelopment Studies; 2010.

6. Dayrit M. Health and Population in The Macapagal-Arroyo Presidency and Administration, Record and Legacy 2001–2004. *The Third UP Public Lectures on the Philippine Presidency and Administration.* Diliman, Quezon City The University of the Philippines Press; 2004.

7. National Health Accounts. World Health Organization; 2009. http://www.who.int/nha/en/. Accessed July 12, 2011.

8. World Health Organization WPRO and SEARO. *Health financing strategy for the Asia Pacific region (2010–2015).* Manila: World Health Organization; 2010.

9. World Health Organization. *World health statistics 2011.* Geneva: World Health Organization; 2011.

10. Porter ME, DeVera M, Huang B, Khan O, Qin Z, Tan A. *Medical tourism in the Philippines: Microeconomics of competitiveness: Firms, clusters and economic development.* 2008. http://www.isc.hbs.edu/pdf/Student_Projects/Philippine_Medical_Tourism_2008.pdf. Accessed April 13, 2012.

11. Joint Foreign Chambers AP. A business perspective. *Arangkada Philippines.* 2010. http://www.investphilippines.info/arangkada/tourism-medical-travel-retirement/. Accessed April 13, 2012.

12. Time Series on Population (Mid-Year Estimates). The Statistics Singapore; 2011. http://www.singstat.gov.sg/stats/themes/people/hist/popn.html. Accessed July 10, 2011.

13. Ministry of Health Singapore. Hospital services. 2011. http://www.moh.gov.sg/content/moh_web/home/our_healthcare_system/Healthcare_Services/Hospitals.html. Accessed June 6, 2011.

14. Department of Statistics Singapore. *Yearbook of statistics Singapore, 2011.* Singapore: Department of Statistics, Ministry of Trade & Industry; 2011.

15. World Health Organization. *World health statistics 2010.* Geneva: World Health Organization; 2010.

16. Wibulpolprasert S, Sirilak S, Ekajumpaka P, Wattanamano N. *Thailand health profile 2008–2010.* Nonthaburi, Thailand: Bureau of Policy and Strategy, Ministry of Public Health; 2011.

17. Pachanee C, Wibulpolprasert S. Incoherent policies on universal coverage of health insurance and promotion of international trade in health services in Thailand. *Health Policy Plann.* July 1, 2006;21(4):310–318.

18. Economic and Social Commission for Asia and the Pacific. *Medical travel in Asia and the Pacific: Challenges and opportunities.* Bangkok: United Nations Economic and Social Commission for Asia and the Pacific; 2008.

19. Chee HL. Ownership, control, and contention: Challenges for the future of healthcare in Malaysia. *Soc Sci Med.* 2008;66(10):2145–2156.

20. Ministry of Health Malaysia. Ministry of health Malaysia. 2011; http://www.myhealthcare.gov.my. Accessed April 13, 2012.

21. Government of the Philippines. Philippines Tourism Act of 2009 Section 37d; 2009.

22. del Mundo J. Personal Communication. Manila 2011.

23. Department of Tourism Philippines. Tourism Statistics 2011. http://www.tourism.gov.ph/Pages/default.aspx. Accessed July 4, 2011.

24. Department of Tourism Philippines. Visitor arrivals by country of residence and purpose of visit; 2007.

25. Medical Tourism in Singapore. 2011. http://www.healthtourisminasia.com/singapore.htm. Accessed June 7, 2011.

26. Accredited healthcare providers. Department of Tourism Philiipines; 2011. http://www.tourism.gov.ph/pages/accreditedhealthcareproviders.aspx. Accessed August 10, 2011.

27. Lee CG. Health care and tourism: Evidence from Singapore. *Tourism Manage.* 2010;31:486–488.

28. Smith RD, Chanda R, Tangcharoensathien V. Trade in health-related services. *Lancet.* 2009;373(9663):593–601.

29. Association of Private Hospitals Malaysia. Health tourism. 2011. http://www.hospitals-malaysia.org/portal/index.asp?menuid=39.

30. Pafford B. The third wave-medical tourism in the 21st century. *South Med J.* 2009;102(8):810–813.

31. Arunanondchai J, Fink C. Globalization for health: Trade in health services in the ASEAN region. *Health Promot Int.* 2007;21:59–66.

32. Rad NF, Som APM, Zainuddin Y. Service quality and patients' satisfaction in medical tourism. *World Applied Sciences Journal.* 2010;10 (Special Issue of Tourism and Hospitality):24–30.

33. Kanchanachitra C, Lindelow M, Johnston T, et al. Human resources for health in southeast Asia: Shortages, distributional challenges, and international trade in health services. *Lancet.* January 25, 2011;377(9767):769–781.

34. NaRanong A, NaRanong V. The effects of medical tourism: Thailand's experience. *Bull World Health Org.* 2011;89:336–344.

35. NaRanong A, NaRanong V, Jindarak S. Thailand Medical Hub: Thailand Development Research Institute; 2009.

36. Department of Health Republic of the Philippines. Administrative Order No. 2007-00412007.

37. Republic of the Philippines. Republic Act No. 1939, June 22, 1957, Section 6. 1957.

38. Docquier F, Bhargava A. The medical brain drain: A new panel data set on physicians' emigration rates (1991–2004). The World Bank; 2006. http://econ.worldbank.org/WBSITE/EXTERNAL/EXTDEC/EXTRESEARCH/0,,contentMDK:21085107~pagePK:64214825~piPK:64214943~theSitePK:469382,00.html. Accessed June 8, 2011.

39. Heng LC, Whittaker A. Guest editors' introduction to the special issue: Why is medical travel of concern to global social policy? *Glob Soc Policy.* 2010;10(3):287–291.

40. Padilla BS. Regulated compensation for kidney donors in the Philippines. *Current Opinion in Organ Transplantation.* April 2009;14(2):120–123.

41. Flores K. Personal communication. Manila 2011.

Chapter 5

Socialized Medicine Meets Private Industry: Medical Tourism in Costa Rica

Courtney A. Lee

As the global medical tourism industry expands, a growing number of Latin American nations are becoming involved in promoting medical tourism as a national economic strategy. This chapter explores the development of the medical tourism industry in Latin America, with a particular focus on Costa Rica. My analysis, based on a year of ethnographic research, examines the social, political, economic, and ethical implications of the emergence of a private health care industry in a country with a strong and successful history of socialized health care.

There are currently about 10 nations in Central and South America that actively promote medical tourism, and the number of facilities in Latin America with Joint Commission International (JCI) accreditation, a credential popular with hospitals targeting international patients, grew from

This research is part of doctoral dissertation research in the Health and Behavioral Sciences Department at the University of Colorado Denver. The project was funded by the National Science Foundation (Doctoral Dissertation Improvement Grant #0852414), the Wenner Gren Foundation, and the Health and Behavioral Sciences Department at the University of Colorado Denver.

10 in 2006 to 44 in 2011.[1] The Latin American region largely focuses on cosmetic and elective surgeries for medical tourists, and although actual data on medical tourism are scarce, it is widely acknowledged that plastic surgery and dentistry constitute the great majority of procedures performed for medical tourists in the region. These types of procedures tend to be the least profitable for hospitals because they are often performed on an outpatient basis; the physician typically brings equipment and supplies, and the patient recuperates in a recovery home instead of at the hospital. Consequently, some Latin American countries have made concerted efforts to promote other, more lucrative, medical interventions beyond the scope of elective cosmetic procedures. Specialties that countries in the region are promoting to supplement their core medical tourism industries include in vitro fertilization (IVF) in Colombia and Panama; bariatric surgeries in Argentina; orthopedic procedures in Costa Rica and Brazil; gastric bypass surgery in Mexico and Panama; dental crowns, caps, implants, and veneers in Costa Rica and Mexico; stem cell procedures in Ecuador, Mexico, Argentina, and Brazil; and "liberation therapy" (also known as venoplasty or vein opening) for the treatment of multiple sclerosis in Costa Rica, Cuba, and Mexico. Cuba is widely regarded as a popular medical tourism destination specializing in a wide array of procedures and treatment programs. Though it is difficult for Americans to travel there because of U.S. trade and diplomatic policy, many Canadians, Europeans, and individuals from other regions seek medical care at Cuban facilities.

DATA CHALLENGES AND QUESTIONABLE STATISTICS

Inconsistent definitions and methods for reporting and collecting medical tourism data make it extremely difficult to provide an accurate estimate of the number of medical tourists traveling to Latin American destinations for health care. Within Costa Rica, estimates vary wildly, from just over 2,200 patients per year to as many as many as 100,000 per year.[2-6] The reality is probably somewhere in between these figures, most likely on the lower end. Media reports within Costa Rica estimate that 36,000 medical tourists visited the country in 2010, but the sources for this figure are unclear, and the number of international patients reported by individual facilities again suggests that this estimate may be high.[7]

MEDICAL TOURISM AND LOCAL WORLDS

Alongside the scarcity of reliable data on medical tourism, there is also very little scholarly research on the effects of medical tourism or local perceptions of medical tourism in destination countries. Powerful players with interests in the industry—including investors, insurance companies, hospital administrators, facilitator companies, development agencies, and trade associations—have made substantial ideological and financial investments in medical tourism. This has translated into upbeat, optimistic media reports of medical tourism and its benefits and muted criticisms. Though recent academic research has begun to examine the topic more critically, there are very few firsthand accounts that assess the impacts of medical tourism within a particular context. This chapter is based on research that examines medical tourism in the context of the "local worlds" of Costa Ricans and addresses this emerging industry through a social lens, rather than an economic or clinical one.

RESEARCH METHODS

To study the impacts of medical tourism within the Costa Rican context, I conducted more than 50 interviews with stakeholders at various levels of the medical tourism industry in and around San José, Costa Rica, between October 2009 and October 2010. Ethnographic data collected included semi-structured qualitative interviews and focus groups with government officials (5); physicians or ex-physicians, including both public and private sector, and those who work in both (25); nurses (2); medical students and residents (7); hospital administrators (4); medical tourism facilitators (5); and academics (3). In addition, I observed and conducted surveys with 200 patients in both public and private health care facilities. Categorizations of participants listed here are only approximate, as most interviewees filled more than one professional role, or had worked in several settings throughout the course of their careers. Interviews and surveys conducted in Spanish were translated into English before analysis.

HEALTH SYSTEMS IN LATIN AMERICA

Before discussing the results from this case study, to understand local impacts on health systems, it is important to situate the research within the broader Latin American and Costa Rican contexts. Although the global medical tourism industry is becoming more standardized across nations with the emergence of international facilitating organizations, accreditation schemes, and insurance companies, it cannot be assumed to have a homogenous effect across destination countries that are very different politically, culturally, socially, historically, and economically. In any discussion of the impacts of medical tourism on local health systems, it is important to consider the different configurations of health systems and regulatory policies.

While nations in the Latin American region developed along different trajectories, general similarities among their health systems do exist. Primary among these is the orientation of these health systems toward social medicine. Though defining social medicine can be complicated—and within the discussion of U.S. health care reform, the phrase has become politically loaded—social medicine generally refers to a state-supported system of health care delivery. While this means that the government *could* fully control the delivery and financing of health care, in practice, socialized medicine represents a range of strategies, from complete government ownership of facilities and employment of health care providers to public financing of private insurance and providers. In Latin America, the principles underlying social medicine—beliefs that social and economic conditions impact health, that the health of the population should be a matter of social concern, and that society should promote health and provide health care services—have played prominently in health system development.[8] Because of this, Latin American countries historically have placed high priority on social welfare programs, particularly education and health; and those programs have often focused on the poor. These nations have seen remarkable improvements in health indicators over time, with the average life expectancy for Latin America and the Caribbean increasing from 57 years in 1960 to 70 years in the year 2000. Nonetheless, there remain significant intra-regional differences in health indicators and achievements. For example, in the year 2000, Costa Rica and Cuba had the highest life expectancies in the region at 78 and 77 years, respectively, while Bolivia and Guyana had the lowest at 63 years—a striking 15-year gap.[9]

COSTA RICA AS A CASE STUDY

Costa Rica, bordered by the Pacific Ocean to the west and Caribbean Sea to the east, is about 19,700 square miles in size (it could fit inside of West Virginia) with a population of about 4.5 million people. It is one of the world's longest standing democracies and has one of the most successful universal health care systems. Costa Rica's socialized health care system makes it an interesting case study for examining the interaction between medical tourism, a global private industry, and local health care delivery, which is almost exclusively a public endeavor.

Although its national gross domestic product (GDP) is far eclipsed by the industrialized nations of the world, Costa Rica's health indices are the best in Latin America, with the exception of Cuba, and rival those in many of the world's most developed nations. These outcomes are the result of a well-developed, publicly funded, comprehensive health care system built on principles of solidarity, universality, and equity. This Central American success story is lauded as a potential role model for other developing nations seeking to achieve "health without wealth."[10,11] The country's per capita income is approximately the same as that of Mexico and one-fourth that of the United States; however Costa Rica's health and equity indicators rank close to the United States' and are well above Mexico's.[12] In 2009,

Costa Rica spent 10.5 percent of its GDP on health care and was ranked 36th in the World Health Organization's rankings of health systems, while the U.S. spent 16.2 percent and was ranked 37th.[13]

History of the Health System

Costa Rica developed its successful health system gradually over time. Prior to 1941, the Costa Rican health system was disjointed, comprised of private or charitable medical care without central organization. In 1941, President Rafael Angel Calderón Guardia created Costa Rica's Social Security Administration (*Caja Costarricense de Seguro Social*, or CCSS), a system for wage earners that gradually expanded to cover to the rest of the population over the next 50 years. In 1949, Costa Rica ratified a constitution that abolished the national army and enabled funding to flow toward social programs such as education and health. With these investments, steady health sector improvement continued; and in 1973, the General Health Law placed all health treatment services, including primary care facilities and hospitals, under the control of the CCSS. This legislation also set provisions for the continued expansion of the CCSS until it eventually became a universal health insurance system. In accordance with the development of universal health coverage, the University of Costa Rica, a public medical school with strong links to the CCSS and one of the most prestigious universities in the region, was formed. All medical residents in the country sign a contract to work for CCSS for a number of years in exchange for their medical education and training.

Today, the CCSS dominates health insurance, employment, and provision, with 29 hospitals (compared to 6 hospitals in the private sector) and an extensive network of clinics around the country, including 940 primary health care teams called EBAIS (*Equipos Básicos de Atención Integral de Salud*). More than 48,000 people and the large majority of the nation's physicians work for the CCSS.[14,15] CCSS funding comes from mandatory taxation on wages from employers (9.25%), employees (5.5%), and the state (0.25%).

The Role of the Private Sector in Health Care

In Costa Rica, the role of the private sector in the national health care system has been "more limited, home grown, and pragmatic"[16(p60)] than in other Latin American countries. The focus has remained on solidarity, equity, and universal access. Costa Ricans have fiercely defended the CCSS from privatization, calling it a "Robin Hood system" in which subsidizing the poor is part of citizens' social responsibility. The health care system and CCSS play a prominent role in national ideology within Costa Rica and are routinely cited as a source of pride and as a "pillar" of the nation.

CCSS is widely acknowledged to provide the best care available for illnesses and injuries because it will perform every test required and take all necessary medical measures to treat patients, regardless of the cost. For the large majority of Costa Ricans, the costs of private care are too high, and the private sector remains out of reach. However, long wait times in the public sector have led patients with financial means to seek care in the private sector, and studies have shown that up to 30 percent of the population now uses private health care in some capacity.[17-19] Only upper class Costa Ricans and foreigners can afford to regularly receive their health care within the private health care system, but middle class patients use the private sector as a limited health care strategy—for example, they might get diagnosed within the private sector to avoid a long wait time in CCSS but upon diagnosis, use the CCSS for treatment and medicines, especially if it is a serious or costly treatment. This results in a strain on the public health care sector, which will be discussed in more detail below.

Current Challenges to the System

Structural Adjustment Programs

The major achievements of the Costa Rican universal health care system have not been without significant challenges. The economic crisis of the 1980s hit the Latin American region hard, resulting in significant intervention by the World Bank and International Monetary Fund (IMF). Structural Adjustment Programs (SAPs) based on neoliberal economic principles were implemented throughout Latin America to reduce the large public debts that governments had accrued. This meant decentralization, privatization, and drastic reductions in social programs, which constituted a large part of public expenditures in the region, in exchange for loans. However, despite the loan terms, and likely due to their historical orientation toward social medicine, only a few countries in Latin America even partially privatized the management or delivery of their publicly financed health services during the reform period.[20] The majority made less drastic reforms by increasing private sector involvement in health care through contracts with the public sector or in other ways.

In Costa Rica, the World Bank reform program recommended several strategies: expanding primary care, separating the purchaser and provider, working with private sector entities, and decentralizing the administration and delivery of health care. Of these objectives, CCSS administrators chose to focus almost exclusively on the expansion of primary care. In particular, they opted to establish EBAIS basic health teams throughout the country to distribute services more equitably, a goal that had existed prior to the World Bank's SAP. There was a general lack of interest, however, in decentralization and reorganization of health system management. Although some primary care services were contracted out to public–private cooperatives, this never really resulted in decentralizing CCSS's power, and CCSS maintained institutional control over the cooperatives that continues today. The World Bank admits that decentralization did not succeed in Costa Rica and reported that its efforts to promote it within CCSS were undermined by internal opposition.[21]

Compared to other countries in the Latin American region, Costa Rica showed weak commitment to neoliberal SAPs, and Costa Rican health authorities weighed heavily on the side of equity—specifically, more equitable geographic distribution of health services—over efficiency in complying with the terms of the structural adjustment loans. Essentially, Costa Ricans took what they wanted from the reform and left the rest.[15]

Trade Agreements and Health Care

In conjunction with SAPs in Latin America, global and international trade agreements such as the General Agreement on Trade in Services (GATS), the North American Free Trade Agreement (NAFTA), and the Central American Free Trade Agreement (CAFTA) removed restrictions on trade (medical tourism is considered trade in health services under GATS), and allowed foreign private corporations to become involved in health service provision within Latin American countries. Such agreements and reforms have caused the state, which has been so central to health care within Latin America, to be displaced and has, as Ellen Shaffer et al. described it, "transformed the capacity of governments to monitor and to protect public health."[22(p23)]

In a controversial 2007 referendum, Costa Rica very narrowly backed the Central American Free Trade Agreement by a vote of 51.6 percent. The agreement took effect in January of 2009, with Costa Rica being the last of the participating nations to ratify, and the only nation to decide via referendum. There was very strong opposition to CAFTA because of its alignment with neoliberal principles that are at odds with Costa Rican values. Even after the referendum passed, resistance to CAFTA remained, and accusations that the referendum was corrupt persisted. Fourteen national laws needed to change in order to accommodate CAFTA, including, most notably, a law that opened previously public industries within Costa Rica to the global market. Within the health care arena, this opened the national health insurance scheme (*Instituto Nacional de Seguros,* or INS) to competition from international private insurance companies. Because of potential violations of intellectual property rights that are part of CAFTA's terms, this may also impact the ability of CCSS to use generic medicines.

The previous and current political administrations in Costa Rica supported CAFTA and the opening of Costa Rican industries to the global market, including the promotion of medical tourism. In 2008, the government declared medical tourism an "activity of national interest" because of its potential to bring revenues to the health sector and bolster auxiliary industries like recovery homes, transportation, and tourism. The Ministry of Tourism estimates that each medical tourist stays 11 days in the country and spends between $6,500 and $7,000: more than four times what a regular tourist would spend.[7] The government's declaration has resulted in government promotion of medical tourism both nationally and abroad, encouragement of private hospitals and clinics to seek international accreditation, support for international agreements with insurance companies and employers, and foreign and national investment in the medical infrastructure.

Internal Pressures

In addition to these global pressures on the Costa Rican health system, internal pressures have also created new challenges for the social security system. An aging population and larger immigrant population have increased the cost of health care, while at the same time, CCSS has had difficulty collecting mandated fees, particularly from the self-employed or those not employed in the legitimate economy. Because of the way the system is structured, anyone who enters a CCSS facility for emergency services will not be turned away, even if they lack the required insurance. Additionally, it is not uncommon for someone to wait until being diagnosed with a serious or chronic illness to enroll in and begin paying for social security insurance because if a Costa Rican citizen begins paying for CCSS insurance today, he or she can begin receiving services tomorrow, regardless of his or her health status and no matter the cost. This has created a situation in which medical care provided to an individual by the CCSS often exceeds what he or she has paid into the system.

In addition, private hospitals often refer patients to the CCSS for the most complicated or critical surgeries. Private providers typically make these referrals because a patient can't afford to pay for the treatment, the procedure is not considered profitable, or because they want to avoid high death or complication rates that might put off the rich patients and foreigners they are targeting for business. Likewise, the EBAIS primary care clinics operated by CCSS and the neighborhood cooperatives (which are funded by CCSS but have private sector administration) tend to refer patients to CCSS hospitals more than is necessary (i.e., when they could instead be treated on an outpatient basis or within the clinic), contributing to extremely high patient volumes in the CCSS hospitals. In Costa Rica, more than 43 percent of the services provided in the public health sector are hospital services, compared with 11.1 percent in private sector.[18] This means that the highest number of patients and the most expensive procedures and treatments all remain within the public hospitals, placing a heavy burden on the system.

Medical Tourism and Costa Rica's Contradicting Visions

The above discussion provides social and political contexts for the countries where medical tourism takes place in Latin America. These factors are often overlooked in discussions of medical tourism that assume this practice will have uniform (and typically positive) effects across destinations. However, questions remain about whether disparities in domestic and international health agendas might exacerbate health disparities by removing the state as a buffer between citizens and global forces and exposing vulnerable populations to forces of the international political economy. The investigation of medical tourism in the particular context of Costa Rica highlights the contradictions at play—Costa Rica is a country that repeatedly rejects neoliberal principles in its health care system, yet adopts them in the signing of CAFTA; that resists encroachments on CCSS by the private health sector but declares medical tourism, an industry fully entrenched in the private sector, an activity of national interest; and a country that is struggling to find its niche in the global economy while at the same time fervently defending the social principles upon which it is founded. My research explores these juxtapositions and takes as its focus the contradictory ideologies that give space for the emergence of medical tourism, an industry seemingly at odds with principles of universal health coverage subsidized by the public sector. Ironically, it is the successes of the Costa Rican socialized health system that allow for medical tourism to exist there in the first place.

There are concerns among Costa Ricans and researchers who work there that Costa Rica may be moving in the direction of "passive privatization" with the recent opening of the state insurance monopoly to private industry, a steadily increasing use of private sector medical services, and the expansion of private hospital groups.[23] This raises questions about the impact that this shift might have on the national health system, potentially creating a contradictory "dual track" of medical care—a private sector primarily driven by profit versus a public sector responsible for the health of all of its citizens.[24–26]

With these two polar conceptions of health systems—socialized health care at one end, in which health is a social right and the state is the guarantor; and market systems on the other, in which health is a commodity to be purchased individually; we begin to see the ideological contradiction of Costa Rica as a popular medical tourism destination.

ETHNOGRAPHIC FINDINGS: LOCAL EXPERIENCES OF MEDICAL TOURISM IN COSTA RICA

A picture of the initial and predicted effects of medical tourism on Costa Ricans and their health system emerged in more than 50 structured interviews conducted in and around the capital city of San José, home to government agencies, the University of Costa Rica, the major CCSS public hospitals, and the three largest private hospitals that cater to medical tourists. Interview respondents, including physicians, nurses, government officials, and medical tourism facilitators, offered their opinions of the industry and assessed potential impacts of medical tourism on Costa Rica's socialized health system. An overview of the results follows.

The State of the Medical Tourism Industry in Costa Rica

Medical tourism in Costa Rica centers on elective surgeries, primarily plastic surgery and cosmetic dentistry, though the industry is attempting to expand the market for orthopedic procedures, bariatric and weight loss surgeries, liberation therapy for multiple sclerosis, and corporate wellness exams, as well as other procedures considered to be more imperative and more profitable.

Medical tourists come to Costa Rica primarily from North America, specifically the United States, which is viewed as the primary target for attracting medical tourists. Those seeking care in Costa Rica are for the most part uninsured, underinsured, or seeking a procedure that insurance will not cover. Although CAFTA's provisions opened the insurance market to international competition, and a few insurance companies have begun to cover medical tourism options, the bulk of medical tourists to Costa Rica pay out of pocket. This is likely because elective surgeries, which insurance plans will not cover, remain the most popular procedures.

Key Stakeholders and the Health Care Cluster

The term "health care cluster" is used to describe the group of stakeholders who promote medical tourism in Costa Rica. Figure 5.1 shows the health care cluster in Costa Rica, as laid out by the former Minister of Competiveness and Regulatory Improvement, Jorge Woodbridge.[27] Table 5.1 illustrates his vision for the government's role. Costa Rica also has its own medical tourism promotion agency, PROMED (the Council for International Promotion of Costa Rican Medicine), established in 2008 to represent the joint interests of the major players from the private sector in the medical tourism industry, communicate with the public sector, and ensure sustainable growth of the industry.

In popular perception, these organizations are often seen as a step in the right direction in terms of presenting a unified front for medical tourism, but as doing very little in practical terms to advance the industry. Some participants see these organizations as gatekeepers, who work only to protect the financial interests of a small group of power holders who profit from medical tourism. One young physician said that she paid nearly $3,000 to join a physician group that promotes medical tourism and supposedly directs medical tourists to member physicians. When asked if she had received any foreign patients through the physician group, she said with a roll of her eyes, "Zero. Absolutely nothing." Another private sector physician remarked that "even though PROMED is a non-profit, they can say, 'I'm in the group and if you want to come in, then I want

Figure 5.1
The Health Care Cluster

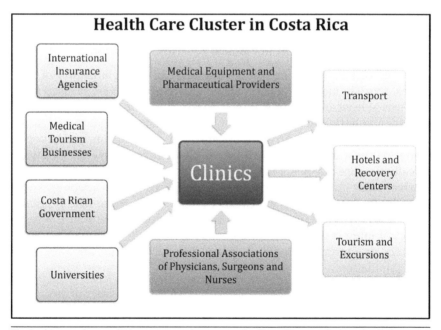

The health care cluster, which supports and promotes the Costa Rican medical tourism industry.
Source: Woodbridge J. Un Clúster Médico en Costa Rica: Oportunidades, estrategias y compromisos. http://www.competitividad.go.cr/bibliotecaimages/documentos/Cluster%20Medico.pdf. Accessed April 13, 2012.

Table 5.1
The role of the Costa Rican government

Ministry of Competitiveness
  • Strategic coordination
Ministry of Health
  • Oversight of quality standards
CCSS and Universities
  • Development of human resources
Institute of Costa Rican Tourism
  • Country image and international promotion campaign
PROCOMER
  • Promotion of exports of medical services
CINDE
  • Attract investment in research and medical sciences

Note: The Costa Rican government supports and promotes the medical tourism industry in a variety of ways.

something from you.' They can move their chips so you cannot be in the group. It is very political."

Role of the Government in Medical Tourism Promotion

In spite of some criticisms about the level of disorganization of the medical tourism industry, most interview participants were pleased that there was at least an attempt by Costa Rican entities to organize and promote the industry. Interestingly, many participants felt that the government should have very little involvement in medical tourism beyond promoting the industry and the image of Costa Rica in general. This was typically because of a belief that the government should not get involved in private industry, either because of faith in free market ideology (not surprisingly, this view was expressed more often by those who profited significantly from medical tourism), or because of a belief that it was a conflict of interest of sorts for the government to be spending time and resources promoting a private industry instead of caring for the Costa Rican population.

Local Hopes for Medical Tourism

In making his case for medical tourism, Minister Woodbridge summarized the anticipated benefits for Costa Rica as follows:

  • Increased flows of direct foreign investment and export of services;
  • More and better opportunities for professionals in medicine;

- Highly competitive health care prices for Costa Ricans;
- Higher standards and continuous improvement of hospital standards (benefiting national as well as foreign patients);
- Higher profits for the health care industry and its value chain (hotels, restaurants, travel agencies, airlines, pharmaceutical, equipment, doctors, etc.); and
- Creation of a Corporate Social Responsibility Fund financed by private institutions to develop social health projects.[27]

These arguments in support of medical tourism, which are quite similar to standard arguments provided by proponents of the industry, are mainly economic and operate on the assumption that increased revenue will go to support the public sector and complement public health efforts, and in this way trickle down to the poor.[28] The extent to which this is actually happening is addressed later in the chapter.

Most stakeholders I interviewed, especially in the private sector, had high hopes for the growth of medical tourism and the opportunities it presents for the country. Participants shared the Ministry of Competitiveness's optimism about the potential for the medical tourism industry to improve standards of living. One physician, who also started a medical tourism facilitation company, described medical tourism as a valuable tool for helping Costa Rica become a developed country:

> I really like to dream. Because I am an example of that dream and I came from a middle low class, public school, public high school, and public university and nowadays I am on the top of medical tourism in Costa Rica, so Costa Rica is a country of opportunities. . . . We really believe that medical tourism, because of the level of income for the country, is the main tool to reach the development that we have been waiting for for many years.

In a subsequent discussion, he even stated that he thought medical tourism might play a role in the reduction of prostitution and sex tourism in Costa Rica.

Though not all stakeholders interviewed had such lofty goals for medical tourism, most did see at least some potential advantages to promoting the industry at a national level. The most oft-cited potential advantage of medical tourism was increased national revenue. The most current national figures project that medical tourism brought $288 million in revenue to Costa Rica in 2010,[7] though because of the data collection and reporting issues mentioned above, this is difficult to confirm. Even though increased revenue was recognized as a principal positive effect of medical tourism, none of the participants interviewed offered evidence of any direct benefit to the CCSS or public system.

Local Anxieties about Medical Tourism

Among those with a high level of investment in medical tourism, there is concern about being outcompeted by nearby nations, particularly Panama, Colombia, and—if trade opens up—Cuba, which can offer medical care at lower prices than those in Costa Rica. This fear of being left behind by the industry has resulted in various changes in medical tourism practices. Physicians often feel that they must reduce their prices to remain competitive. Some saw cutting prices in order to receive a larger volume of international patients as an effective strategy for promoting medical tourism "in bulk," but other physicians felt exploited in these situations. One private sector surgeon said, "I have been working with facilitators . . . they are always saying, 'We will bring you patients.' But the problem is the prices. I think they are trying to prostitute our practice. So for example, if I do a surgery, the hospital reduces the prices a little bit, but why do we, the physicians, have to go lower and lower? I don't know, I think it's prostitution."

On the other hand, because prices of medical procedures are unregulated, some see medical tourism as an opportunity to charge higher fees, since some medical tourists can afford to pay them.

In addition, there are concerns that if the number of foreign patients does grow substantially, as many hope, this would mean a decrease in access to private health care for Costa Ricans, who would be unable to pay the higher prices. "They would consider it very expensive," one government official stated. "I mean someone from the U.S., they might think $5,000 for a surgery is cheap, but for a Costa Rican, it is very, very expensive."

An executive at an international medical tourism facilitator company shared in the hopes for industry growth but at the same time had concerns that it might be for some a *Field of Dreams* scenario, asking, "What if they build it and then they [the medical tourists] don't come?" This is of particular concern with the stakeholders building and investing so much in the industry during the current economic crisis.

The fact that there are 47 million uninsured Americans came up numerous times in interviews as an indication that medical tourism would grow in Costa Rica. One physician who worked in a private hospital stated hopefully: "I mean, there are plenty of patients in North America for all of us. We don't have space available for all the people that need help in the States . . . we are still not even approaching 0.001% of those patients that need medical services [in the United States]." His comment not only illustrates Costa Ricans' expectations for the industry but also touches on a question raised by other participants: whether Costa Rica has the capacity to accommodate a medical tourism "boom." Costa Rica is a country of 4.5 million people marketing to a population of 47 million. At the time that this research was conducted, there were only three JCI-accredited private hospitals working with medical tourists. Although more facilities targeting medical tourists are in the works, some participants wondered if Costa Rica could support a surge of medical tourists. While some expressed anxiety about what will happen if "they don't come," many also are concerned about what will happen if they *do* come. Does Costa Rica have enough facilities to accommodate substantially more medical tourists, and even if it does, would that accommodation come at the expense of Costa Rican residents?

An answer to these questions may come with the realization of a large medical tourism undertaking in the Guanacaste region of the country on the Pacific coast, a very popular tourist region where most of the county's beaches are located. Two of the three major private hospitals in the country plan to expand to open hospitals in the region, and the third plans to open a clinic there. Unlike the existing hospitals in San José, the Guanacaste facilities will cater almost exclusively to medical tourists and residents of a retirement community for North Americans that is simultaneously being constructed in the area. While there are many expectations for this multi-million-dollar development, there are also doubts among those working in the industry about whether "they will come."

Meanwhile, some interview participants worried not about whether this development in Guanacaste will be a profitable venture but whether the project will worsen inequities in this area and further contribute to the development of a "local-free" zone to which only foreigners have access. Guanacaste has a history of highly inequitable tourism development. The region, one of the poorest in Costa Rica, developed rapidly without a clear plan for sustainability and is today rife with disparities—golf courses sit next to local communities without access to clean water, and all-inclusive resorts have risen in communities of primarily impoverished farmers who lack the education to work in these facilities. While many local Costa Ricans were displaced in the name of this tourism development in the Guanacaste province, most of the profits have remained with private investors. An academic at the University of Costa Rica cautioned against further exacerbating such a situation with medical tourism, stating, "My point is that we cannot open the issue of medical tourism if we're not opening it with a vision that is regulated responsibly, with clearly defined policies, but also in a way that engages 'production chains' that service communities, so that the situation that we've seen in Guanacaste is not repeated any more. I think it is a terrible lesson learned there, and yet it still continues to be repeated."

Health and Human Resources Migration within Costa Rica

Many physicians who practice full time in the CCSS also work after hours in the private sector. There are no laws or restrictions against doing so, and physicians commonly supplement their CCSS salaries in this manner. Some participants suggested that this is a strategy that enables the CCSS to keep their physicians happy with less pay. As one participant put it, it is a way to "live in the best of two worlds." Though there are no recent statistics, it seems that the practice of working in both sectors is increasing. In the early 1990s, approximately 10 percent of health professionals worked in the private sector; by the late 1990s, this proportion had risen to 24 percent.[17] Although the great majority of Costa Ricans continue to use the CCSS for health care, and the majority of physicians work for CCSS, increasing patient volume in the private sector, including the infusion of medical tourists in some specialties, makes it increasingly attractive for physicians to practice there.

The majority of the physicians I interviewed worked, or had worked, in both sectors, and many expressed a desire to eventually acquire enough clients to be able to leave the public sector altogether and move into the private sector, where they could earn a significantly higher salary and have more control over their time. The fact that the same physicians work in both the public and private sectors and can flow relatively freely between the two has led to some abuse of this dual position. For instance, physicians in the private sphere may take monetary bribes, known as *biombos*, from private patients to push them to the top of the wait list in a CCSS facility. In these cases, the patient benefits by not having to pay for expensive private services and avoids the often long wait times for treatment in the CCSS, while the physician makes extra money "off the books." In fact, as one economist interviewed pointed out, not only do the doctors move between sectors, but the patients do too: "As a physician, you are hired by Caja [CCSS], but at 3:00 when you finish your day [in the public sector], you go across the street to your private office. And your patients in one sphere could be the same patients as in the other. And then . . . well only angels will keep good accounting of the situation."

Although participants expressed personal satisfaction with working for CCSS and fulfilling their social obligation to Costa Ricans, most who specialized in services that are in demand by medical tourists said that they would like to work with medical tourists, primarily for the salary boost. This may be contributing to a divide in which public sector physicians are expected to work for moral incentives, while physicians who treat foreigners work for private gain, often receiving much higher remuneration, as was seen in research in Cuba.[24] A physician working for CCSS might make somewhere between $US1,500 and $US3,000 per month, whereas a plastic surgeon or orthopedist working in the private sector might make up to $US10,000 for one surgery. A private sector surgeon I spoke with said that for every surgery he does in his private practice, he receives the equivalent of his entire month's salary from the

CCSS. Not all specialties are so lucrative though, and the majority of physicians enjoy the stability and benefits that come with their CCSS positions and work only a couple evenings per week in the private sector to bolster their wages.

Still, the phenomenon known as "internal brain drain," wherein physicians opt to practice in the more profitable private sector over the public sector, is of concern with regard to the continuing development of medical tourism in Costa Rica. Particularly in certain specialties like anesthesiology, CCSS has seen major shortages due to the number of physicians who were trained in the public sector but then found it more profitable to break their contract with CCSS and move directly into private practice, where they could make more money. This option is not possible for all specialists, since some would not have the client base to move into private practice early in their careers. Nonetheless, the public subsidization of physicians who eventually end up practicing in the private sector is worrying, especially in a system that is already financially strained. Several participants expressed this concern. One administrator at CCSS who believed that medical tourism would certainly have an impact on CCSS through the loss of human resources stated, "the amount of professionals that are in the private sector are enough, that came from our [public] classrooms." Another participant, an academic, expressed a similar frustration:

> And on the subject of human resources in the health field, this is creating a big conflict because with my taxes and all of us who pay taxes here in Costa Rica, we are paying for the training of medical specialists and many of these medical specialists are not even going to work in the public health system! They will work in the private system where wage standards are very, very different, very different, than in the public health system . . . I mean, my colleagues have confessed to me and said, "Look, I gave up working for the social security system because even when I had 25 years of working with CCSS and I was almost ready to retire, my salary did not exceed $2,500, so I prefer not to continue with this salary but instead to earn in private practice $20,000 per month." This really changes things.

The Current Reality of Medical Tourism in Costa Rica

Interview and survey responses suggest that most stakeholders do feel that there might be national benefits for promoting medical tourism; however, as yet, none of these potential benefits can be discerned. This may be because the medical tourism "boom" that many anticipated has yet to happen in Costa Rica. Despite extensive discussion about what could and could not happen in the future, with a few exceptions—notably plastic surgeons and a small number of other physicians who have profitable medical tourism practices—not even the most enthusiastic stakeholders reported substantial impacts, either positive or negative, within Costa Rica to date.

One of the most important findings of this research is that there appears to be no mechanism in place to ensure that medical tourism directly benefits CCSS or public health care. This is especially noteworthy since the Costa Rican government, CCSS, and universities are all viewed as having a role to play in the promotion and support of the medical tourism industry (see Figure 5.1 and Table 5.1). The "Corporate Social Responsibility Fund" that Minister Woodbridge suggests will connect medical tourism to social health does not exist as of this writing, and medical tourism is not taxed differently than any other industry, though a few participants felt that it should be. Profits from medical tourism have so far remained almost exclusively with private sector hospitals and physicians. Some believed that there was a need for the government to take a stronger regulatory approach in dealing with medical tourism and its profits in order to maximize potential advantages and minimize harmful impacts. One Ministry of Health official stated:

> I think that the government should regulate it more . . . the government should have some part of what medical tourism generates in terms of money and distribute it to the people who really need it. . . . I mean to put it into social programs that reduce inequity. I think that money should be distributed in a better way, but all the money is staying with the hospitals. And nobody is thinking about it. Or at least nobody in the government. Of course there is a lot of money involved here—it is a very good business and many people. . . . Well it's very nice for them to keep it quiet. To not do something with it.

Medical tourism represents a new configuration of health care provision in a globalized world, and there is currently a lack of consensus about whose responsibility it is to ensure that medical tourism, along with other global industries, is regulated in a socially responsible way. There is currently no global oversight for industries such as medical tourism. Additionally, the growing standardization on the "sending" side of the medical tourism industry has not been matched in "receiving" countries, making the industry subject to varying national regulations and costs.

Ethical and Ideological Conflicts

Overarching the more tangible impacts that medical tourism has or may have on the health care system in Costa Rica are the ethical and ideological implications that medical tourism has in a context such as Costa Rica. The socialized health system, founded on principles of solidarity, equity, and universal access, is a national symbol of Costa Rican values. During the year that I lived in San José, not one Costa Rican I spoke with complained about the fact that wealthier Costa Ricans subsidize health care for the poor, or questioned this logic. In fact, assessments of the CCSS system, in spite of its current challenges and shortcomings, were overwhelmingly positive. Costa Ricans love the CCSS system and are deservedly proud of its achievements. One physician put it this way:

> The focus of health should always be directed to equity, solidarity, universality. And to attend to the user who needs it the most who has fewer resources. Because we have seen that economic issues are related to health—the less I have, the more probability I have of getting sick. So there will be many more problems in the larger population when we don't take care of the poor. The health system can't favor, or lean towards, the elite population. It should work in favor of the simpler population that is in need of services. Those for me are the principles that should always govern us.

When this social mentality is positioned alongside a model of private for-profit health care, these messages of solidarity get convoluted. This is underscored by the fundamental conflict over whether health care is to be viewed as a right, accessible to all; or a business, to be outsourced as other businesses have been. One public sector nurse summarized this point well, stating that it is not the direct impacts of medical tourism that concern her at present, but the incremental shifts in thinking that it represents.

> I think that what is happening now with this type of tourism, is that it's making the private sector grow. They are building hotels right next to these hospitals, or in the hospitals and . . . well, you can see the connection. So the private hospitals are focusing on growth, but it is only for a certain group that has acquisitive capacity to be able to do it, and has foreign capital. In a certain way, I don't know if I can say that it is *all* negative, but this brings changes to our culture. Because medical tourism, since it is for people with higher income, and above all for foreigners—this changes the idiosyncrasies, the individual character of our culture, as well as the determined spaces meant for certain sectors. So it becomes more elite focused . . . and things happen that are for this other population, not for Costa Ricans. So there are cultural changes that also come with this process, and it is very important to take these into account.

In addition to ideological shifts in thinking that medical tourism presents, a few participants felt that it is at its core an unethical or exploitive practice, in that it promotes taking advantage of the lower health care costs in Costa Rica rather than fixing the problems of the health systems from which medical tourists are coming. One participant, an academic, said:

> I don't like medical tourism. I don't know; I don't like it. Because I think it is making use of lower costs here than in the country where the people are from. Which I don't know if that is fair . . . if you take resources away here from Costa Ricans, then you are doing something wrong, and you just do it because those people coming here can pay so much money.

CONCLUSION

Today, Costa Rica is caught between two competing visions of national development—one that adheres to the principles of socialized medicine that have allowed for the noteworthy achievements of the past, and another that emphasizes neoliberal growth and establishing a position within the global marketplace. Confronted with industries like medical tourism, which is one, but not the only, example of this neoliberal vision, the state finds itself in a contradictory role—promoting a national ideology based on social medicine for Costa Ricans within the public sector, while at the same time opening its borders to foreigners who come to consume private sector services that local Costa Ricans cannot afford.

In thinking about medical tourism, it must be noted that this practice exists precisely because there are significant inequities between sending and receiving nations. Medical tourism occurs across lines of economic and social class divisions, and in fact depends upon these divisions, as well as entrenched inequalities within and between nations, for its prosperity.

Despite considerable concerns about the effects of medical tourism in Costa Rica, participants acknowledged that there might be constructive ways in which the industry can impact local health systems. At this point, however, these benefits seem to be little more than hypothetical; to date, it's impossible to identify any direct benefit for the public health system.

To maximize the positive effects and reduce the harms of medical tourism, it is important to consider regulatory measures and oversight of the industry. These measures should ensure socially responsible practices that sustain the health care achievements that Costa Rica has made in the past century, rather than dismantle them. Examples of such regulation could include special taxation on medical tourism, channeling a percentage of medical tourism profits directly into the public health sector, monitoring human resource needs more closely in order to provide for both sectors, requiring the private sector to contribute to the training of physicians through the CCSS, or utilizing private sector resources to ease the current burden on the public sector.

Ethnographic perspectives are an important means to bring to light "local worlds" that are often overshadowed by powerful stakeholders and to help broaden understanding of the effects of medical tourism on local health systems and perceptions of health care. This chapter is meant to be a step in this direction, voicing the concerns and experiences of local Costa Ricans who live within this system in flux. To this end, more critical attention is needed on the practice of medical tourism and the ways in which it interacts with and impacts existing health systems in Latin America and elsewhere.

REFERENCES

1. Joint Commission International. JCI Accredited Organizations. 2011; List of all JCI accredited organizations. http://www.jointcommissioninternational.org/JCI-Accredited-Organizations/. Accessed April 13, 2012.

2. Aérea de Turismo Receptor. *Número, porcentaje y variación porcentual de la cantidad de viajeros que llegaron a Costa Rica por vía aérea por motivo de salud según año.* 2009.

3. Arce S. Costa Rica intenta atraer al turismo médico corporativo. *La Nacion.* May 2, 2011.

4. Arguedas J. Crece el turismo de salud en Costa Rica. *ImpreZona.* 2009. http://www.impre.com/imprezona/2009/2/5/crece-el-turismo-de-salud-en-c-107477-1.html. Accessed April 13, 2012.

5. Council for International Promotion of Costa Rican Medicine (PROMED). *El Turismo de Salud.* 2010.

6. Ministerio de Producción. *Turismo Médico: Un cluster incipiente y potencial para Costa Rica.* 2010.

7. Brenes CQ. Turismo medico da fuertes latidos: industria vincula unas 600 empresas u generó $288 millones en 2010. *El Financiero.* June 26, 2011.

8. Waitzkin H, Iriart C, Estrada A, Lamadrid S. Social medicine then and now: Lessons fom Latin America. *American Journal of Public Health.* 2001;91(10):1592–1601.

9. Soares R. Life expectancy and welfare in Latin America and the Caribbean. *Health Economics.* 2009;18(S1):S37–S54.

10. Morgan L. Health without wealth? Costa Rica's health system under economic crisis. *Journal of Public Health Policy.* 1987;8(1):86–105.

11. Morgan L. Political will" and community participation in Costa Rican primary health care. *Medical Anthropology Quarterly.* 1989;3(3):232–245.

12. Unger J-P, de Paepe P, Buitrón R, Soors W. Costa Rica: Achievements of a heterodox health policy. *American Journal of Public Health.* 2007;98(4):636–643.

13. World Health Organization. *The world health report 2000—Health systems: Improving performance.* 2000.

14. CCSS. Trabajadores de la Caja y Salarios según sexo por años de servicio. 2010.

15. Clark M. Health sector reform in Costa Rica: Reinforcing a public system. In: Kaufman R, Nelson J, eds. *Crucial needs, weak incentives: Social sector reform, democratization, and globalization in Latin America.* Washington, DC: Woodrow Wilson International Center Press and Johns Hopkins University Press; 2004.

16. Homedes N, Ugalde A. Privatización de los servicios de salud: las experiencias de Chile y Costa Rica. *Gaceta Sanitaria.* 2002;16(1):54–62.

17. Connolly G. Costa Rican health care: A maturing comprehensive system. *Global Health Council.* 2002:11.

18. Herrero F, Durán F. El Sector Privado en el Sistema de Salud de Costa Rica. In: (CEPAL) CEpAL, ed. *Santiago de Chile.* 2001.

19. University of Costa Rica. *Encuesta Nacional de Salud (ENSA).* San José: University of Costa Rica. 2006.

20. Homedes N, Ugalde A. Why neoliberal health reforms have failed in Latin America. *Health Policy.* 2005;71:83–96.

21. World Bank. *Implementation Completion Report (CPL 36540) on a Loan in the Amount of $US 22 Million to the Republic of Costa Rica for a Health Sector Reform Project.* Washington, DC. 2003.

22. Shaffer ER, Waitzkin H, Brenner J, Jasso-Aguilar R. Health policy and ethics: Global trade in public health. *American Journal of Public Health.* 2005;95(1):23–34.

23. Clark M. The Recentralization of Health Care Reform in Costa Rica. Occasional Paper prepared for the Center for Inter-American Policy and Research (CIPR). July 21, 2010.

24. Brotherton PS. We have to think like capitalists but continue being socialists: Medicalized subjectivities, emergent capital, and socialist entrepreneurs in post-Soviet Cuba. *American Ethnologist.* 2008;35(2):259–274.

25. Rylko-Baur B, Farmer P. Managed care or managed inequality? A call for critiques of market based medicine. *Medical Anthropology Quarterly.* 2002; 16(4):476–502.

26. Wilson A. Medical Tourism, Neoliberal Populism and the Body Economy in Thailand. Paper presented at: American Anthropological Association. 2006; Atlanta.

27. Woodbridge J. *Un Clúster Médico en Costa Rica: Oportunidades, estrategias y compromisos.* http://www.competitividad.go.cr/bibliotecaimages/documentos/Cluster%20Medico.pdf. Accessed April 13, 2012.

28. Turner L. First world health care at third world prices: Globalization, bioethics, and medical tourism. *Biosocieties.* 2007;2:303–325.

Part II

Border Crossings: Risks, Controversies, and Consequences

Chapter 6

Unseen Travelers: Medical Tourism and the Spread of Infectious Disease

Jill R. Hodges and Ann Marie Kimball

Medical tourism entails two activities known to spread infections—travel and hospital procedures. Combined, and absent the necessary safeguards, these activities have the potential to accelerate the global spread of disease. Potentially compounding the risks are patients with compromised or suppressed immune systems traveling to and from destinations with relatively high rates of infectious disease, including new multidrug-resistant agents that defy standard forms of detection and treatment. The emergence and spread of the gene that produces the multidrug-resistant enzyme known as NDM-1 illustrates the challenges that can arise when patients (and their bacteria) cross borders, but disease surveillance and control mechanisms do not.

In September 2009, a multinational team of researchers, Dongeun Yong et al., published a study describing a new type of enzyme that equips bacteria to disarm a wide range of antibiotics, including the carbapenems, one of the last lines of defense against common respiratory and urinary tract infections.[1] The enzyme was detected in January 2008 in bacteria from a 59-year-old man with a urinary tract infection who was being treated at a hospital in Örebro, Sweden. The patient, a Swedish man of Indian origin, had type 2 diabetes, and had in the previous month undergone surgeries at two hospitals in India during a visit. He developed a pressure ulcer and was referred for further treatment to the facility in Sweden. There, clinicians determined he had a strain of the bacteria *Klebsiella pneumoniae* that carried an enzyme that made it resistant to all but a few antibiotics. Further examination showed that he also had another bacteria, *Escherichia coli*, with the same severe resistance, suggesting that the *bla*NDM-1 gene that produced this resistant enzyme could shuttle on plasmids among different types of bacteria, making it even more difficult to detect and treat. Researchers concluded that the gene had originated in India, and designated the enzyme New Delhi metallo-beta-lactamase-1 (NDM-1)—a label that was to become highly controversial when the spread of NDM-1 was linked to medical travel. In their conclusion, the authors, who were from institutions in South Korea, the United Kingdom, and Sweden, stated that they planned to study the extent to which NDM-1 was present inside and outside health care settings in India, noting, "In a country where there is little control on antibiotic prescriptions, the rapid dissemination of such a plasmid is alarming."[1(p5053)]

Nearly a year later, another multinational team that included some of the original researchers, as well as scientists from India and Pakistan, published a second study that examined laboratory reports to assess the presence of bacteria carrying NDM-1 in India, Pakistan, and the United Kingdom.[2] NDM-1, which was first detected in the United Kingdom in 2008, had by 2009 become the most commonly detected carbapenem-resistant agent among intestinal bacteria there. The study found that at least 17 of the 29 UK patients with bacteria carrying NDM-1—nearly 60 percent—had traveled to India or Pakistan within the last year, and that 14 of those 17 patients had received medical treatment during their travels. Some of the patients had fallen ill or been in accidents while traveling, and others had traveled specifically for procedures such as cosmetic surgery or kidney and bone marrow transplants. The study also found evidence that bacteria carrying NDM-1 were present not just in hospital facilities in India but in the general community. In their discussion, the authors challenged a news article citing a study that projected that the United Kingdom's National Health Service could save money by developing an arrangement that gave patients the option of traveling to India for certain health services rather than waiting to receive them in the United Kingdom.[3] Instead, the authors suggested, such a practice could result in greater costs due to infections. They concluded, "we would strongly advise against such proposals" and called the potential for spreading bacteria carrying NDM-1 "clear and frightening."[2(p602)]

The article, published in *The Lancet Infectious Diseases*, was accompanied by a commentary expressing concern about the spread of multidrug-resistant bacteria, including those with NDM-1.[4] The commentary noted the potential risks of spread via medical tourism and called for worldwide monitoring and international surveillance studies for multidrug-resistant bacteria, particularly "in countries that actively promote medical tourism" and recommended screening of patients who have undergone medical procedures in India.[4(p578)] The United Kingdom's Health Protection Agency issued a National Resistance Alert 3 advising clinicians to recognize exposure to health care in India and Pakistan as "major risk factors" for acquiring carbapenemase-resistant bacteria and other countries, including the United States, France, and Canada, took similar steps.

Meanwhile, Indian government officials took issue with the study linking the UK cases to India and with the accompanying warnings about traveling to India for medical care, noting among other things that India is not unique in its struggle against multidrug-resistant pathogens.[5] A commentary in the *Indian Journal of Public Health* pointed out that the fact that the NDM-1 enzyme was first identified in India did not necessarily mean it originated there.[6] The authors noted that the UK patients presumed to have acquired bacteria carrying NDM-1 in India had not been tested for bacteria with the enzyme prior to their travel, leaving open the possibility that they had acquired it at home or elsewhere. In the end, while questioning the validity of the evidence linking the resistant bacteria to India, the Indian government acknowledged the importance of addressing the spread of drug-resistant agents and convened a task force to enhance and enforce policies on antibiotic use and to develop a national surveillance system for drug-resistant agents.[5]

Since its initial identification in January 2008, NDM-1 has been detected in a variety of bacteria in hundreds of patients in more than 30 countries, including Canada, Japan, the United States, Israel, Turkey, China, Australia, France, Taiwan, and Norway.[7] Figure 6.1 illustrates the potential dissemination paths of some of the early reported cases. To date, most cases have been linked to travel to the Indian subcontinent or the Balkans and many have involved some type of exposure to medical facilities. But a study by Timothy R. Walsh et al. published in *The Lancet Infectious Diseases* in April 2011 confirmed earlier suspicions that NDM-1 is not only present in medical facilities but also in the community.[8] Researchers found bacteria carrying the enzyme in both standing water on the street and tap water, presenting the possibility for exposure in the general environment for not only medical tourists but also any companions who travel with them.

While disease transmission has always been a concern in medical tourism, the investigations into the emergence and spread of NDM-1, a newly identified multidrug-resistant agent, made the potential risks more

Figure 6.1
Importations of NDM-1

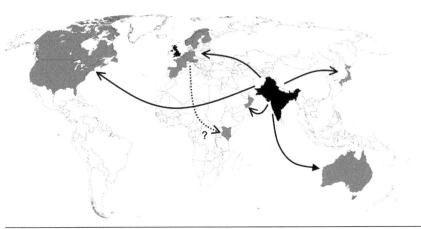

Schematic representation of the epicenter (black) and early reported/potential importations (gray) of New Delhi metallo-ß-lactamase-producing organisms. A number of these importations were linked with medical travel.
Source: Benjamin A. Rogers, Zohreh Aminzadeh, Yoshiro Hayashi, David L. Paterson. Country-to-country transfer of patients and the risk of multi-resistant bacterial infection. *Clinical Infectious Diseases.* 2011;53(1):49–56. By permission of Oxford University Press.

explicit. These cases serve to illustrate many of the health, economic, and political issues that arise when travel and medical care intersect—issues that we will explore in greater detail in this chapter. We will begin with a brief discussion of the growing problem of multidrug-resistant agents in this context, then discuss how travel and medical care contribute to the spread of these agents and others. We conclude with an examination of the systems that are currently in place and the work that remains to better understand and address the risks of acquiring and spreading disease that arise when patients cross borders for medical care.

OVERVIEW: MICROBIAL MELTING POT

Although the extent and nature of medical travel is not precisely documented, it's established that people travel to and from every continent for a range of medical services, many of which involve some kind of invasive procedure, such as heart valve replacement, hip resurfacing, knee replacement, breast augmentation, and kidney transplants. And while all invasive medical procedures entail some risk of infection, medical tourism theoretically brings additional risk by intermingling populations with different commensal bacteria—or bugs that live in and on their hosts in a harmless, or in some cases mutually beneficial, relationship. Medicine broadly categorizes microbes into two groups: commensals, the "normal" bugs that all people carry—on our skin, in our mouths, and throughout our intestinal tracts—and pathogens, the harmful bacteria that cause disease through infection. That divide is becoming increasingly blurred as practices such as traveling for medical care become more common, since one person's commensal bacteria can be another individual's exotic pathogen.

When patients travel for medical care, they carry both the commensal and pathogenic bacteria residing in their systems (and communities) into geographically distant settings. The patient is, in turn, then exposed to the resident bacteria in the hospital or clinic he or she visits, to the commensals living in and on his or her health care provider team, and in and on individuals in the community at large. Finally, these microbes may hitch a ride back to the home of the patient, potentially introducing new and unknown bacteria into the community or clinic where the patient next seeks care. In other words, at any point in the circular migration of patients traveling for medical care, microbes may travel from one location where they constitute a harmless bacteria, or at least a known and treatable infection, to another where they are unknown, making diagnosis and treatment much more problematic.

EMERGING ANTIBIOTIC DRUG RESISTANCE

Of particular concern is the emergence and proliferation of antibiotic-resistant strains of common bacteria. Resistance has been an issue ever since antibiotics came into widespread use with the introduction of penicillin more than 60 years ago, but concern has heightened in recent years as rapidly multiplying microbes have evolved to challenge one class of antibiotics after another and threatened to outpace the development of new and more effective drugs. Almost every bacterial pathogen has developed resistance to at least one antibiotic, and some are resistant to nearly all. Meanwhile, the ever-increasing flow of people and animal products around the globe has served to expand the resistant agents' trajectories.

By definition, drug-resistant infections can be difficult, if not impossible, to treat. Consequently, their transmission via medical travelers presents a potentially significant expense and concern for hospitals and public health systems not only in sending countries, as in the case of the apparent NDM-1 transmission from India to Sweden discussed above, but also for hospitals and health systems in receiving countries. One sobering example is the report by Chee Kiang Phua et al. of the first case of extensively drug-resistant tuberculosis (XDR-TB) in Singapore, which arrived with a patient from Indonesia in January 2010.[9] The patient, a 41-year-old woman, arrived at the emergency department of a public hospital in

Singapore with a cough and fever. She was eventually diagnosed with extensively drug-resistant tuberculosis that required five months of intensive multidrug treatment, hospitalization in a special isolation facility, and lung surgery at a total cost of more than S$100,000 (US$78,000) before she was able to return home. Singapore, a popular medical tourism destination known for its high quality care, is located in a region with a number of countries with relatively high rates of TB, including Indonesia. The patient in this case had been diagnosed and treated for various forms of TB on three occasions in Indonesia beginning in 2003 before seeking treatment in Singapore for the extensively drug-resistant strain. In addition to this case, there has been at least one anecdotal account of a patient seeking services in Singapore for a condition other than TB who was incidentally found to have resistant TB.[10] This is not surprising in light of the TB rates in some of Singapore's neighboring countries, and may be somewhat of a harbinger for other medical destinations in similar locations. Such incidental disease represents a challenge to receiving institutions and their attendant public health systems even in countries like Singapore, which has scrupulous isolation and hospital infection control policies.

Key drivers of drug resistance include use of antibiotics when they are not effective or necessary (commonly referred to as overuse), lack of access to drugs when they are needed (underuse), failure to complete a full course of antibiotics or use of substandard or counterfeit drugs (misuse), and excessive antibiotic use in food animals to promote growth. In many regions, antibiotics are widely available without prescription, contributing to overuse or misuse as a result of inappropriate drug choice or dosage.[11] Even in places where antibiotics require prescriptions, such as the United States, they often are overprescribed or misused. And the more drugs that are circulating in the environment, the more opportunity bacteria have to evolve in ways that lead to increased resistance.

In a review article, Benjamin Rogers et al. provide a comprehensive look at the transmission and introduction of antimicrobial strains across borders via what they term "intercountry patients," a group that they define to include medical tourists, disaster and military evacuees, and ex-patriots.[12] The authors note that the pathogens' resistance patterns vary by region, complicating their detection and treatment. They document cases that show that that multidrug-resistant bacteria emerge in and spread from high- as well as low-resource settings, and note that "Healthcare–associated multiresistant bacterial infection is greatly heterogeneous, and not necessarily divided along lines of economic development and industrialization."[12(p49)]

While the continually changing profiles of resistant bacteria and the lack of a global surveillance system can make it difficult to identify high prevalence areas with precision, some regions are known to have high burdens of resistant strains. A review by Shio-Shin Jean and Po-Ren Hsueh of resistance patterns in Asia, which encompasses a number of popular medical tourism destinations, including Thailand, India, and China, describes Asia as "one of the epicentres of antimicrobial resistance."[13(p291)] Among the factors that contribute to these high burdens are limited sanitation, health care, and surveillance infrastructures, as well as misuse of antibiotics.

Although it is difficult to fully assess the extent to which drug-resistant pathogens and other dangerous bacteria may be traveling in or on patients who are hospitalized abroad, given the rising levels of antibiotic resistance and the growing number of cases in which resistant pathogens have been linked to medical travel, the potential risks are important to consider and address. In the next sections, we will look specifically at the risks of disease transmission through travel and medical care before returning to a discussion on mitigating the risks when these two activities are combined.

FOREIGN EXCHANGE: TRAVEL AND THE SPREAD OF INFECTIOUS DISEASE

The spread of disease via international travel is well established. Human travel was key to the rapid global spread of severe acute respiratory syndrome (SARS), which spanned more than two dozen countries and resulted in 774 deaths in 2003[14,15]; and influenza A (H1N1), which spread to more than 200 countries and caused more than 18,000 deaths in 2009–2010.[16,17] Travelers have been the vectors for international transmission of many other emergent infections, among them influenza, measles, and polio. An analysis of travel patterns and the spread of influenza in the United States found that as travel volumes increase, the spread of influenza accelerates.[18] Another analysis showed that the spread of influenza A (H1N1), which originated in Mexico, reflected travel patterns of spring vacationers to that country—16 of the 20 countries that had the highest volumes of visitors to Mexico in 2008 had confirmed cases of influenza A (H1N1) imported from Mexico in 2009.[19] As many as half of the more than 100 million people who travel annually from nontropical areas to developing countries develop some kind of health problem during their travels, including infectious diseases ranging from flu to malaria.[20]

Patients traveling for medical care are exposed to a host of pathogens each step of their journeys, from the taxi to the airport to the hotel where they stay for their recovery. Often, as a result of their health conditions or medical procedures, these patients may have compromised immune systems. In addition to being more vulnerable to infections such as tuberculosis and malaria, patients with certain conditions such as HIV cannot effectively use vaccinations to prevent infections such as hepatitis B and influenza.

Exposure During Transit

Many medical tourists travel by air, often for many hours. Flights from Chicago to Bangkok are typically 20 hours or longer; flights from London to Mumbai are 8 hours or more. For the most part, the risk of disease transmission on commercial aircraft is minimal. A World Health Organization (WHO) report on International Travel and Health notes that in general, research indicates that "there is very little risk of any communicable disease being transmitted on board an aircraft."[21(p23)] Nonetheless, international aircraft travel, in which passengers typically are confined for a period of hours in close quarters, presents opportunities for disease transmission.

Air travel has been associated with the spread of SARS, measles, tuberculosis, and A/H1N1 influenza, among other pathogens. In their 2005 review article on commercial air travel and disease transmission, Alexandra Mangili and Mark Gendreau note that all four modes of disease transmission—contact, common vehicle, vector, airborne—potentially come into play with air travel.[22] Contact entails transmission via body-to-body contact or contact with an intermediate vehicle such as a doorknob, tray table, or armrest. Common vehicle involves transmission via a contaminated source such as food or water. Vector signifies transmission via insects or vermin, and airborne transmission results when a pathogen is aerosolized, or dispensed, through the air, for instance when an infected person sneezes or coughs.

Of greatest likelihood and concern on aircraft is airborne transmission of respiratory infections. Many later model commercial aircraft are equipped with high efficiency particulate air (HEPA) filters that help prevent the circulation of infectious microbes. However, HEPA filters are effective only when in use. In one case, for example, after an aircraft carrying 54 people, including a passenger who was ill with influenza, sat for three hours without the ventilation system operating, 72 percent of the passengers who remained on board during the delay developed symptoms of influenza in the following three days.[23] While more recent aircraft are equipped with HEPA filters, older planes may not be. Moreover, the protocol for changing the filters is based on air miles traveled, in line with other maintenance—not by the level of function of the filter.

Passengers sitting close to an infected person are at risk, regardless of the air filtration process. After a three-hour flight from Hong Kong to Beijing carrying a passenger with SARS, 16 passengers subsequently developed confirmed cases of SARS, including 8 of 23 passengers sitting in the three rows in front of that passenger.[24] In addition to proximity, factors that influence the spread of infection on aircraft include the degree to which the infected person has symptoms, such as fever or cough, the virulence of the agent, the duration of the exposure, and the health of the people who are exposed—these last two considerations are of particular concern to medical travelers.

Proximity to other passengers and duration of exposure can be an even more significant factor on buses and trains, which often have more crowded conditions and longer trips. Indeed, 13 passengers and crew on a train traveling through China developed the A (H1N1) virus after being exposed to a passenger who made the 40-hour journey while sick with the virus.[16] An investigation found that passengers who rode in the same car and those who rode the train for longer periods had a greater risk of developing the virus. Cruise ships, with their closed environments and extended journeys, also present exposure risks. But while some minor cosmetic procedures are currently available at sea, and there has been discussion about expanding the range of offerings, cruise ships are not at present a high volume destination or transit source for medical tourists.

Although the speed of airline travel reduces passengers' exposure times, it carries other risks. A plane flight may be over before an infected person exhibits any symptoms, so other passengers may be unwittingly exposed. Rapid travel via air can also serve to spread infections further and faster. Theoretically, passengers who are considered a threat to public health can be denied boarding provided there is an applicable national or airline policy in place. But as WHO's Tuberculosis and Air Travel: Guidelines for Prevention and Control[25] notes, in addition to the challenges of identifying passengers whose health status may pose a threat, these provisions can be difficult to apply given privacy concerns and differing national policies. In 2007, a man who flew from the United States to Europe with what was believed to be extensively resistant tuberculosis (XDR-TB) provoked worldwide concern as authorities sought to stop him from boarding another commercial flight and potentially exposing more passengers. He ultimately flew to Montreal, Canada, and drove a rented car back into the United States, where he was then isolated in a medical facility.[26] Meanwhile health officials contacted several hundred passengers to advise them of the exposure and tested those who were at greatest risk. In the end, it was determined that the man had a less-resistant form TB, and follow-up tests showed that none of the passengers developed TB.

Community-Based Exposure

In addition to exposure during air travel, patients traveling for medical care are subject to potential exposure to infectious disease in the communities they visit. They may be exposed to foreign pathogens in the water they drink, the food they eat, the soil they touch, the air they breathe, and the insects that bite them. The movement of people across borders has long been linked to the acquisition and spread of foreign bacteria, from the dissemination of Yellow Fever from the Caribbean to the Americas in the 1600s and 1700s, to the more recent cases of international transmission of SARS, influenza A (H1N1) and bacteria carrying NDM-1. Depending on their health and medical needs, medical travelers may visit for several days or weeks before or after their medical procedures. As the term "medical tourism" suggests, a number of travel companies, medical providers, and governments promote the opportunity to combine medical services and a vacation. While there are no definitive data indicating how often patients actually include leisure activities or destinations in their medical care, medical needs in some cases require that they spend at least some time abroad before returning home. Patients who undergo surgery, for instance, are not advised travel by air until they are at least 24 to 48 hours past general anesthesia and able to withstand pressure changes in the cabin. A variety of factors contribute to travelers' risk of community-acquired infections; risk increases with longer stays and exposure to rural areas, for instance. Travelers who are visiting friends and family tend to be at higher risk because they're more likely to stay longer, visit remote areas and consume local food and water, and less likely to take precautions such as getting vaccinations.[21] Medical tourists' health status may make them more vulnerable than the average traveler to disease, particularly if their condition or procedure entails immunosuppression.

Many of the primary destinations for medical travel are countries where the prices for medical procedures are lower—and infectious disease rates are generally higher, due to limited resources for public health services and clean water and sanitation infrastructure. This problem could be exacerbated if, as some fear, governments' focus on medical tourism results in fewer resources or medical personnel available to treat local populations. One review found that 22 to 64 percent of people who travel to the developing world report some health problems, and that each day abroad increases the risk of illness 3 to 4 percent.[27] Two of the most common medical travel destinations, India and Thailand, are countries where infectious diseases of global concern such as TB and malaria are endemic. Asia accounted for 55 percent of all new TB cases in 2009,[28] and WHO classifies several popular medical tourism destinations as high burden countries for the disease, including Brazil, India, and Thailand.

Along with potential exposure to major diseases of historic concern, such as TB and malaria, travelers may encounter in the community any number of more pedestrian but unfamiliar pathogens. While acquisition of NDM-1 was originally linked to exposure to medical care, further research showed that the resistant agent was present in bacteria in drinking and standing water in the community.[8] In an analysis of the international spread of antimicrobial resistance, Ziad Memish and colleagues describe how travel and migration have contributed to the emergence and spread of resistant pathogens across borders.[29] They cite examples of two *Methicillin-resistant Staphylococcus aureus* (MRSA) outbreaks in Canada linked to a village in India and cases of multidrug-resistant typhoid in the United States tied to six different developing countries. The authors observe that even when they are taking prophylactic antibiotics, travelers acquire *Escherichia coli,* suggesting that they are encountering strains that are resistant to the drugs. They also note that individuals carrying the resistant bacteria do not always show symptoms and can travel home and expose others to the resistant organism before the disease is detected. A study of 247 patients in the Calgary Health Region in Canada with multidrug-resistant *E. coli* determined that 72 percent of the infections were acquired in the community rather than in a hospital setting, and that international travel was a "major risk factor" associated with developing the infection.[30(p444)]

In addition to exposure to pathogens that develop and spread in the local community, medical travelers and their companions also may be exposed to unfamiliar flora or other infections carried by fellow patients— not only in the hospital but also in hotels and resorts popular with convalescing patients. Some medical tourism facilitators funnel patients to common hotel facilities that have medical personnel on staff or other amenities for people traveling for medical care. For example, outside Seoul, Korea, the government is building Jeju "Health Care Town," a community of medical and resort facilities designed for international patients. In such environments, medical travelers may be exposed to people from other hemispheres, introducing the possibility of off-season exposure to influenza—that is, exposure before the influenza season has arrived in their area of the world and appropriate vaccines have been developed and administered.

Although we are not aware of any documented cases of patients traveling for medical procedures contracting infection at their hotels, hotels have in the past been a confirmed source of infection, most notably Legionnaires' disease and SARS. SARS moved from China to Hong Kong in 2003 after a doctor from Guangdong infected with the respiratory disease stayed at a Hong Kong hotel for only one night. At least 17 guests were infected; and they, in turn, carried the disease to Canada, Singapore, and Vietnam.[31] Legionellosis, or Legionnaires' disease, another respiratory infection spread through airborne particles, has been the source of a number of hotel-based outbreaks, beginning with the 1976 incident at an American Legion convention in Philadelphia in which some 200 people fell ill with a respiratory disease and 29 people died.[32]

FOREIGN BODIES: HEALTH CARE–ASSOCIATED INFECTIONS

While there is always some risk of encountering and acquiring infections as a result of international travel, this risk may increase when the traveler undergoes medical procedures, another established source of infection transmission. Infections are the most common complication resulting from hospital care, affecting hundreds of millions of people every year and causing extended hospital stays, avoidable illness, and death. WHO defines health care–associated (or nosocomial) infections as those that "affect patients in a hospital or other health care facility and are not present or incubating at the time of admission."[33] This definition includes infections that are acquired in the hospital but appear after the patient is discharged and infections among hospital staff. Pathogens travel via myriad transmission routes in health care facilities, including contaminated water and medical devices, such as ventilators and catheters, and contact with health care providers, who may carry the infections from one patient to the next on their hands, clothing, or medical instruments.

The most common health care–acquired infections are urinary tract infections in high-income countries and surgical site infections in low-resource settings. The financial and health tolls of these infectious are enormous. In 2002, an estimated 1.7 million patients in the United States developed health care–acquired infections, and nearly 99,000 patients died from those infections.[34] In more recent years, despite advances in infection control, health care–associated infections continue to affect roughly 1 in 20 patients hospitalized in the United States.[35] In Europe, health care–associated infections cause an estimated 37,000 deaths annually and add €7 billion (US$9.4 billion) in direct costs.[33]

Since most countries do not systematically track health care–acquired infections, the true global burden of these infections is unknown. But a WHO Patient Safety program analysis of studies on health care–acquired infections published from 1995–2010 concluded that the prevalence appears to be substantially higher in low- to middle-income countries (an estimated 10–15 of every 100 hospitalized patients at any given time) vs. high-income countries (7–8 of every 100 hospitalized patients).[36] The rates for patients in intensive care units are even more alarming—nearly a third (30 percent) in high-income countries, and as much as two to three times that in low- and middle-income countries are affected by at least one nosocomial infection. In addition to health care–acquired infections, patients face the prospect of receiving infected blood during a transfusion. According to WHO, 39 of 164 countries (nearly one-fourth) that responded to its 2008 survey on blood safety indicated that they do not follow WHO recommendations to routinely screen donated blood for HIV, hepatitis B and C, and syphilis,[37] and even those who do screen may not do so in an effective manner.

Although the rate of health care–acquired infections is generally higher in developing countries, it is not known whether this applies to the particular medical facilities in these countries that cater to patients traveling for medical care, since even when individual institutions collect data on these infections, the data are not generally publicly available. Many facilities targeting international patients may have superior infection control—some are newly constructed, with state-of-the-art ventilation and isolation technology, and some feature individual patient rooms and smaller patient-to-health provider ratios. On the other hand, in countries with high rates of endemic infectious disease, there is the possibility that health care providers who work at both public facilities serving the general population and private facilities serving international clientele may in effect serve as vectors ferrying bacteria among the hospitals where they work.

Post-Surgical Stowaways

Regardless of the relative risk of infection when a patient seeks medical care at a facility at home or abroad, case reports illustrate that patients who travel across borders can and do contract nosocomial infections and seek treatment for these infections upon returning home. In Sweden, an analysis of 444 MRSA cases linked to international travel found that more than half of those cases (55%) were health care acquired.[38] In 2004, physicians consulting the Emerging Infections Network (EIN), a listserv for infectious disease specialists, noted that 20 women who had traveled from the United States to the Dominican Republic for cosmetic surgery had developed *Mycobacterium abscessus* wound infections. The U.S. Centers for Disease Control and Prevention (CDC) and the New York City Department of Health and Mental Hygiene subsequently determined that 8 of these women had the same strain of infection and had traveled to the same clinic in Santo Domingo for surgery.[39] Investigators suggested that one source of the infection might have been the tap water that at least one patient used to cleanse her surgical wound as instructed by her doctor.

In another instance, a patient who traveled from Australia to India for knee surgery developed a *Mycobacterium fortuitum* infection that ultimately required four subsequent operations to address the resulting problems.[40] In describing the case, authors Ian Cheung and Anthony Wilson point out some of the potential challenges that arise when patients travel to distant locations for medical care. While in this case the patient's infection was detected relatively early, they note "it is not hard to imagine delayed microbiological diagnoses, given that mycobacterial infections are very uncommon in Australia, nor is it hard to imagine the potential difficulties in chasing up relevant data from an index hospital located overseas."[40(p667)] The authors also noted that the patient's physician in Australia had recommended against surgical interventions, and they questioned whether after arranging and paying for a trip for medical care in India, the patient might have become invested in pursuing surgery regardless of whether it was clinically appropriate.

As the discussion in this section underscores, regardless of where the procedure takes place, in opting for an invasive medical procedure, a patient is exposing him or herself to the possibility of contracting a health care–associated infection. But in addition to the usual risks of nosocomial infection, patients who cross borders for medical care also potentially expose themselves to infections that they would not normally encounter. This includes not only the community- and hospital-acquired infections in the destination country, but also those of other international patients seeking care at the same facilities and with the same providers. Patients converging from around the world all potentially carry with them the possibility of introducing a new or exotic pathogen into the hospital flora, which may in turn be spread in that local community or contracted and carried by other patients to other parts of the world. Detection and treatment of these infections upon patients' returns can be compromised not only when their physicians are unaware of their travels but also by a lack of communication or documentation about the treatment the patient received abroad.

Extreme Exposure: Transplants Abroad

The relatively small but significant practice of cross-border organ transplants entails particular risks and concerns in relation to disease transmission. The medical issues are further complicated by the quandaries that face clinicians who oppose the commercial or potentially coercive nature of cross-border organ transplants with respect to organ vendors and may be reluctant to treat patients when they return with complications. Chapter 7 addresses the ethical issues around traveling for transplants; the discussion in this chapter will focus on related infection risks.

Transplants have been linked with the transmission of hepatitis, HIV, malaria, Creutzfeldt-Jakob disease, rabies, and tuberculosis, among many other infections.[41] Transplant patients face enhanced infection risks in at least two respects. First, patients' immune systems are suppressed to help ensure their bodies accept the transplant, and second, they are exposed in an extreme fashion to whatever pathogens may be present in the donated organ or blood products. Risks for patients who cross borders for transplants are potentially heightened because they may require additional immunosuppression to accept an organ that is less rigorously typed for genetic matching and because they may be traveling to areas with high disease burdens for their transplant procedures. In a review of transplantation and tropical diseases, Carlos Franco-Paredes et al. note an increase in tropical infections among transplant recipients due, in part, to patients traveling to regions with a high prevalence of infectious tropical diseases for transplants.[42] They remark that these infections often go undiagnosed because most clinicians typically do not screen for tropical diseases outside of regions where they are endemic. When the infections go undiagnosed, they may spread undetected when the patient returns home and seeks follow-up care at a local hospital. One case study documents the spread of hepatitis B virus (HBV) in two hospitals outside London linked to a patient who had traveled to India for a kidney transplant.[43] The patient, an elderly man with chronic renal failure and colorectal cancer, traveled to India for the transplant in February 2001. The patient did not demonstrate hepatitis symptoms upon his return to the United Kingdom, and the infection was not discovered until more than six months later, after three members of his household developed acute HBV. A subsequent examination of blood samples taken in the course of his treatment showed that he had tested negative for hepatitis before leaving for India but tested positive after his return. Further investigation revealed that four patients at two different hospitals where the patient had been treated, along with the wife of one of the patients, had contracted identical strains of HBV. Investigators concluded that it is "highly likely" that the transplant patient contracted HBV in India, where the prevalence of the virus was estimated to be 2 to 8 percent.

Overall, the evidence on infection rates for cross-border transplants is mixed, and to date the issue has not been adequately and systematically studied. But early studies suggest that patients who travel internationally for transplants are more likely to contract infectious disease than those who have procedures in their home countries. A study comparing 36 patients from Kosovo, Macedonia, and Albania who went to Pakistan for kidney transplants with 22 patients who received transplants in Macedonia determined that 33 patients (90%) who traveled developed urinary tract infections, compared to 4 patients (18%) who were treated in Macedonia.[44] A study comparing 93 Saudi patients who traveled for transplants—primarily to Pakistan (49%) and the Philippines (28%)—with 72 who received transplants locally found that those who received transplants abroad had higher rates of hepatitis C (7.5% vs. 0%) and cytomegalovirus, (15.1% vs. 5.6%), a common virus that does not usually cause symptoms but can result in serious illness in people who are immunosuppressed. However, the study showed similarly high rates of urinary tract infections in both groups (43% and 41.7% respectively).[45] A study comparing 74 Saudi and Egyptian patients who went to China for transplants with 120 patients who received transplants in their respective home countries between January 2003 and January 2007 also found that the patients who traveled for transplants developed more infections. Four of the Chinese patients who had previously tested negative for hepatitis B developed the virus (vs. none of the patients who had the procedure at home), and seven patients who went to China developed complications due to infections (vs. one of the patients who had the procedure at home).[46] The authors noted that although the patients who stayed home fared better overall, the disparate results may have, in part, reflected the fact that the patients who went abroad included those who had been denied transplants at home based on their age or health status.

Jagbir Gill and colleagues compared outcomes of 33 patients from the United States who received transplants abroad and were subsequently seen at UCLA upon their return with 66 similar patients who had received transplants in the United States. They found that while the rate of infectious complications between the two groups was similar, roughly 50 percent, patients who received transplants outside the United States were more likely to develop serious infectious complications requiring hospitalization.[47] In a study of 10 patients who underwent kidney transplants outside the United States and received follow-up care in Minnesota, Muna Canales and colleagues determined that 4 of the 10 had developed life-threatening infections.[48] Canales et al. state that the reason for higher infection rates among patients who travel across borders for transplants has not been established, but that "Some have speculated that early overimmunosuppression of recipients (in compensation for poor matching), poor hygiene and operative practices, and inadequate education of patients regarding the risks of infection after transplantation may be culpable."[48(p1661)]

Another contributing factor could be the screening of organ donors, a particular challenge in the case of urgent transplants, such as those involving nonliving donors. Screening practices vary from one location to the next; and donors, many of whom are destitute or otherwise vulnerable people in developing countries, may have undetected health conditions or asymptomatic infections. In China, which formerly served as a major source of organs for medical travelers, many transplanted organs for foreign recipients came from executed prisoners before China took steps to stop the practice. (For details, see chapter 7.)

Experimental Exposures: Stem Cells and Animal Tissues

Assessing the risks and health outcomes of transplants abroad becomes even more complex when they involve controversial or largely unproven procedures such as certain stem cell therapies and transplants from animals. The majority of these procedures are offered without systematic protocols, primate studies, or regulation. In the case of unproven therapies, patients may undergo infection risks without any potential benefits.

Darren Lau and colleagues reviewed the stem cell offerings on the Internet in 2007 and concluded they were "overoptimistic" in light of current evidence.[49(p594)] Only about a quarter (26%) of the 19 websites reviewed by Lau et al. mentioned any risks associated with the procedures.

In response to shortages of human organs available for transplant, researchers have been exploring the potential for transplantation of tissues from other mammal species, with the pig as the leading contender for donation. This prospect raises concerns about introducing new pathogens in humans. Pigs, for instance, carry in their genetic material endogenous retrovirus known as "PERV" or Porcine Endogenous Retrovirus. In 2004 the World Health Assembly passed a resolution on xenotransplantation that urges member states to establish regulation and surveillance mechanisms and to collaborate on global strategies to prevent infections (Resolution WHA57–18 2004). As part of this effort, representatives from nations around the world gathered in Changsha, China, in November 2008 to outline requirements for clinical trials on xenotransplantation. The *Changsha Communiqué*, which summarizes the proceedings, includes recommendations that source animals be extensively tested for pathogens and warns of the potential development of new and serious infections that could spread to the wider community. Among the group's recommendations is a stipulation that "Member States should ensure that public health officials are aware of the infection risks of xenotransplantation, including those associated with patients travelling to receive xenotransplantation products outside their territories and have plans in place to timely identify and respond to any such infection."[50(p.3)]

RISK REDUCTION STRATEGIES AND ACTIVITIES

A number of systems are in place to address the emergence and global spread of infectious disease in this growing global market for health services—examples include WHO Patient Safety, global surveillance networks, and international accreditation bodies. But more work remains, particularly with respect to surveillance efforts, which are fragmented and uneven. In this section, we will examine several promising initiatives currently underway and identify opportunities for future work.

WHO Patient Safety

In 2004, WHO created the World Alliance for Patient Safety to address adverse events related to medical care such as medication errors, surgical errors, unsafe blood products, and health care–associated infections. The initiative, now known as WHO Patient Safety, provides research, training, and strategies for health care providers and patients in both high- and low-resource settings. It also runs global campaigns targeting key issues. The "Clean Care Is Safer Care" challenge, launched in 2005, includes the annual Save Lives: Clean Your Hands campaign promoting hand hygiene in health care, a relatively simple but remarkably effective strategy for reducing infections.

Disease Surveillance

As the WHO Patient Safety Report indicates, the ability to monitor for health care–acquired infections varies substantially from one country to the next. Currently, there is no reliable, publicly available information on the rates of nosocomial infections in many regions of the world, much less at specific hospitals that medical travelers might consider. A WHO Global Patient Safety Challenge survey found that only 23 of 147 (15.6%) developing countries surveyed in 2010 had working national surveillance systems of health care–acquired infections.[36] Only a few regions, such as the United States and the European Union, compel individual facilities to collect and report the incidence of infection, and even fewer require that information to be publicly reported. This confidentiality is intended to encourage facilities to track, report, and learn from these incidents without fear of being stigmatized. Consequently, even when these data are collected, they generally are not comparable across facilities; regions; and especially, borders. Ideally a global network of data on hospital infections would be available to track the movement of infections across health care facilities and borders. The Argentina-based International Nosocomial Infection Control Consortium has, in fact, initiated a system to track and aggregate such data using standard definitions and methodologies. This network, modeled on the National Nosocomial Infections Surveillance system of the U.S. CDC, is voluntary. To date, more than 140 health care facilities in 36 countries have submitted data. Since the hospitals are not publicly identified, it is not possible to determine whether they include hospitals frequented by medical tourists. Nonetheless, this is a significant source of aggregated data that is likely to become increasingly robust and useful for health care providers and their patients as they contemplate medical travel.

As we have discussed, to fully assess and reduce the risk of the spread of infections resulting from patients traveling across borders, it is important to consider not just health care–acquired infections but also the prevalence and emergence of infectious diseases in the community at large in both the originating and destination countries. A growing number of international networks are in place to track and disseminate this information, from WHO's Global Outbreak Alert and Response Network (GOARN) to GeoSentinel, a network of travel and tropical medicine clinics located across six continents, to automated event-based reporting systems such as

HealthMap. Emily Chan et al. analyzed 398 disease outbreaks from 1996 to 2009 and found that in general, outbreaks are being detected and publicly reported more quickly, although the degree of improvement varied by region.[51] The median time between the start and detection of outbreaks decreased from 29.5 days in 1996 to 13.5 days in 2009, and the median time between when outbreaks are discovered and publicly reported decreased from 40 days in 1996 to 19 days in 2009. But while the growing array of surveillance tools show promise for detecting and curbing the global spread of infectious disease, they ultimately do not capture the full spectrum of risks for medical travelers. GOARN, for instance, focuses on reporting "outbreaks of international importance," such as influenza epidemics, and is not geared to capture incidents such as a single patient returning with a multidrug-resistant pathogen. GeoSentinel, a global network of travel/tropical medicine clinics, may detect some of these smaller incidents and provide a general sense of infections in different regions, but its scope is limited to the patients who present to reporting clinics and laboratories. HealthMap, which mines and aggregates thousands of reports of disease outbreaks from official and unofficial sources, from eyewitness and media reports to government notices, provides a dynamic graphic depiction of outbreaks around the globe. But much of HealthMap's reports come from news media,[52] and as such are only as timely and accurate as media accounts upon which they are based.

On a global basis, screening and diagnostic capacities remain inconsistent, especially in lower income areas where the scant resources are more likely to go toward treating patients than monitoring disease. WHO's Global Alert and Response program and others are working to equip low-resource nations with the technical resources and expertise they need to monitor disease. Regional efforts such as the European Centre for Disease Prevention and Control's European Antimicrobial Resistance Surveillance Network (EARS-Net) are making progress toward establishing common diagnostic and reporting standards to enable cross-border analyses of disease trends and outbreaks. But even the most sophisticated techniques are unlikely to detect early cases of recently imported or evolving strains of multidrug-resistant agents that medical travelers may acquire and spread, such as NDM-1. In the end, as growing numbers of patients traverse the globe for care, it is not clear who can or should be responsible for identifying and tracking individual patients' disease exposures in the course of their health care journeys.

Beyond the technical challenges that surveillance poses, there are political and economic factors to consider. The national governments that are responsible for collecting and sharing disease data with a global network are the same governments that have invested significant resources in promoting their medical tourism industries and who therefore may be reluctant to report adverse events that would discourage medical tourists

from visiting their countries. During the 2003 SARS outbreak, official restrictions and travelers' fears led to a 50–70 percent decrease in travel to
the affected regions in the months following the outbreak.[53] In 1994, India
declared a plague outbreak in the city of Surat based on the appearance
of clusters of patients admitted to several area hospitals with pneumonia-
like symptoms. Ultimately it was determined that there was no evidence
of person-to-person transmission, and the outbreak was limited to poor
people living in certain areas. But despite the relatively minor scope of
the outbreak and the fact that WHO requested other nations to refrain
from travel or trade restrictions, international panic led to both, and the
precipitous drops in trade and travel contributed to more than $2 billion in
losses to the Indian economy.[54] So in considering what rises to the level of
a reportable event, hospitals and health ministries may factor in potential
economic repercussions along with health concerns. Theoretically, that is
where safeguards such as accreditation and regulation have potential to
play a meaningful role.

Accreditation and Regulation

Many of the major hospitals targeting international patients are accredited by international quality organizations that require protocols to
promote infection reduction and control, such as the Joint Commission
International (JCI) based in the United States, and Quality Healthcare Advice Trent Accreditation, based in the United Kingdom. JCI standards, for
instance, require tracking, monitoring, and reporting infectious diseases
to public health agencies. But while accreditation requires that these infection control measures are in place, it does not necessarily ensure that they
are consistently employed. So although accreditation may help encourage
and implement infection control, it is by no means a guarantee. Chapter 11
explores this and other aspects of accreditation in greater depth.

In addition to accreditation, another potential safeguard is the International Health Regulations (IHR). The second edition of the IHR, which
took effect in 2007, requires countries to develop the capacity to conduct
surveillance for and report to WHO a "public health emergency of international concern," or in other words, an event "that may cause international disease spread." If WHO determines such a threat exists, it may
issue recommendations to curb the spread of disease, such as quaran-
tine or travel restrictions for affected or potentially affected individuals.
These regulations provide more comprehensive protection than the previous version of the IHR in effect since 1981, which pertained to only three
diseases—yellow fever, plague, and cholera. If member countries, in fact,
achieve the core capacities, this could certainly reduce the risk of community infection acquisition during "spa" time. But the regulations, which
apply only in the event of an outbreak of major consequence, are unlikely

to come into play as individual patients crisscross borders for medical care carrying exotic pathogens, sometimes without symptoms. In an interview with the WHO Bulletin on the rise of drug-resistant pathogens, University of Calgary microbiologist John Conly suggested that the emergence of an agent like NDM-1 does constitute a public health event of international concern under the IHR.[55] But a study of what public health experts deemed "notifiable events" under the IHR found that most experts did not consider a cluster of cases of a new strain *Klebsiella pneumoniae* resistant to all currently available antimicrobials to require reporting under the IHR.[56] Another challenge is enforcement. As a summary of a 2006 Institute of Medicine workshop on global disease surveillance put it, "Countries do not share surveillance data without government approval, participants observed, and the IHRs do not presently impose sufficient consequences to overcome economic barriers to reporting disease."[57(p26)] Those consequences typically amount to the threat of being named as an offender in a WHO bulletin.

CONCLUSION

At present, the evidence that patients seeking medical care abroad may amplify the transnational spread of infections is primarily limited to case reports and small-scale retrospective studies. Patients' travel patterns are not systematically tracked on a global—or even national or regional—level. And absent definitive data about who is going where for what health procedures, it is difficult to determine what proportion return with infections or other complications. More systematic research will help reveal the nature and the extent of the risks and inform approaches to reduce those risks. Meanwhile, given the documented evidence of the spread of infection that results from both travel and from medical care, along with recent examples such as the emergence in spread of NDM-1 and extensively drug-resistant TB, it's reasonable to infer that a mix of the two will lead to elevated risks. The churn of patients and their companions cycling in and out of international medical facilities and back to their home communities establishes a potentially highly efficient pathogenic breeding and distribution system. In light of growing concerns about the spread of antimicrobial-resistant agents, it's imperative to consider and mitigate this risk.

The classic public health approach calls for addressing the risk on three levels: prevention, detection, and control. Prevention entails everything from establishing safe practices such as hand washing in medical facilities; to curbing the inappropriate use of antibiotics; to bolstering water, sanitation, and public health infrastructures. Detection includes establishing systems to identify new multidrug-resistant agents in early stages of emergence. This challenge, which often taxes even the best-resourced facilities, regions, and nations, becomes even more complex when it involves the rapid cross-border circulation of medical tourists. Organizational, regional, and national surveillance systems scan for different types of agents and resistance patterns depending upon a variety of factors, including previously identified pathogens, commonly used antimicrobials, and laboratory protocols and capacities. If a patient acquires a particular type of resistant agent in one region where that agent may be more common and therefore subject to surveillance but does not experience symptoms until returning home, where that agent has never been detected, chances are that it will take longer to detect and address, allowing more opportunity for spread. The final step, control, involves steps such as isolating infected patients and their companions; or at the extreme, temporarily halting travel to and from a particular region altogether. Consequently, public reporting of disease outbreaks is fraught with political and economic considerations.

All of the parties involved in medical tourism—patients, facilitators, medical care providers, ministries of health and tourism—have a role to play in curbing the emergence and spread of disease. Patients who undertake international travel for medical procedures need to be educated and invested with the responsibility to take precautions to avoid adverse events, including receiving the proper vaccinations before going abroad, attending to the cleanliness of the food and water they ingest and use to cleanse their wounds, conducting due diligence regarding the care providers and procedures they select, watching for and insisting upon hand hygiene, and refraining from unsafe or exploitive transplant procedures. But patients' ability to make informed decisions is limited by the availability and reliability of information about care providers and procedures, which may in turn be influenced by the commercial interests of the facilitators, care providers, and even national ministries that provide this type of information.

Similarly, patients can serve as a critical communication link between their physicians at home and abroad to help raise awareness of potential infections or complications—if they receive the necessary documentation and support. A survey of practices in cardiology departments at 315 hospitals in the Czech Republic, France, Poland, and Spain that treat cross-border patients found that the hospital doctors "rarely" made contact with the patients' primary care doctors in their country of residence. They also found that while oral discharge instructions usually were available for foreign patients, written instructions were available in the patients' language less than half the time (41.7%).[58] In any case, persuading patients to assume these responsibilities can be difficult, since they sometimes opt for medical care abroad against the recommendations of their local physicians and may be reluctant to divulge that they have done so. Physicians can help by routinely asking questions about treatment or travels abroad when a patient presents with infection and by respecting patients' right to make their own health care decisions based on their own needs and priorities. The European Union Directive on the Application of Patients' Rights in Cross Border Health Care, which outlines patients' rights when they seek health care in other EU member countries, provides an excellent template for establishing the supports necessary to enable patients to engage safely in cross-border care. Among other things, the Directive adopted in 2011 includes provisions for national contact points for information on quality and safety.

While the individuals and organizations involved in medical tourism all have roles to play in reducing the risk of the emergence and cross-border spread of disease, a global health care market ultimately requires a global infrastructure to address the accompanying risks. This infrastructure requires internationally compatible electronic health records systems and more effective global means for tracking antimicrobial resistance and nosocomial pathogens. The current fragmented systems do not allow the correlation of transnational traffic for medical services with the migration of resistant agents. As Hajo Grundmann, project leader of the European Antimicrobial Resistance Surveillance System (EARS-Net), noted in an editorial, while developing a coherent international tracking system is a huge and complex undertaking, the national and regional tracking systems currently in place provide a sturdy foundation to build such a database.[59]

The current international initiatives and agreements such as WHO Patient Safety and the International Health Regulations also have the potential to advance and support some of these efforts. But these agreements remain largely confined to public sector partners, while many of the major players in medical tourism are private entities. The private sector interests operating in high-volume provider countries also will need to be engaged, either through global bodies such as WHO or the World Trade Organization or in collaboration with a public/private partner such as JCI. Engaging private entities may be a difficult proposition in light of the current market structure, in which international medical centers may have little or no legal or financial responsibility when adverse events occur after patients have returned home. Nonetheless, recent history provides examples of trade-related health concerns serving as the impetus for engaging private partners. The profound economic toll from the SARS outbreak—estimated at a $30 billion impact on China's economy alone—spurred transnational trade communities such as the Asia-Pacific Economic Cooperation (APEC) forum and the Association of Southeast Asian Nations (ASEAN) to redouble their efforts toward more rapid, accurate, and networked surveillance systems. The European Union's treaty-based legal structure has enabled the creation of one of the most integrated regional surveillance systems to date, Eurosurveillance, which focuses on Legionnaires' disease, enteric diseases, and antimicrobial resistance (EARS-Net).

These initiatives provide promising evidence of what can result when the links between global health and trade are made explicit. In the future, this kind of cross-sector collaboration will be essential in understanding and addressing the risks of medical travel and the international spread of disease. Because as the number of patients crossing borders for care increases, no single entity, public or private, will be capable of effectively addressing the potential emergence and global spread of drug-resistant agents on its own. Global cooperation at an unprecedented scale for prevention, detection, and control will clearly be required to better protect and promote population safety.

ACKNOWLEDGMENT

This chapter includes research conducted for the World Health Organization Workshop on the movement of patients across international borders.

REFERENCES

1. Yong D, Toleman MA, Giske CG, Cho HS, Sundman K, Lee K, Walsh TR. Characterization of a new metallo-beta-lactamase gene, bla(NDM-1), and a novel erythromycin esterase gene carried on a unique genetic structure in Klebsiella pneumoniae sequence type 14 from India. *Antimicrob Agents Chemother.* 2009;53(12):5046–5054.

2. Kumarasamy KK, Toleman MA, Walsh TR, et al. Emergence of a new antibiotic resistance mechanism in India, Pakistan, and the UK: A molecular, biological, and epidemiological study. *Lancet Infect Dis.* 2010;10(9):597–602.

3. Lakhani N. NHS "could save millions" by flying patients to India—experts urge Department of Health to consider using hospitals outside Europe. *The Independent.* January 17, 2010.

4. Pitout JDD. The latest threat in the war on antimicrobial resistance. *Lancet Infect Dis.* 2010;10(9):578–579.

5. Srivastava RK, Ichhpujani RI, Khare S, Rai A, Chauhan LS. Superbug—the so-called NDM-1. *Indian J. Med. Res.* 2011;133(5):458–460.

6. Kant S, Haldar P. Is NDM-1 actually being imported to UK from India? *Indian J Public Health.* 2010;54(3):151–154.

7. Guo Y, Wang J, Niu G, et al. A structural view of the antibiotic degradation enzyme NDM-1 from a superbug. *Protein Cell.* 2011;2(5):384–394.

8. Walsh TR, Weeks J, Livermore DM, Toleman MA. Dissemination of NDM-1 positive bacteria in the New Delhi environment and its implications for human health: An environmental point prevalence study. *Lancet Infect Dis.* 2011;11(5):355–362.

9. Phua CK, Chee CBE, Chua APG, et al. Managing a case of extensively drug-resistant (XDR) pulmonary tuberculosis in Singapore. *Ann. Acad. Med. Singap.* 2011;40(3):132–135.

10. Singapore Ministry of Health. Impact of MDRTB cases among medical tourists in Singapore. Asia-Pacific Economic Cooperation EINet Presentation, Trade and Travel Impacts of Infectious Diseases, November 10, 2011.

11. Morgan DJ, Okeke IN, Laxminarayan R, Perencevich EN, Weisenberg S. Non-prescription antimicrobial use worldwide: A systematic review. *Lancet Infect Dis.* 2011;11(9):692–701.

12. Rogers BA, Aminzadeh Z, Hayashi Y, Paterson DL. Country-to-country transfer of patients and the risk of multi-resistant bacterial infection. *Clin. Infect. Dis.* 2011;53(1):49–56.

13. Jean S-S, Hsueh P-R. High burden of antimicrobial resistance in Asia. *Int. J. Antimicrob. Agents.* 2011;37(4):291–295.

14. Peiris JSM, Guan Y, Yuen KY. Severe acute respiratory syndrome. *Nat. Med.* 2004;10(12 Suppl):S88–97.

15. World Health Organization. Summary of probable SARS cases with onset of illness from November 1, 2002, to July 31, 2003. World Health Organization. http://www.who.int/csr/sars/country/table2004_04_21/en/index.html. Published 2004. Accessed July 17, 2011.

16. Cui F, Luo H, Zhou L, et al. Transmission of pandemic influenza A (H1N1) virus in a train in China. *J Epidemiol.* 2011;21(4):271–277.

17. World Health Organization. Pandemic (H1N1) 2009—update 112. World Health Organization. http://www.who.int/csr/don/2010_08_06/en/index.html. Published 2010. Accessed July 17, 2011.

18. Brownstein JS, Wolfe CJ, Mandl KD. Empirical evidence for the effect of airline travel on inter-regional influenza spread in the United States. *PLoS Med.* 2006;3(10):e401.

19. Khan K, Arino J, Hu W, et al. Spread of a novel influenza A (H1N1) virus via global airline transportation. *N. Engl. J. Med.* 2009;361(2):212–214.

20. Torresi J, Leder K. Defining infections in international travellers through the GeoSentinel surveillance network. *Nat. Rev. Microbiol.* 2009;7(12):895–901.

21. World Health Organization. *International travel and health 2011 edition.* World Health Organization; 2011. http://www.who.int/ith/en/. Accessed July 17, 2011.

22. Mangili A, Gendreau MA. Transmission of infectious diseases during commercial air travel. *Lancet.* 2005;365(9463):989–996.

23. Moser MR, Bender TR, Margolis HS, et al. An outbreak of influenza aboard a commercial airliner. *Am. J. Epidemiol.* 1979;110(1):1–6.

24. Olsen SJ, Chang H-L, Cheung TY-Y, et al. Transmission of the severe acute respiratory syndrome on aircraft. *N. Engl. J. Med.* 2003;349(25):2416–2422.

25. World Health Organization. Tuberculosis and Air Travel—Guidelines for Prevention and Control. World Health Organization. www.who.int/tb/publications/2008/WHO_HTM_TB_2008.399_eng.pdf. Published 2008. Accessed July 17, 2011.

26. Gerberding J. Recent Case of Extensively Drug Resistant TB: CDC's Public Health Response. Testimony before the Committee on Appropriations Subcommittee on Labor-HHS-Education, United States Senate. Wednesday June 6, 2007.

27. House HR, Ehlers JP. Travel-related infections. *Emerg. Med. Clin. North Am.* 2008;26(2):499–516, x.

28. World Health Organization. Global Tuberculosis Control 2010. World Health Organization. http://www.who.int/tb/publications/global_report/2010/en/index.html. Published 2010. Accessed July 18, 2011.

29. Memish ZA, Venkatesh S, Shibl AM. Impact of travel on international spread of antimicrobial resistance. *Int. J. Antimicrob. Agents.* 2003;21(2):135–142.

30. Laupland KB, Church DL, Vidakovich J, Mucenski M, Pitout JDD. Community-onset extended-spectrum beta-lactamase (ESBL) producing Escherichia coli: Importance of international travel. *J. Infect.* 2008;57(6):441–448.

31. Zhong N-S, Wong GWK. Epidemiology of severe acute respiratory syndrome (SARS): Adults and children. *Paediatr Respir Rev.* 2004;5(4):270–274.

32. Fraser DW, Tsai TR, Orenstein W, et al. Legionnaires' disease: Description of an epidemic of pneumonia. *N. Engl. J. Med.* 1977;297(22):1189–1197.

33. World Health Organization. WHO Health Care–Associated Infections Fact Sheet. World Health Organization. www.who.int/gpsc/country_work/gpsc_ccisc_fact_sheet_en.pdf. Published 2011. Accessed July 18, 2011.

34. Klevens RM, Edwards JR, Richards CL Jr, et al. Estimating health care–associated infections and deaths in U.S. hospitals, 2002. *Public Health Rep.* 2007;122(2):160–166.

35. Centers for Disease Control and Prevention. Healthcare–associated Infections (HAIs): The Burden. Centers for Disease Control and Prevention. http://www.cdc.gov/HAI/burden.html. Published December 13, 2010. Accessed September 8, 2011.

36. World Health Organization. Report on the Burden of Healthcare–Associated Infection Worldwide. World Health Organization. www.who.int/gpsc/country_work/summary_20100430_en.pdf. Published 2011. Accessed September 8, 2011.

37. World Health Organization. Blood Safety Fact Sheet. 2011. http://www.who.int/topics/blood_safety/en/. World Health Organization. Published 2011. Accessed July 13, 2011.

38. Stenhem M, Ortqvist A, Ringberg H, et al. Imported methicillin-resistant Staphylococcus aureus, Sweden. *Emerging Infect. Dis.* 2010;16(2):189–196.

39. Furuya EY, Paez A, Srinivasan A, et al. Outbreak of Mycobacterium abscessus wound infections among "lipotourists" from the United States who underwent abdominoplasty in the Dominican Republic. *Clin. Infect. Dis.* 2008;46(8):1181–1188.

40. Cheung IK, Wilson A. Arthroplasty tourism. *Med. J. Aust.* 2007;187(11–12):666–667.

41. Martín-Dávila P, Fortún J, López-Vélez R, et al. Transmission of tropical and geographically restricted infections during solid-organ transplantation. *Clin. Microbiol. Rev.* 2008;21(1):60–96.

42. Franco-Paredes C, Jacob JT, Hidron A, et al. Transplantation and tropical infectious diseases. *Int. J. Infect. Dis.* 2010;14(3):e189–196.

43. Harling R, Turbitt D, Millar M, et al. Passage from India: An outbreak of hepatitis B linked to a patient who acquired infection from health care overseas. *Public Health.* 2007;121(10):734–741.

44. Ivanovski N, Masin J, Rambabova-Busljetic I, et al. The outcome of commercial kidney transplant tourism in Pakistan. *Clin Transplant.* 2011;25(1):171–173.

45. Alghamdi SA, Nabi ZG, Alkhafaji DM, et al. Transplant tourism outcome: a single center experience. *Transplantation.* 2010;90(2):184–188.

46. Allam N, Al Saghier M, El Sheikh Y, et al. Clinical outcomes for Saudi and Egyptian patients receiving deceased donor liver transplantation in China. *Am. J. Transplant.* 2010;10(8):1834–1841.

47. Gill J, Madhira BR, Gjertson D, et al. Transplant tourism in the United States: A single-center experience. *Clin J Am Soc Nephrol.* 2008;3(6):1820–1828.

48. Canales MT, Kasiske BL, Rosenberg ME. Transplant tourism: Outcomes of United States residents who undergo kidney transplantation overseas. *Transplantation.* 2006;82(12):1658–1661.

49. Lau D, Ogbogu U, Taylor B, et al. Stem cell clinics online: The direct-to-consumer portrayal of stem cell medicine. *Cell Stem Cell.* 2008;3(6):591–594.

50. World Health Organization. The Changsha Communiqué: First WHO Global Consultation on Regulatory Requirements for First Xenotransplantation Clinical Trials. World Health Organization. http://www.who.int/entity/transplantation/xeno/ChangshaCommunique.pdf. Published 2008. Accessed September 8, 2011.

51. Chan EH, Brewer TF, Madoff LC, et al. Global capacity for emerging infectious disease detection. *Proc. Natl. Acad. Sci. U.S.A.* 2010;107(50):21701–21706.

52. Keller M, Blench M, Tolentino H, et al. Use of unstructured event-based reports for global infectious disease surveillance. *Emerging Infect. Dis.* 2009;15(5):689–695.

53. World Health Organization. The World Health Report 2003—Shaping the Future. World Health Organization. http://www.who.int/whr/2003/en/index.html. Published 2003. Accessed August 24, 2011.

54. Cash RA, Narasimhan V. Impediments to global surveillance of infectious diseases: Consequences of open reporting in a global economy. *Bull. World Health Organ.* 2000;78(11):1358–1367.

55. Conly J. Antimicrobial resistance: Revisiting the "tragedy of the commons." *Bull. World Health Organ.* 2010;88(11):805–806.

56. Haustein T, Hollmeyer H, Hardiman M, Harbarth S, Pittet D. Should this event be notified to the World Health Organization? Reliability of the international health regulations notification assessment process. *Bull. World Health Organ.* 2011;89(4):296–303.

57. Lemon SM. *Global infectious disease surveillance and detection: Assessing the challenges—finding solutions: Workshop summary.* Washington, DC: National Academies Press, 2007.

58. Groene O, Suñol R. Factors associated with the implementation of quality and safety requirements for cross-border care in acute myocardial infarction: Results from 315 hospitals in four countries. *Health Policy.* 2010;98(2–3):107–113.

59. Grundmann H, Livermore DM, Giske CG, et al. Carbapenem-non-susceptible Enterobacteriaceae in Europe: Conclusions from a meeting of national experts. *Euro Surveill.* 2010;15(46). http://www.ncbi.nlm.nih.gov/pubmed/21144429. Accessed July 12, 2011.

Chapter 7

Perilous Voyages: Travel Abroad for Organ Transplants and Stem Cell Treatments

Dominique Martin

A recent Bloomberg report on the international human organ market tells a story that has become sadly familiar over the last few decades.[1] An older American man, suffering from kidney failure and desperate to receive an organ transplant, traveled abroad to Nicaragua, a country where his wealth, as a retired bus supervisor, seemed unfathomable to a poorly educated 23-year-old man working as a construction laborer. The two men met through the boy's employers, who happened to be the American's local relatives by marriage, and they agreed to a deal that appeared to offer great benefits for them both. The sick but wealthy older tourist would purchase a life-saving organ from the healthy young man, who would in return receive the promise of a better future—"a job and an apartment in New York." After meeting with local transplant professionals and passing dubious screening procedures in which statements of voluntariness and altruistic motivations were signed and approved, both men underwent surgery. Within months, both men were dead. The Nicaraguan man died from operative complications, and the American organ recipient died from acute graft rejection.

Almost as alarming as such tales of "transplant tourism" are accounts of "stem cell tourism," in which equally desperate patients suffering from a range of chronic, debilitating, or life-threatening diseases seek access to unproven therapies using a variety of stem cells in foreign countries. Stem cells "have both the capacity to self-renew (make more stem cells by cell division) as well as to differentiate into mature, specialized cells."[2] The therapeutic potential of these abilities has been widely publicized, fostering the idea that if these cells can be inserted into the human body, they will seek out damaged or defective cells or organs and repair or replace faulty tissue with healthy, functional new cells. This simplistic conception of therapeutic stem cell science is often employed by providers of stem cell-based treatments to justify their claims. However, with the exception of haematopoietic stem cells used in the treatment of hematological disorders, therapeutic use of stem cells remains highly experimental, and scientists anticipate it may take more than a decade for therapeutic products to be developed.[3] Nevertheless, patients travel to China, India, Russia, and elsewhere to clinics where treatments have been described by some international health experts as "unethical and potentially dangerous."[4(p967)] Many patients raise thousands of dollars by mortgaging homes and organizing charitable drives to fund these journeys. Evidence of patient benefits from these unproven therapies remains largely anecdotal, while reports of infection,[5] tumor development,[4] and death[6] have prompted groups such as the International Society for Stem Cell Research (ISSCR)[7] and the European Medicines Agency[8] to issue public warnings about unproven stem cell treatments. National ministries of health have also stepped in to close some of the centers offering such treatments, citing violations of laws prohibiting the sale of unproven treatments or unlicensed use of stem cells in humans.[6,9–10]

Travel for commercial organ transplantation and travel for unproven stem cell treatments are both niche markets within the vast global cross-border health care industry. Human organ transplantation has been well recognized for a number of decades as a highly effective treatment for many patients with end stage organ failure, whereas the stem cell therapies offered in the cross-border market for a range of diseases remain largely unproven and represent a relatively recent phenomenon. Despite this fundamental difference between the two forms of travel, they share many important features. Both markets are driven by the desperation of patients suffering debilitating chronic and life-threatening diseases for which curative treatments are scarce or nonexistent in domestic health care systems as a result of organ shortages or the current limitations of medical science. The transplantation of organs or stem cells abroad offers these patients hope of improvement in their clinical condition, if not a cure, for which they are willing to pay substantial amounts—up to $180,000 for a liver transplant[11] or more than $47,000 on average for stem cell treatments,[12] in addition to travel costs. The industries are thus highly lucrative for the health care professionals involved, as well as for organ brokers, hospitals, clinics, and other associates. Both markets require the procurement of human biological materials from deceased or living organ providers,[13] from the patient herself in the case of autologous stem cell use, or from fetal tissue or biological materials obtained from living adults. In some cases, stem cells are even obtained from animals. Evidence suggests that recipients of organ or stem cell transplants abroad are at risk of serious complications and even death. And both industries have been linked to criminal activities in the form of organ theft, organized crime,[14] and fraud.[15]

Concerns about these practices have motivated national and international efforts to develop guidelines and legislation and enforce regulations governing organ and stem cell transplantation activities. In 2008, for example, the World Health Organization (WHO) produced updated Guiding Principles on Cell, Tissue and Organ Transplantation,[16] and an international gathering of experts developed the Declaration of Istanbul on Organ Trafficking and Transplant Tourism.[17] The same year, the ISSCR published Guidelines for the Clinical Translation of Stem Cells.[18] Despite these efforts, which have sought to minimize the trade and encourage more restrictive regulations, ongoing travel for these procedures has prompted calls by transplant professionals and ethicists to consider the introduction of domestic organ markets[19] and encouraged patients to lobby for more experimental stem cell trials within domestic settings.[20]

This chapter provides an overview of international travel for transplantation of organs and stem cells, exploring in particular the pursuit of commercial organ transplantation and unproven stem cell treatments. After reviewing and defining the terms used to describe these practices, I examine each market before outlining the potential benefits and concerns associated with each activity. Finally, I review current international efforts to guide and regulate travel for transplantation.

FORGET ABOUT "TOURISM": DEFINING THE SERIOUS BUSINESS OF TRAVEL FOR TRANSPLANTATION

Although some domains of international travel for health care remain closely associated with the traditional tourism industry, the term "medical travel" is increasingly being used in lieu of the popular term "medical tourism," particularly when discussing practices such as travel for transplants and stem cell procedures. The term "tourism" may inadvertently bias readers against travel for transplantation, or conversely trivialize activities that are of exceptional importance to participants in the field.[21] For the purpose of this discussion, international travel for organ transplantation is best defined as voluntary travel outside one's domestic health care jurisdiction for the purpose of accessing organ transplantation. Similarly, "stem cell travel" may be broadly defined as travel by a patient outside his or her own health care jurisdiction for the purpose of accessing a therapeutic intervention involving the transplantation of stem cells.

There are numerous varieties of travel for organ or stem cell transplantation. However, most accounts of "transplant tourism" and "stem cell tourism" refer to particular kinds of travel for transplantation. These consist of practices that are widely regarded as problematic or controversial and which are the target of policy debate and regulatory measures. In particular, they refer to travel for organ transplantation that involves trade in organs, and travel for stem cell treatments that are unproven. These categories of transplant travel will be the focus of examination in this chapter.

Although various kinds of travel for organ transplantation may require the patient to pay for some, if not all, of the costs of transplantation services, commodification of the transplanted organ occurs when it acquires "an overt or covert monetary price"[22(p959)] through profitable transfer between individuals. In these cases, organ providers may be paid, and brokers or professionals involved in the removal, transfer, or transplantation of organs may charge for supplying the organ over and above the routine fees for the provision of transplantation services. As well as meeting these charges, organ recipients may also pay to secure an organ ahead of other patients. All such instances constitute commodification of the organ and are examples of transplant commercialism, which the Declaration of Istanbul defines as "a policy or practice in which an organ is treated as a commodity, including by being bought or sold or used for material gain."[17(p855)] Travel for commercial organ transplantation thus refers to organ transplant travel in which the transplanted organ is effectively commodified.

The types of stem cell therapies associated with stem cell tourism are characterized by the fact that most, if not all, are considered of "unproven" benefit to patients. Stem cell therapies described as unproven usually

- lack independent scientific evidence of their efficacy and offer no means for independent researchers to examine this;
- rely on anecdotal reports or "testimonials" by patients as "proof"; and
- are underpinned by the implausible theory that the stem cells in question—regardless of their origin—will migrate to the diseased area—regardless of the mechanism and site of cell transplantation—and repair, renew, or replace the diseased tissue—regardless of the nature of the disease.

In this discussion, travel for unproven stem cell treatments is defined as travel for the purpose of accessing therapeutic interventions involving the transplantation of stem cells for which there is no credible independent evidence available to support the claim that the intervention is beneficial in the treatment of a particular disease, and/or the treatment is not offered in the context of a formal clinical trial that conforms to minimum ethical and scientific standards of research. Although defining minimum standards for research can be problematic, Cynthia Cohen and Peter Cohen offer a plausible account in their review of travel for stem cell treatment in Russia and India. They note that many stem cell treatments offered to travelers in these countries

> lack transparency, follow no publicly available protocol, and have not undergone peer review and publication, thereby failing to provide data sufficient to allow other investigators to attempt to replicate their claimed benefits and safety. Moreover, few of those conducting them seek informed consent from persons who will undergo these putative treatments. Consequently, they do not constitute legitimate clinical research aimed at providing safe and efficacious stem cell interventions to a broad range of patients. They are unproven.[23(p39)]

OVERVIEW OF TRAVEL FOR COMMERCIAL ORGAN TRANSPLANTATION

The first reports of patients traveling abroad to purchase organ transplants date from the beginning of the 1980s, when the advent of the immunosuppressant drug cyclosporine enabled more people to receive transplants from unrelated providers. This development facilitated transplantation in general and contributed in particular to the increased use of living unrelated providers. In 1983, a deregistered Virginian doctor, H. Barry Jacobs, proposed brokering of organ sales between poor immigrants and wealthy Americans in need of kidney transplants. In 1985, a Pulitzer Prize winning investigation by Andrew Schneider and Mary Pat Flaherty[24] revealed widespread commercialism within the American transplantation system, including the export of as many as 300 organs annually to foreign countries, and the allocation of deceased donor organs to foreign patients over local patients in return for higher fees. The investigation also revealed evidence of patients traveling from a variety of countries to hospitals in Britain, India, Japan, and elsewhere for transplants, sometimes purchasing an organ on site; and sometimes traveling with a paid, unrelated organ provider. Both this exposé and Jacobs's proposal were influential in the development and evolution of legislation governing organ transplantation in the United States.[25] As awareness of organ markets spread, numerous countries enacted legislation prohibiting payment for organs. Markets have persisted, however, in a variety of locations, even those in which organ trading has been legally prohibited. India, for example, prohibited organ markets in 1994, but trade continues to flourish in some Indian regions. Persistence of this practice prompted the recent approval of an amendment to the law, which includes more stringent penalties for those involved in the organ trade.[26] Most organ markets, with the exception of legal markets in Iran and Saudi Arabia, have remained open to foreign patients, although some countries such as China have sought to at least prioritize access to transplantation services for domestic patients.[27]

In the 1990s, anthropologists and medical professionals began reporting on travel for commercial organ transplantation in South America, South Africa, and the Indian subcontinent. Nancy Scheper-Hughes, one of the founders of Organs Watch, has played a key role in publicizing the international organ market since the late 1990s, revealing trade in Brazil, Turkey, Eastern Europe, South Africa, and the Philippines.[28-29] In particular, she has revealed the globalized nature of travel for organ transplantation, with interconnected networks of organ brokers and transplant surgeons in various countries. She describes, for example, regular "transplant junkets" for Israeli patients who traveled with Israeli surgeons to third party countries such as Turkey and South Africa to procure kidneys from vendors from Brazil and Moldova.[29] Other researchers report hundreds of transplant travelers from Saudi Arabia, Taiwan, and various countries throughout the world.[30-32]

As Table 7.1 demonstrates, there are numerous variations on travel for organ transplantation. Some patients may travel abroad with an altruistic living donor to access transplantation services that are unavailable in their own country (Category 1A). The Tanzanian government, for example, sends living related donor-recipient pairs to India to undergo organ procurement and transplantation, due to a lack of surgical expertise in Tanzania.[33] Other patients benefit from humanitarian programs that offer a small number of deceased donor organs to foreign patients (Category 3), such as the now defunct Australian program that provided cadaveric liver transplants to Japanese children in the late 1980s.[34] However, most types of transplant travel involve payment to organ providers or financially motivated allocation of deceased donor organs. Precise numbers of commercial transplant travelers throughout the world remain unknown, although the WHO estimates up to 10 percent of global transplants—as many as 10,000 organs—involve patients who have traveled abroad and purchased an organ.[30] At its peak, it was reported that possibly half of China's organ transplants obtained from executed prisoners were sold to foreign patients,[30] potentially representing more than 5,000 cases a year.[32] With the exception of the Chinese market, which was curtailed following the 2007 law against transplant tourism,[32] most transplant travelers acquire organs such as kidneys and partial livers from living vendors (Category 2) in countries like Pakistan, India, the Philippines, and Colombia.[30,32,35-36]

The Current Market

The most popular destinations for transplant travelers have shifted with the evolution of legislation and the enforcement of regulations that render access to local markets more or less difficult for foreign patients. For example, at its peak, the kidney trade in Pakistan earned it a reputation

Table 7.1
Types of international travel for organ transplantation

Type	Description	Subtypes	Examples
I	Transplantation and unpaid living related donation abroad.[1]	A. Due to lack or cost of health care services in the country of origin[1], patients may undergo transplant abroad, *bringing with them* their unpaid, related living organ donor. B. A patient may travel abroad to undergo transplantation in the country of origin of their unpaid LRD due to barriers preventing the donor traveling and/or undergoing organ procurement in the recipient's country.	Tanzania sends recipient-donor pairs to India for transplantation.
2*	Transplantation and purchase of an organ from a living vendor abroad.	A. A patient travels abroad for transplantation, *bringing with them* their own paid living organ provider. This organ vendor may be from the recipient's country of origin or from a third party country. B. A patient travels abroad for transplantation and purchases an organ from a living vendor in the destination country.	A wealthy Bangladeshi and his unrelated paid organ provider pretend to be relatives in order to have organ procurement and transplantation performed in Singapore. An Australian travels to Pakistan to purchase a kidney.
3	Transplantation abroad through compassionate access to deceased donor organs.	A. Foreign patients may be included in a national organ waiting list and allowed access to donated organs from unpaid deceased donors. Inclusion is not subject to financial considerations on the part of transplant service providers or other parties and foreign patients are equitably allocated organs in accordance with transparent eligibility criteria that apply to domestic patients. B. Foreign patients may be allowed access to organs as part of a regional organ sharing program to optimize efficient use of available organs and treat urgent cases. Usually this would involve direct export and import of organs (i.e., not transplant travel) rather than travel by the patients themselves.	A foreign tourist suffers unexpected liver failure from acute infection while traveling in Australia, and is allocated a life-saving transplant.

C. Foreign travelers who suffer unexpected organ failure and require emergency transplantation may be allocated an organ from the deceased donor pool. This is not strictly speaking "travel for transplantation," as patients have not traveled for the purpose of undergoing transplantation.

4*	Transplantation and purchase of an organ from an unpaid deceased donor abroad.	A.	A patient may travel abroad and purchase access to the waiting list for deceased donor organs. This may involve "queue jumping" (immediate organ allocation) or simply a place in the waiting list with allocation subject to equitable (nonfinancial) criteria.
		B.	A patient may travel abroad and purchase an organ obtained from an unpaid deceased organ provider in the absence of formal or effective organ allocation protocols and waiting lists.
5*	Transplantation and purchase of an organ from a paid deceased organ provider abroad.	A.	Patients might travel to a country where organs are effectively sold by deceased organ providers—either through futures markets or payment to deceased estates.

[1]Where patients are assessed in a foreign country, it may be difficult to establish the authenticity of the relationship between donors and recipients, and to exclude concealed payments. Some instances of transplant travel may be incorrectly identified as type A.

*Types 2, 4, and 5 constitute Travel for Commercial Organ Transplantation.

Note: Patients travel for organ transplants under a variety of arrangements, some involving commercial transactions such as organ sales or purchased access to a spot on a waiting list.

as a "global kidney bazaar" in which nearly 2,000 kidneys were sold each year to foreign patients.[37] Pakistan's 2007 Ordinance on Human Tissue and Organ Transplantation, which prohibits payment for organs as well as transplants to foreigners, is believed to have substantially reduced transplant travel to Pakistan,[37] although trade has recently resurged.[38] Similarly, the Philippines and China have now implemented legislation with the aim of decreasing incoming transplant travel.[27,35] Egypt, which has also been a major destination in recent years, introduced prohibitory legislation in 2010, although it remains to be seen whether the legislation will prove effective in the light of recent political upheavals there.[39]

The true extent of past and current travel for commercial organ transplants is largely unknown. The illicit nature of such travel and the disapproval with which it is widely held likely underpin the reluctance of patients and professionals involved to report their experiences. Although studies have enabled rough quantifications of trade in some regions, most researchers rely on organ vendors or transplant travelers to volunteer information from which conclusions may be extrapolated. The Colombian Ministry of Health, for example, recently reported an 85 percent reduction in transplants to foreign patients since implementing a law in 2005 giving preference to domestic patients.[40] The statistics report only 16 foreign patient transplants in 2010, and a total of 321 over the last 6 years.[40] However, a recent study of the organ trade in the Colombian cities of Bogota and Medellin that included a survey of 151 organ vendors suggests at least 61 percent of organs sold there go to foreign patients.[36] It further reported only 17 percent of vendors were aware of the legal prohibition of organ selling.[36] Similarly, despite the significant drop in organ transplant travel to China in the last few years, returning patients continue to report having purchased an organ transplant in that country.[11]

Could International Trade in Organs Be Beneficial?

Case studies of commercial transplant travelers reveal understandably defensive attitudes regarding the purchase of organs overseas. Travelers argue that they have no other option than to buy an organ to save their own lives. Recognizing that their organ vendors are likely to be poor and desperate, they express hope that the transaction will also benefit the vendor. A newspaper article quoted an Australian woman, for example, stating that the impoverished Filipino rickshaw driver who sold his kidney to her would "be like extended family for me. It's a win-win situation. He is giving me life and I am giving him a new lifestyle."[41] She stated that she would ensure he "was compensated" at five times the going rate for a kidney and cared for by the doctors. Whether she was able to fulfill this pledge is unknown. The nature of most commercial transplant travel is such that patients are kept separate from organ vendors, and there is little protection of vendor rights.

Numerous advocates of regulated organ markets have argued that national markets will help to prevent harmful transplant travel. The argument that regulated markets may help reduce harmful practices may, of course, be extended to international markets, and it is not implausible to suppose that the introduction of new national markets would encourage growth in cross-border organ markets. In fact, some commentators have already suggested international trade in organs could be effectively used to address organ shortages and health care costs in some countries while offering financial advantages to receiving countries and their organ vendors. Ethicist J.S. Taylor, for example, argues that kidneys from poor living providers might justifiably be exported from India to wealthier countries.[42] More recently, MedToGo International, a medical travel company, provoked controversy by proposing organized transplant travel from Arizona to Mexico.[1] Although the plan was dismissed by Arizona policy makers, it highlights the probability that decriminalization of organ markets would be swiftly embraced by potential brokers and patients in many countries. The appeal of commercial transplant travel, like that of medical travel more generally, is that of quicker access to cheaper health care in foreign countries. At a practical level, the MedToGo proposal, like that of Barry Jacobs in 1983, seems a logical solution to organ shortages in wealthier countries.

Arguments in favor of allowing organ sales include claims that financial incentives will increase organ supplies; that vendors will benefit financially—perhaps escaping from extreme poverty; that participants in sales are exercising their right to liberty and ought not to be prevented from doing so; that prohibition only encourages more harmful market practices; and that efforts to meet needs for organ transplantation in the absence of payment have failed. Each of these claims represents potential arguments that may be made in favor of allowing or encouraging travel for commercial organ transplantation in a regulated or unregulated form, or at least ending efforts to curtail the practice. I shall address these arguments shortly. First, however, I will examine the evidence surrounding existing travel for commercial organ transplantation in order to identify the concerns that have prompted growing efforts to prevent or discourage such travel.

The Other Side of the Coin—Selling Kidneys

Renal transplants comprise the majority of organ transplants performed worldwide, roughly 69,300 annually, 46 percent of which are from living providers.[43] Unsurprisingly, most of the transplant travel market involves renal transplants. Not only do hundreds of thousands of people suffer end stage renal failure, with ever-increasing incidence, but many patients can also be kept alive using dialysis, thus buying time to arrange transplants. Renal patients are also more likely to be fit to travel overseas for transplant than those suffering heart, liver, or lung failure, for example. Finally, the key factor is that many healthy individuals can have a kidney removed with relatively minimal risks to their well-being, if they are appropriately screened and receive adequate follow-up care. Thus, it's far easier for people to buy a kidney on demand from a stranger than it is to procure one from a system or program organized to allocate organs from deceased providers. In contrast, partial liver removal remains more hazardous and occurs less frequently among both paid and unpaid living providers.

A number of studies of living kidney vendors in India,[44] Pakistan and Iran,[45] the Philippines,[35] Egypt,[46] and Colombia[36] have been published, revealing the motivations for and impact of selling a kidney. Although commercial transplant travel compromises a variable proportion of the markets studied, it is reasonable to assume that vendors selling to foreign patients share the same experience as their peers selling to domestic patients in the same market. The evidence of both illegal and legal kidney markets is overwhelmingly negative. It shows that vendors are disproportionately drawn from extremely poor and socially disadvantaged communities, driven to sell as a result of debts or desperation to provide necessary health care or education to children and relatives. Suffering high rates of illiteracy, vendors may fail to comprehend whatever information is provided to them regarding the procedure and aftermath of kidney provision. Some are coerced into selling. Unlike providers in living donation programs, vendors often fail to receive appropriate screening tests, with the result that those at increased risk of harm from provision—who would normally be excluded from donation programs—are "allowed" to sell. Following the removal of their kidneys, vendors are frequently denied essential postoperative care and ongoing follow-up to prevent, identify, and manage complications.

The result, for most kidney vendors, is that they are left worse off after selling, spiraling further into debt. They suffer psychological distress and social stigma, and experience ill health that can prevent them from working. The payment they receive is sometimes less than the promised amount—as little as $1,200 in Pakistan[45] and $1,700 in Colombia.[36] Whatever the precise amount, it generally proves insufficient to enable a sustained improvement in their financial situation.

Commodifying Cadavers?

Organs from deceased providers are less readily available to transplant travelers than kidneys (or partial livers) from living vendors. This is largely due to the fact that most deceased provider programs rely on altruistic donors who provide organs to a public pool, with strict allocation protocols that require a formal waiting list based on medical rather than financial criteria. Organs in such programs can rarely be purchased on demand by foreign patients, although concerns have recently been expressed about this possibility in the United Kingdom.[47] In addition, the ethics committee of the United Network for Organ Sharing (UNOS) in the United States recently discussed the need for greater transparency in monitoring incoming transplant travel—that is, foreign patients undergoing transplantation in the United States.[48] The limited access to deceased donor organs that is allowed to foreign patients in the United States, as in other countries such as the United Kingdom and Australia, is intended to help foreign patients in urgent need of transplantation and to avoid wastage of organs, not to promote commercial interests. In order to access public deceased donor organs, patients must be wait-listed and available to receive suitably matched organs if and when they become available. For patients residing in a foreign country, this makes travel for organs from deceased providers highly impractical.

China was a notorious exception to the rule that deceased provider organs cannot be made available to a specific patient on demand. For a number of years, organs were procured from prisoners executed in China and sold to local and foreign patients for transplantation.[49] But since 2006, the Chinese government has prohibited the sale of organs to transplant travelers and sought to establish better oversight and regulation of the domestic market, including plans to reduce reliance on organs from executed prisoners.[27]

International outrage over the use of executed prisoner organs is multifactorial and extends far beyond criticism of the death penalty per se. First, there is the concern that the criminal justice process is corrupted by the interest in facilitating organ procurement. Second, critics of China's use of executed prisoners to provide organs argue that prisoners are effectively coerced into providing their organs. Although the government insists that prisoners voluntarily "donate," and some Chinese commentators[50] have claimed it represents an expiatory act for criminals, many international medical groups argue it is impossible to guarantee freedom of consent for prisoners, especially when they are facing execution.[51] Third, and perhaps most important, the practice of timing executions to facilitate organ removal is antithetical to the fundamental principle of deceased organ provision—namely, that while someone might be considered a potential provider, the diagnosis of death must always precede the removal of organs, and the diagnosis of death must be distinctly separate from organ procurement to avoid conflicts of interest that might lead to compromised care or effective murder for the purpose of organ procurement.[51]

Dangers for Transplant Travelers Purchasing Organs Abroad

Criticism of travel for commercial organ transplantation has traditionally emphasized the harms suffered by those who provide organs, especially where the autonomy of organ vendors is threatened, but transplant
travelers are also at risk. Foreign patients must pay considerable fees to
arrange and undergo transplantation abroad, up to $180,000 for a liver
transplant in China,[11] for example, and as much as $125,000 for a kidney
transplant in Peru.[1] These costs are frequently inflated, with fees ostensibly
for organ vendors, for example, frequently diverted to swell middlemen
profits rather than rewarding the individual to whom transplant travelers
are most grateful. Furthermore, the desperation of patients suffering life-
threatening organ failure may be exploited by unscrupulous scam artists[52]
or transplant professionals who demand higher pay at the last minute to
secure organs.[11]

Studies show that commercial transplant travelers suffer higher rates
of postoperative complications, graft failure, and infection.[31] A review of
Pakistani commercial organ transplant recipients suggests numerous factors that may result in poorer outcomes for recipients of organs from paid
providers.[53] These include higher rates of infectious diseases such as HIV
and hepatitis among organ vendor populations, poorer screening and
matching mechanisms in receiving countries, inadequate perioperative
care, and compromised continuity of care for highly complex transplant
patients in the cross-border, often illicit, setting of commercial transplant
travel. Furthermore, a number of commercial transplant travelers have
been assessed as unfit for transplantation in their own health care jurisdictions. Thus, the population of prospective transplant travelers may be in
worse health and consequently more likely to have poorer outcomes. Of
note, the costs of complications suffered by transplant travelers are likely
to be borne by the health care systems of their own countries.

Reviewing the Arguments

The arguments for and against markets in human organs have been
fiercely debated and reviewed in a vast body of academic literature and
public media. I shall review these briefly in the context of travel for commercial organ transplantation. First, as a practical matter, it should be
noted that efforts to create a regulated international system of commercial
organ transplantation are likely to fail, given the challenges of enforcing
minimum standards of care and payment for organ vendors in the cross-
border setting. The extent of global poverty is such that a pool of willing
organ vendors will readily be found among the most disadvantaged and
disenfranchised communities. Lacking alternative economic options, such
individuals are likely to suffer similar experiences to those of vendors in
current unregulated markets. The argument that the poor will benefit

from better selling opportunities is equally flawed, as it implies that efforts to secure basic human rights and to eradicate poverty can justifiably be made conditional on the provision of organs to foreign benefactors. Furthermore, the introduction of effective market regulations, such as fitness eligibility criteria for organ vendors, is likely to result in the creation or persistence of black markets in which those excluded from the regulated market participate, possibly at lower prices, due to the availability of regulated market organs.

Second, encouraging travel for commercial organ transplantation may have negative ramifications for sending and receiving countries. The former are likely to become dependent on foreign supplies of organs, detracting from local efforts to establish reliable and sustainable organ procurement programs. The latter may become economically dependent in part on the export of organs, and may struggle to meet domestic organ transplant needs if foreign buyers outprice local patients. The commercialization of transplantation and organ provision may also undermine trust in the integrity of health care professionals as well as transplant programs and subvert efforts to promote equitable allocation of organs.

Third, the claim that prohibition of commercial transplant travel impairs individual liberty or autonomy and is unjustifiably paternalistic must be considered in a wider social context than that of individual transactions between desperate patients and poor vendors. While for two individuals it is conceivable that the commercial transfer of an organ may, in some cases, offer a genuine improvement in their respective lives and constitute a valid expression of their autonomy, it does not automatically follow that public policies endorsing such exchanges are justifiable. It is the role of politicians, health care professionals, and members of society to develop policies that serve the interests of communities, not simply individuals, when these policies relate to matters that are intrinsically social, not self-regarding, concerns. The nature of organ transplantation and health care in general is such that transplant services can be effectively and efficiently delivered to those in need only when systems are established to: encourage optimal community participation in organ provision programs, reduce the need for transplantation through treatment and prevention of organ failure, and coordinate the transfer of organs between matched providers and recipients. Similarly, poverty is generally conditioned by a number of interacting social factors and cannot be effectively addressed without public investment in education, health care, and employment opportunities, among other areas. The sale and purchase of organs for transplantation by individuals—whether regulated or not—is surely not the best solution to growing rates of organ failure or endemic poverty. In the conclusion to this chapter, I will review efforts to address the challenges of travel for commercial organ transplantation.

OVERVIEW OF TRAVEL FOR UNPROVEN STEM CELL TREATMENTS

There are numerous kinds of stem cells and many different therapeutic interventions that may involve the transplantation of such cells into patients. In routine medical practices, adult stem cells are removed from bone marrow and transfused into patients suffering from hematological malignancies or immunological disorders. These haematopoietic cells can help to restore the systems that produce vital blood cells when these have been destroyed. Extensive scientific research is currently underway in efforts to use both adult and embryonic stem cells to restore, renew, or repair defective organs, cells, or tissue in patients with many diseases and injuries. With the exception of certain blood disorders and haematopoietic stem cells, research has not yet translated into treatments widely accepted by the scientific community. Although the focus of public debate has often fallen on the issue of using human embryos in research, a wealth of television programs, newspaper, and magazine articles have all fueled the fires of speculation regarding the promise of stem cell therapies. While politicians and scientists have continued to debate, regulate, and pursue stem cell research, with relatively limited progress announced in the form of effective treatments, some medical practitioners have quietly set up shop as purveyors of unproven stem cell therapies, and thousands of patients have flocked to their doors at clinics throughout the world, in countries including China, India, Russia, Turkey, Germany, the Dominican Republic, and Ukraine.[23,54]

In the last five years, reports of patients traveling abroad for unproven stem cell treatments, patients dying, and clinics engaging in outright fraud have caught the attention of international experts and policy makers. Efforts to discourage such travel and to close down dangerous or fraudulent providers of stem cell interventions have been motivated by concern for patients and fears that such practices will detract from legitimate research efforts. However, the industry shows little sign of slowing down, and patients continue to seek out new or even repeat treatments. In this section, I review travel for unproven stem cell treatments and its major issues.

The Current Market

Currently, one of the most popular locations for unproven stem cell treatments is that of China. More than 200 hospitals in China offer stem cell therapies that may be accessed by foreign patients.[55] One of the biggest providers of unproven stem cell treatments in the world is Beike Biotechnology, which claims to have treated more than 900 foreign patients at its 26 hospitals in China and Thailand.[55] The cost of stem cell treatments from

Beike is usually around $30,000, although once travel costs are factored in, it may cost considerably more. A family from Detroit paid as much as $85,000 for two treatments at Beike for their four-year-old daughter with spastic quadriplegia.[56] Although they had hoped she would gain the ability to hold up her own head, they report satisfaction with an improved "disposition" and the fact she seemed "more relaxed" after her treatment. In China, most stem cell treatments involve the injection of adult or umbilical cord stem cells, as well as intensive physical therapy and the use of complementary medicines such as acupuncture, which may be provided over a period of weeks. In March 2011, the Chinese Ministry of Health introduced regulations governing the use of unproven stem cell treatments that require providers to demonstrate the safety and efficacy of the treatments on offer in clinical trials prior to selling them. The effects of this new order on companies such as Beike and on the extent of stem cell travel to China are as yet unknown.

Russia is another global center for unproven stem cell treatments, with numerous institutions providing treatments in what Cohen and Cohen describe as a grossly under-regulated environment that places patients at significant risk.[23] Reports of skin and animal cells being used to replace the advertised human fetal cell injections, practitioners without medical qualifications, and hundreds of unlicensed clinics in Moscow alone suggest that treatment in Russia is a precarious venture. Despite this, clinics continue to charge considerable fees. One clinic, for example, estimates patients will pay from 20 to 25 percent of the allegedly standard worldwide fee of $250,000.[57]

Relatively small, independent clinics offering unproven stem cell treatments have been set up in countries from Argentina to Ukraine to Thailand (see Table 7.2). While a clinic in the Philippines advertises treatments for as little as $17,000, an email inquiry to India's Moolchand Hospital returned the information from a Mr. Kapoor (August 6, 2011) that four sessions of stem cell treatment were advised to treat spinal cord injury at a cost of "about USD 8,900" per session. Although Moolchand recommended sessions be spaced at monthly intervals, they could be fitted into one month for the patient's convenience. While the majority of treatment centers are located in developing countries outside Western Europe, the United Kingdom, and North America, one of the most famous was, until recently, thriving in Germany. The X-Cell Center claimed to treat 25 patients from the United Kingdom alone every month at prices ranging from $15,000 to $30,000 and was popular with patients from Europe, the United States, and Australia, among other countries. The clinic was closed by the German government in May 2011 following the death of a child and the near death of another child as a result of procedures in which autologous stem cells were transplanted directly into the brain.[6]

Table 7.2
Online examples of clinics offering stem cell treatments for foreign patients

Clinic	Examples of alleged treatment modalities and therapeutic claims
Dr Fernandez Vina Foundation, Argentina http://www.fundacionfernandezvina.org	Embryonic stem cells administered "intracavitary, intravenously and subcutaneously," for example in the treatment of multiple sclerosis; stem cell source is patient's own bone marrow cells, and possibly umbilical cord cells.
Wu Stem Cells Medical Center, China www.unistemcells.com	Various cells used in the treatment of neurological disorders: "neural stem cells and retinal pigment epithelium derived from a spontaneously aborted fetus, and mesenchymal stem cells from either bone marrow (autologous), umbilical cord, or cord blood." Cells are transplanted directly into the brain or fluid surrounding the spinal cord (intrathecal infusion), or infused intravenously (in the case of "diabetes, liver, or rheumatology diseases"), or injected intramuscularly.
Moolchand Hospital Centre for Stem Cell Therapy, India http://www.moolchandhealthcare.com	Umbilical cord cells administered in the treatment of orthopaedic disorders, cardiomyopathy, liver and kidney impairment, cerebral palsy, Parkinson's disease, and motor neuron disease, as well as diabetes. Also used for "rejuvenation."
Fetal Cell Technologies International, Malaysia www.fetal-cells.com	Blood drawn from the patient is sent to the institute where stem cells are specially extracted and turned into Precursor Stem Cells. These are then dispatched to the patient and implanted (using an unexplained technique). Diseases treated include "pre-terminal AIDS," for which a success rate of more than 95% is claimed. Adjunct therapies such as special diets and behavioral therapy may be offered, for example in the treatment of autism. Alternatively, it appears the clinic also offers transplantation of fetal stem cells derived from New Zealand white rabbits.
Integra Medical Center, Mexico http://www.dromargonzalez.com/	Placental tissue obtained following Caesarian section (to avoid bacterial contamination) is implanted subcutaneously in patients.
Stem Cell Institute, Panama http://www.cellmedicine.com/	Cells from patient's adipose tissue or bone marrow, or from umbilical cord blood, are processed and injected into joints, muscles, the spinal cord, or intravenously.
NeuroVita, Russia http://www.neurovita.ru/eng_index.html	Cells obtained from the patient's bone marrow or "separated" from her peripheral blood are injected intrathecally or intravenously where they trigger "the inner mechanism of self curing." Diseases treated include malignant tumors and traumatic epilepsy.

Center of Medico-Biological Technologies, Russia http://www.cmbt.su/eng/	Blood or bone marrow from patient used to obtain cells that are then re-injected. Specializes in sports disorders, but also offers treatments for neurological, sexual, and cardiovascular disorders as well as burns, "life-extension," and infectious diseases among others.
Tissu, Syechelles http://www.tissustemcell.com/	Umbilical cord blood cells injected intravenously, intra-arterially or intrathecally, primarily for neurological disorders, anti-aging, or spinal cord injuries.
Returning Hope, Thailand www.returninghope.com	Stem cells derived from the patient's bone marrow, blood, fat or skin are injected intravenously or directly into organs such as the heart, pancreas, or brain. "Activated" stem cells from fat tissue may also be used to enhance procedures such as breast augmentation surgery.
Thai Regen, Thailand www.thairegen.com	Cells are obtained from the patient's peripheral blood, after being treated with "mobilizing factors" that "cause stem cells from the bone marrow" to enter the bloodstream. After processing, they are administered intravenously, intrathecally, or intra-arterially. Treatment specialties include liver and kidney failure, diabetes, stroke, erectile dysfunction, and spinal cord injuries.
Asian Stem Cell Regeneration Institute, Philippines http://www.stem-cell-regeneration.com	Cells derived from the patient's adipose tissue used to treat various degenerative diseases as well as to enhance cosmetic surgery, via intravenous, intrathecal, or intramuscular injections.
EmCell, Ukraine www.emcell.com	Cells from derived from aborted human embryos infused or implanted subcutaneously to treat numerous diseases including HIV, cancer, ulcerative colitis, anemia, and heart disease.

Note: Stem cell treatments on offer on the Internet target patients suffering from conditions ranging from cancer to erectile dysfunction.

Source: All websites were last accessed September 18, 2011.

The list of diseases and conditions for which institutions offer unproven stem cell treatments to foreigners is remarkably similar, regardless of which website one visits (see Table 7.2). A typical list includes arthritis, autism, cerebral palsy, multiple sclerosis, and spinal cord injury. Diabetes, cancer, Alzheimer's, Parkinson's disease, and motor neuron disease are also frequently cited. The Beike website lists no less than 67 varieties of neurological disorders that can be treated.[58] The approach to treatment is, however, remarkably varied throughout the world. While larger institutions often rely on treatments involving the use of patients' own stem cells, such as autologous bone marrow transplants or adipose tissue procurement and reinfusion, thereby minimizing concerns about infection, smaller clinics facing less public scrutiny offer a fascinating, albeit disturbing, range of therapies.

Travelers' Tales and the Putative Benefits of Unproven Treatments

Global numbers of travelers for unproven stem cell treatment are unknown, and claims by particular institutions regarding their annual patient loads are often unreliable and incomplete. Nevertheless, it is plausible to surmise that at least a few thousand patients travel each year for such treatments abroad, and perhaps many more. In contrast to organ transplant travelers, however, the personal experience of patients seeking unproven stem cell treatments are well known. Unlike organ transplant travelers, who are likely to conceal involvement in commercial transplantation abroad due to concerns about public opinion and legal issues, stem cell patients frequently seek public attention in the context of fundraising efforts to pay for their "journey of hope." Furthermore, there are numerous online forums in which patients discuss and compare experiences with unproven treatments, such as Stem Cell Pioneers.[59] There are also many personal blogs detailing travel abroad for treatment.[54] Such blogs often describe in detail the hopes and expectations of patients prior to traveling, the cultural challenges sometimes encountered, and the financial barriers to travel abroad for treatment. There are often optimistic reports of immediate improvements noted after the treatment—perhaps unsurprising given the need to reassure readers who may have contributed to fundraising efforts. Blogs often tail off after treatment is received, although one American blogger, who initially reported "great results" after paying $50,000 for treatment at a Beike clinic in China, returned to the blog to express disappointment and even regret in the long term. Two years after his treatment, the 50-year-old man, who suffers from a form of muscular dystrophy, wrote: "The positive results I initially received only lasted about 8 months. . . . Would I go again? No. It seems to me that the technology for stem cell treatment [of his condition] is just not there yet."[60]

Such pessimism, however, is a rarity in patient accounts of travel for stem cell treatments. Stem cell travelers are vocal in their defense of the practice, both in personal blogs and on the websites of clinics, in which individual accounts—frequently in the form of video interviews and blogs to enhance authenticity—attest to the benefits of treatment. Despite the dubious science of many treatments, patients and their relatives report "remarkable" improvements, such as enhanced language skills and a "milder temper" for a 16-year-old Norwegian boy with cerebral palsy, and reduced reliance on medications for a 52-year-old American woman with Parkinson's disease.[61] Another Beike website claims that 60 percent of patients report "some improvement" after therapy, based on a study of 20 patients.[62] In online discussions and newspaper interviews, many patients argue in favor of traveling abroad on the grounds that they have "nothing to lose." Many note the importance of "trying" unproven treatments, even where they fail to produce genuine therapeutic benefits. Pursuing these journeys appears to offer intrinsic benefits in the form of hope.

Charles Murdoch and Christopher Thomas Scott suggest that hope "itself could produce a net beneficial outcome" in some instances of stem cell travel.[63] They point to the role of communities and family who band together in support of patients raising funds for treatment, and the online support networks created by patients seeking stem cell cures, and argue that "Patients and their families may feel that doing nothing is tantamount to admitting failure, acknowledging approaching death, or a lifetime of morbidity. Thus, their actions, irrespective of content, may be healing."[63(p20)] Others have noted the potential benefits of complementary therapies offered in association with unproven stem cell treatments, which may be responsible for some of the improvements reported by patients.[64] Finally, as some authors have argued, it is possible that some treatments offered to foreign patients are in fact efficacious, or that some unproven treatments in the future may be shown to offer therapeutic benefits. Murdoch and Scott point out that in some regions, "there may be a medical culture . . . that places less value on clinical trials" and consequently (potentially beneficial) treatments may not meet the standards of proof required by canonical evidence based medicine.[63(p18)]

Medical Innovation Rather Than Unproven Treatment?

Some commentators have sought to moderate the widespread criticism of travel for unproven stem cell treatments by noting the practical challenges of developing and implementing clinical trials for stem cell-based therapies in human beings.[65] Prohibitive costs, and the usual delays of progressive stages of trials before human-based trials are permitted, it is argued, prevent many patients suffering terminal diseases from accessing potentially beneficial novel therapies. Patients for whom no treatment or no curative treatment exists may be willing to incur higher levels of risk than are usually considered ethically justifiable for the chance to benefit from new treatments. The desperation of such patients might even discourage them from participation in randomized double blind clinical trials, for fear of receiving a placebo.

Olle Lindvall and Insoo Hyun[65] argue that some unproven stem cell treatments should be categorized as legitimate "medical innovations" rather than included in the group of unproven treatments habitually critiqued as "stem cell tourism." Medically innovative treatments, they suggest, prioritize patient care over research goals, essentially offering potentially beneficial treatments to "seriously ill patients" who lack treatment alternatives of proven efficacy. Although they note such an approach lacks the benefits of clinical trials that offer information about relative efficacy, long-term risks and so on, Lindvall and Hyun argue that "Patients with precious little time might not care much about expanding knowledge; what they care about is getting better and surviving."[65(p1664)] Nevertheless, they conclude that patients "should continue to be counseled against medical travel for unproven stem cell based therapies at this time."[65(p1665)] Reviewing the challenges of developing minimum standards to identify "medical innovations" in stem cell treatment, as well as the hazards associated with "medically innovative" treatments, Cohen and Cohen suggest:

> The treatments used in such instances should be preceded by studies in nonhumans that indicate not only that they might be efficacious, but also that it seems highly unlikely that they would result in harm to patients. Such treatments should be identified as having a strong scientific rationale and as falling within a class of stem cell treatments directed toward patients who have no other good options and who have been made aware of any known risks that they run.[23(p43)]

Why Worry about Unproven Stem Cell Travel?

There is widespread disapproval of stem cell travel among ethicists, stem cell researchers, policy makers, and health care professionals, not only in countries from which patients travel, but also in those that receive patients. Concerns primarily focus on the harms that traveling patients may experience.[12] These include:

- significant financial burdens;[66]
- lack of therapeutic benefit;[4,7-9]

- risks of treatment including infection, surgical complications, and death;[4-6]
- risks of overseas travel while suffering from severe disease or disability;[63]
- disqualification from future opportunities to participate in legitimate clinical trials due to previous unproven treatments.[4,63]

Patients may be especially vulnerable to exploitation by providers of unproven treatments due to desperation and depression as they suffer from chronic debilitating or life-threatening conditions for which no cure or treatment is available in their own country. Providers may thus more easily charge inappropriate fees, offer inadequate levels of information about the risks and benefits of treatment, and generally exploit patients for their own gain.

Travel for unproven stem cell treatment may also cause harm to other individuals and communities. Stem cell researchers in particular have expressed concern about the impact of unproven treatments on clinical trials and genuine research.[4,63,64] Patients may be less willing to participate in trials in which some patients will be offered placebo treatments, for example. Furthermore, the fraudulent claims of many treatment providers and the nonsensical science offered in support of some unproven stem cell treatments may detract from public trust in stem cell research and discourage investment, thus impairing the progress of stem cell science and regenerative medicine.[4] Stem cell travel might also harm members of the patient's own society through the spread of infection and the cost of treating complications of treatment abroad.

Finally, stem cell travel may involve the use of cells and tissue obtained from other human individuals. Stem cells advertised to traveling patients include those derived from human embryos, umbilical cords, placentas, and adult bone marrow. Little is known of the providers of such tissue, whether they are remunerated or not, whether they have consented to the use of their tissue in the treatments, and whether the procedures used to obtain the materials have caused harm. Each of the procedures involved in obtaining these materials is associated with risk. Abortion, umbilical cord blood procurement, caesarian section, and bone marrow aspiration are all standard medical procedures, but they are associated with risks to women, newborn infants, and adults of both sexes undergoing marrow aspiration. Such risks are customarily applied only when the procedure offers a therapeutic benefit to the provider, an infant, or when a fully informed person consents to donate bone marrow to benefit a loved one or an anonymous patient who is highly likely to gain a significant and genuine therapeutic benefit from bone marrow transplantation.

ADDRESSING TRAVEL FOR COMMERCIAL ORGAN TRANSPLANTATION OR UNPROVEN STEM CELL TREATMENTS

The last decade has seen significant growth in travel for unproven stem cell treatments and widespread travel for commercial organ transplantation. During this period, there has been convergence in international opinion on the regulation of these practices and efforts to address their challenges. The World Health Organization has guided international policy and national legislation through its Guiding Principles on Cell, Tissue and Organ Transplantation[16]—endorsed by the World Health Assembly in May 2010[67]—which condemn commercialism in transplantation services and encourage the voluntary, unpaid donation of human materials for transplantation. International professional organizations such as the International Society of Nephrology (ISN), The Transplantation Society (TTS), and the International Society for Stem Cell Research have promoted awareness of the ethical perils of some forms of travel for transplantation, and both the ISSCR and the Declaration of Istanbul Custodian Group—formed under the aegis of ISN and TTS—have created information pamphlets for prospective transplant travelers to consider before going abroad for treatment.[7,68]

Such groups recognize that patients who travel abroad for commercial organ transplantation or unproven stem cell treatments do not do so with bad intentions. Rather, they are driven by desperate circumstances to seek potentially life-saving treatment in the absence of more accessible treatment in their own countries. Nevertheless, the cost of such travel to patients and to providers of materials for transplantation is often greater than the benefits obtained, and prevention of travel has accordingly become a high priority for those concerned with ethical practice in transplantation worldwide. Prevention is not the sole goal of policy development, however, as prohibition of travel alone fails to address the urgent health care needs of prospective travelers. Consequently, efforts to enhance domestic systems of organ procurement and transplantation are closely affiliated with the campaign against travel for commercial organ transplantation, with the goal of "national self-sufficiency" in transplantation strongly advocated by the World Health Organization, the Declaration of Istanbul, and others.[69] Similarly, the ISSCR seeks to promote research in stem cell treatments.

Efforts to Prevent Unethical Practices

Although significant progress has been achieved in recent years, in particular through the introduction of legislation in numerous countries prohibiting organ trading and trafficking, the successful prevention of harmful transplant travel depends on intervention at a number of points. First, governments should be encouraged to develop and enforce legislation and regulation of activities involving the procurement of human biological materials and their transplantation. Furthermore, they may actively discourage participation of citizens in unethical practices abroad, for example, by collaborating in regional and international efforts to address organ trafficking.[14] Second, health care professionals may be encouraged through their professional societies to conform to ethical standards of practice. The Declaration of Istanbul, for example, has now been endorsed by nearly 100 organizations.[70] Third, members of the transplant travel industry and the medical travel industry more generally are urged to conform to national regulations and to meet international standards of patient care. The ISSCR's recent proposal to publicly review clinics providing unproven stem cell treatments, although shelved for fear of litigation, indicates a potentially effective method of raising consumer awareness.[71] Fourth, initiatives must continue to expose prospective transplant travelers to information and education about the risks and benefits of commercial organ transplantation and unproven stem cell treatments.[7,68] Fifth, efforts must be made to meet the needs of patients suffering organ failure and other diseases within their own health care systems, including developing ethically and scientifically sound stem cell research,[4] and minimizing dependency on outsourcing of treatment and research in countries where ethical standards may be less easily monitored and enforced. Armed with the support of professional societies and the mandate of the World Health Assembly's Resolution on Human Organ Cell and Tissue Transplantation,[67] it is time for national governments to adopt responsibility for the health care marketplace and to examine domestic practices and lead efforts within national borders to ensure that domestic and foreign patients, as well as the providers of human biological materials, receive the best available care.

The root causes of harmful transplant travel are self-evident: inadequate health care services and supplies of organs within domestic systems; socioeconomic inequity both within and between countries; failure to rigorously enforce domestic regulations governing transplantation; and lack of empirical research into the extent of such travel. Money drives the industry, lack of oversight enables it, and, perhaps, unachievable expectations of contemporary science and medicine—"the 'mythos' of regenerative medicine"[63(p19)]—are likely to perpetuate it.

CONCLUSION

Whether travel for commercial organ transplantation or unproven stem cell treatments offers an effective long-term or temporary solution to the needs of desperately ill patients is uncertain at best. In its current form, such travel presents grave dangers to patients and also to others such as organ providers and their communities. For both organ and stem cell transplant patients, travel abroad usually represents a strategy of last resort that offers hope when domestic health care services appear to offer none. The stakes of illness are so high that the risks of transplant travel might seem small in comparison. However, the evidence suggests this assumption is mistaken.

Transplant travelers—whether pursuing organs or stem cell treatments—set out on perilous, lonely voyages. Unprotected in foreign countries, at the mercy of private or even illegal health care providers without effective oversight by health care authorities, travelers may be fortunate enough to successfully achieve some of their health care goals. In doing so, however, they may place others at significant risk. They may also compromise efforts to enhance the development of organ transplantation and stem cell therapies within their own countries or in those of receiving communities. Although travel for transplantation is sometimes defended as an expression of individual liberty, and the (often illusory) hope it offers to patients described as an intrinsic benefit, desperate patients would be better served by united efforts within and between domestic health care systems to develop transplantation services, enhance organ procurement, and promote the development of safe and effective treatments for disease.

REFERENCES

1. Smith M. Desperate Americans buy kidneys from Peru poor in fatal trade. *Bloomberg.* May 12, 2011. http://www.Bloomberg.com/news/2011-05-12/desperate-americans-buy-kidneys-from-peru-poor-in-fatal-trade.html. Accessed June 7, 2011.

2. ISSCR. Glossary of Stem Cell Related Terms. International Society for Stem Cell Research, 2003. http://www.isscr.org/Glossary_of_Stem_Cell_Related_Terms.htm Accessed June 6, 2011.

3. Daley GQ. Stem cells: Roadmap to the clinic. *J Clin Invest,* 2010;120(1):8–10.

4. Gunter KC, Caplan AL, Mason C, et al. Cell therapy medical tourism: Time for action. *Cytotherapy.* 2010;12(8):965–968.

5. Dobkin BH, Curt A, Guest J. Cellular transplants in China: Observational study from the largest human experiment in chronic spinal cord injury. *Neurorehabil Neural Repair.* 2006;20(1):5–13.

6. Mendick R, Hall, A. Europe's largest stem cell clinic shut down after death of baby. *The Telegraph.* May 8, 2011. http://www.telegraph.co.uk/news/worldnews/europe/germany/8500233/Europes-largest-stem-cell-clinic-shut-down-after-death-of-baby.html. Accessed July 8, 2011.

7. A Closer Look at Stem Cells. ISSCR website providing information for patients considering unproven stem cell treatments. http://closerlookatstemcells.org. Accessed July 8, 2011.

8. Tejada P. Warning on Stem Cell Tourism. EURORDIS website. http://www.eurordis.org/content/warning-stem-cell-tourism. Published January 20, 2010. Updated July 2, 2010. Accessed September 7, 2010.

9. Josephs L. Costa Rica puts brakes on popular stem cell tourism. *Reuters.* June 7, 2010. http://www.reuters.com/article/2010/06/07/us-costarica-stemcells-idUSTRE6516UR20100607. Accessed September 7, 2011.

10. Stem cell treatments illegal, Dominican authorities warn. *Dominican Today.* May 24, 2011. http://www.dominicantoday.com/dr/local/2011/5/24/39647/stem-cell-treatments-illegal-domincanauthorities-warn. Accessed July 7, 2011.

11. Echevarria B. The cost of a liver. *El Pais* (English edition). March 16, 2010:4–5.

12. Zarzeczny A, Rachul C, Nisbet M, Caulfield T. Stem cell clinics in the news. *Nat Biotechnol.* 2010;28(12):1243–1246.

13. The term *provider* refers to an individual from whom biological materials are removed for therapeutic use in another person. Where the provider receives payment, she may be referred to as a *vendor.* Where she volunteers to provide material without payment or equivalent material incentives, she may be referred to as a *donor.*

14. Francis LP, Francis JG. Stateless crimes, legitimacy, and international criminal law: The case of organ trafficking. *Criminal Law and Philosophy.* 2010;4(3):283–295.

15. 21st Century Snake Oil. *Sixty Minutes Program.* CBS News. Published April 16, 2010. http://www.cbsnews.com/stories/2010/04/16/60minutes/main6402854_page7.shtml?tag=contentMain;contentBody. Accessed July 7, 2011.

16. World Health Organization. WHO Guiding Principles on Human Cell, Tissue and Organ Transplantation (Updated Edition). Geneva: World Health Organization: 2008. www.who.int/transplantation/TxGP08-en.pdf. Accessed July 7, 2011.

17. Participants in the International Summit on Transplant Tourism and Organ Trafficking convened by The Transplantation Society and International Society of Nephrology in Istanbul, Turkey, April 30 to May 2, 2008. The Declaration of Istanbul on organ trafficking and transplant tourism. *Kidney Int.* 2008;74(7):854–859.

18. ISSCR. Guidelines for the Clinical Translation of Stem Cells. December 3, 2008. www.isscr.org/clinical_trans/pdfs/ISSCRGLClinicalTrans.pdf. Accessed July 7, 2011.

19. Smith L. Sale of human organs should be legalised, say surgeons. *The Independent.* January 5, 2011. http://www.independent.co.uk/life-style/health-and-families/health-news/sale-of-human-organs-should-be-legalised-say-surgeons-2176110.html. Accessed July 7, 2011.

20. Wenley S. Lobbyists anxiously await stem cell trial decision. *Sunday Star Times.* January 16, 2011. http://www.stuff.co.nz/sunday-star-times/features/4542836/Lobbyists-anxiously-await-stem-cell-trial-decision. Accessed April 12, 2012.

21. Turner L. Let's wave goodbye to "transplant tourism." *BMJ* 336, no. 7657 (2008):1377.

22. Epstein M, Martin D, Danovitch G. Caution: Deceased donor organ commercialism! *Transpl Int.* 2011;24:958–964.

23. Cohen CB, Cohen PJ. International stem cell tourism and the need for effective regulation: Part I: Stem cell tourism in Russia and India: Clinical research, innovative treatment, or unproven hype? *Kennedy Inst Ethics J.* 2010;20 (1):27–49.

24. Schneider A, Flaherty M. The challenge of a miracle—selling the gift. *Pittsburgh Press.* November 3–8, 1985.

25. Gross JA. E Pluribus UNOS: The National Organ Transplant Act and its postoperative complications. *Yale J Health Policy Law Ethics.* 2008;8:145–421.

26. Carvalho N. Law against organ trafficking approved. *Asia News.* August 29, 2011. http://www.asianews.it/news-en/Law-against-organ-trafficking-approved-22490.html. Accessed September 7, 2011.

27. Huang J, Mao Y, Millis JM. Government policy and organ transplantation in China. *Lancet.* 2008;372(9654):1937–1938.

28. Scheper-Hughes N, Alter JS, Ayora-Diaz SI, et al. The global traffic in human organs. *Curr Anthropol.* 2000;41(2):191–224.

29. Scheper-Hughes N. Parts unknown: Undercover ethnography of the organs-trafficking underworld. *Ethnography.* 2004;5(1):29–73.

30. Shimazono Y. The state of the international organ trade: A provisional picture based on integration of available information. *Bull World Health Organ.* 2007;85(12):955–962.

31. Delmonico FL. Transplantation: Transplant tourism: An update regarding the realities. *Nat Rev Nephrol.* 2011;7(5):248–250.

32. Budiani-Saberi DA, Delmonico FL. Organ trafficking and transplant tourism: A commentary on the global realities. *Am J Transplant.* 2008;8(5):925–929.

33. Ashok S, Lakshmi K. A hub of medical tourism. *The Hindu.* July 18, 2011. http://www.thehindu.com/news/cities/Chennai/article2237677.ece. Accessed September 7, 2011.

34. Ishikawa M, Kitatani H, Akiyama T, et al. The management and long-term results of Japanese pediatric liver transplant recipients. *Surg Today.* 1994; 24(5):403–409.

35. Padilla BS. Regulated compensation for kidney donors in the Philippines. *Curr Opin Organ Transplan.* 2009;14(2):120–123.

36. Mendoza RL. Colombia's organ trade: Evidence from Bogota and Medellìn. *J Public Health.* 2010;18(4):375–384.

37. Rizvi SAH, Anwar Naqvi SA, Zafar MN, et al. Pakistan abolishes kidney market and ushers in a new era of ethical transplantation. *IJOTM.* 2010;1(4)193–197.

38. Another kidney shop unearthed. *Dawn.* July 1, 2011. http://www.dawn.com/2011/07/02/another-kidney-shop-unearthed.html. Accessed July 7, 2011.

39. Rosenberg D. Egypt clamps down on organ trafficking. August 7, 2011. http://www.jpost.com/MiddleEast/Article.aspx?id=228494&R=R3. Accessed April 12, 2012.

40. Hockman B. Colombia's organ transplant tourism on decline: Govt. *Colombia Reports.* March 23, 2011. http://colombiareports.com/colombia-news/news/15083-colombian-organ-transplants-for-foreigners-continues-to-decrease-govt.html. Accessed April 18, 2011.

41. Weaver C. Woman pays $65 000 for kidney. *Daily Telegraph.* March 2, 2008:23.

42. Taylor JS. Stakes and kidneys: Why markets in human body parts are morally imperative: Aldershot, England: Ashgate Publishing; 2005.

43. Global Observatory on Donation and Transplantation. Organ donation and Transplantation: Activities, Laws and Organization 2010. www.transplant-observatory.org/Data%20Reports//2010%20Report%20final.pdf. Accessed September 7, 2011.

44. Goyal M, Mehta RL, Schneiderman LJ, Sehgal AR. Economic and health consequences of selling a kidney in India. *JAMA.* 2002;288(13):1589–1593.

45. Rizvi AHS, Naqvi ASA, Zafar NM, Ahmed E. Regulated compensated donation in Pakistan and Iran. *Current Opinion in Organ Transplantation.* 2009;14(2):124–128.

46. Budiani Saberi D, Mostafa A. Care for commercial living donors: The experience of an NGO's outreach in Egypt. *Transpl Int.* 2010;24(4):317–323.

47. Macrae F. Foreign patients pay £1m for liver transplants at top NHS hospital. *The Daily Mail.* June 13, 2011. http://www.dailymail.co.uk/health/article-2002805/Foreign-patients-pay-1m-liver-transplants-NHS-hospital.html. Accessed July 7, 2011.

48. Organ Procurement and Transplantation Network website. OPTN/UNOS Ethics Committee Report to the Board of Directors. June 28–29, 2011. http://optn.transplant.hrsa.gov/CommitteeReports/board_main_EthicsCommittee_7_1_2011_10_37.pdf. Accessed September 7, 2011.

49. Danovitch GM, Shapiro ME, Lavee J. The use of executed prisoners as a source of organ transplants in China must stop. *Am J Transplant.* 2011;11(3):426–428.

50. Wang M, Wang X. Organ donation by capital prisoners in China: Reflections in Confucian ethics. *J Med Philos.* 2010;35(2):197.

51. Rothman DJ, Rose E, Awaya T, et al. The Bellagio Task Force report on transplantation, bodily integrity, and the international traffic in organs. *Transplantation Proc.* 1997;29:2739–2746.

52. Scheper-Hughes N. Commodity fetishism in organ trafficking. In Scheper-Hughes N, Wacquant LJD eds., *Commodifying bodies.* London: Sage Publications; 2002:31–62.

53. Rizvi SAH, Naqvi SAA, Zafar MN, et al. Commercial transplants in local Pakistanis from vended kidneys: A socio economic and outcome study. *Transpl Int.* 2009;22(6):615–621.

54. Ryan KA, Sanders AN, Wang DD, Levine AD. Tracking the rise of stem cell tourism. *Regen Med.* 2010;5(1):27–33.

55. McMahon DS, Thorsteinsdottir H, Singer PA, Daar AS. Cultivating regenerative medicine innovation in China. *Regen Med.* 2010;5(1):35–44.

56. Feighan M. Family looks to China for child's treatment. *The Detroit News.* June 7, 2011.

57. Neuro Vita Clinic. Frequently asked questions. http://www.neurovita.ru/eng_faq.html#q10. Accessed September 18, 2011.

58. Shenzhen Beike Biotechnology Co., Ltd. Treatable Diseases. Stem Cell Treatment Now. http://stemcelltreatmentnow.com/index.php/treatment/treatable-diseases.html. Accessed September 7, 2011.

59. Stem Cell Pioneers. www.stemcellpioneers.com Accessed September 18, 2011.

60. Kleve R. New Post-2 Years Post Treatment. April 24, 2011. Russ Kleve Stem Cell Treatment. http://russkleve.blogspot.com. Accessed September 18, 2011.

61. Beijing Puhua International Hospital Stem Cell Treatment Center. Patient's Experience. Stem Cells Puhua. http://www.stemcellspuhua.com/experience.shtml. Accessed September 18, 2011.

62. Adult Stem Cell Technology. SCI Treatment. http://spinalcordinjuryscitreatment.com/. Accessed September 18, 2011.

63. Murdoch CE, Scott CT. Stem cell tourism and the power of hope. *Am J Bioeth.* 2010;10(5):16–23.

64. Cohen CB, Cohen PJ. International stem cell tourism and the need for effective regulation: Part II: Developing sound oversight measures and effective patient support. *Kennedy Inst Ethics J.* 2010;20(3):207–230.

65. Lindvall O, Hyun I. Medical innovation versus stem cell tourism. *Science.* 2009;324(5935):1664–1665.

66. Lau D, Ogbogu U, Taylor B, Stafinski T, Menon D, Caulfield T. Stem cell clinics online: The direct-to-consumer portrayal of stem cell medicine. *Cell Stem Cell.* 2008;3(6):591–594.

67. World Health Organization. Resolution on Human Organ and Tissue Transplantation (WHA 63.22). http://apps.who.int/gb/ebwha/pdf_files/WHA63/A63_R22-en.pdf. Accessed December 28, 2010.

68. Declaration of Istanbul Custodian Group. Patient Brochure. Declaration of Istanbul. http://www.declarationofistanbul.org/images/stories/Patient_brochure_A4_LoRes.pdf. Accessed September 7, 2011.

69. Third WHO Global Consultation on Organ Donation and Transplantation: Striving to Achieve Self-Sufficiency, March 23–25, 2010, Madrid, Spain. *Transplantation* 2011 91 (Supplement 11S) S27–S114.

70. Declaration of Istanbul Custodian Group. List of endorsing organizations. Declaration of Istanbul. http://www.declarationofistanbul.org/index.php?option=com_content&view=article&id=74&Itemid=56. Accessed September 7, 2011.

71. Ledford H. Stem-cell scientists grapple with clinics. *Nature.* 2011;474(7353):550.

Chapter 8

Cross-Border Assisted Reproductive Care: Global Quests for a Child

Andrea Whittaker

An increasing number of couples and individuals are traveling across international borders to undergo a range of assisted reproductive treatments in a quest to conceive children. These journeys have been variously labeled as "fertility," "procreative" or "reproductive tourism," "cross-border reproductive care," and even "reproductive exile."[1,2] They involve traveling to obtain surrogacy services, donor eggs or donor sperm, or for treatments through IVF (in vitro fertilization) and associated technologies, including IUI (intrauterine injection), ICSI (intracytoplasmic sperm injection), and procedures such as PGD (preimplantation genetic diagnosis). Although exact statistics on the number of people traveling for this care are unavailable, surveys suggest that the number is increasing.

In this chapter, I describe the main hubs for reproductive travel, the motivations and experiences of people traveling for cross-border reproductive care, and the implications for the countries and women involved in providing these services. The majority of patients undertaking cross-border care are doing so due to regulations in their home countries that limit their access to services. For some groups of people, cross-border reproductive care may be the only option they have to pursue their quest for children. But these forms of medical tourism are also mired in controversy.

As this chapter outlines, there are a range of risks to patients, including the absence of adequate malpractice protections in some jurisdictions, and a variety of legal complexities. Ethical questions also arise, particularly when destination clinics operate within developing countries. The growth of a trade oriented to foreigners may affect the availability of specialists and access within a destination country's own health system for its local population. In many countries there is a lack of transparency regarding the conditions under which egg donations are made and traded. Exploitation of poorer women to carry surrogate pregnancies is also a risk. As more people cross borders to seek assisted reproduction services or to service the trade, better regulation is needed to protect those at risk.

Cross-border travel has been long associated with assorted other reproductive services. For example, many Chinese women cross the border to give birth in Hong Kong to achieve permanent residency status for their children, and women seeking to terminate pregnancies travel from Ireland, where such procedures are banned, to the United Kingdom for these services. Other services that fall under a broad rubric of reproductive travel include travel for pelvic, gynecological, and testicular surgeries. However, within common parlance, cross-border reproductive travel has come to be associated with assisted reproductive treatments (see Box 8.1 for a description of these treatments).

8.1 List of Acronyms and Terms

ARTs: Assisted reproductive technologies.

EHSRE: European Society of Human Reproduction and Embryology.

IVF: In vitro fertilization; generally, a term for any technique in which egg cells are fertilized outside the woman's body.

ICSI: Intracytoplasmic sperm injection, an in vitro fertilization procedure in which a single sperm is injected directly into an egg. It is distinguished from conventional IVF in which many sperm are placed with an egg in a dish and compete to be the first to enter the egg.

PGD: Preimplantation genetic diagnosis, the testing of IVF embryos before implantation by removing one or more cells for analysis. It may also refer to the testing of eggs before fertilization.

Surrogacy: Procedures in which a woman carries and delivers a child for another couple or person.

Gestational surrogacy: Procedures in which a woman carries a pregnancy to delivery after having been implanted with an embryo, as opposed to "traditional surrogacy" where the surrogate is also the genetic source of eggs.

Commercial surrogacy: Arrangements in which the surrogate receives some form of financial compensation for carrying and delivering the child (other than reasonable medical costs and expenses). In contrast, where no compensation is involved other than reasonable costs, this is called "altruistic surrogacy."

WHAT DOES CROSS-BORDER REPRODUCTIVE TREATMENT INVOLVE?

Cross-border travel for assisted reproductive treatments usually involves a period of preparation prior to travel and then a range of tests and procedures at the destination clinic. Although it differs depending on the medical history of the patients and their particular treatment needs, for some patients this can mean multiple steps and trips and extended stays in the destination country. In some cases, some of the required tests or preparatory steps may be done under the supervision of a doctor in the home country in coordination with the clinic in the destination country. In such a case, a woman undergoing IVF must stay at the destination clinic for approximately two to three weeks. If she chooses to complete all of her preparation and testing for a cycle in the destination clinic, she may need to stay for up to three months.

For example, when a woman undertakes a "cycle" in IVF, treatment takes place across approximately 21 to 28 days. It entails suppressing a woman's normal menstrual cycle; inducing ovulation, which usually involves daily injections of pituitary hormones to produce a number of eggs; the "harvesting" of those eggs using an ultrasonically guided needle ("oocyte retrieval"); fertilization of the eggs by sperm; growth in vitro in the laboratory across a number of days; selection of the embryos and further testing in the case of PGD; further hormonal stimulation for some women to induce the production of endometrial lining; and transferring (usually two) resulting embryos directly into the uterus. Two weeks later, further testing (which may occur back in the home country) reveals whether implantation of the embryo has been successful. Men's involvement in the whole IVF cycle usually ends with sperm testing and sperm collection through masturbation or a surgical procedure. In some cases a male partner may not travel but have sperm collected in his home country and couriered overseas for use. Due to the fact that IVF treatment often does not result in a successful pregnancy, some couples undergo treatment multiple times.

Couples who travel for surrogacy services or egg donors may need to spend less time in the destination clinic. A woman using a surrogate but her own eggs will undergo most procedures at home, excluding the transfer of the embryos. When a couple uses donor eggs and a surrogate, a male partner may travel alone to deposit sperm, and the only further trip that may be made occurs when the couple receives the newborn child.

Although popular accounts of cross-border-assisted reproduction describe it as "reproductive tourism," in many cases traveling overseas is not viewed as an opportunity for a pleasurable tourism experience in addition to treatment. For this reason, I refer to it using the more neutral term of "cross-border reproductive travel." As one informant in a study in Thailand noted, "because traveling for doing this [is] not traveling like a tourist, you know, I mean, but because we want to have a baby, we just, I'm gonna do it, I want to do it, I have to do it."[2(p370)] While many medical facilitation companies offering packages for reproductive treatments do include side trips to local attractions and promote the opportunity to relax and undertake some tourism as an added bonus of the care offered,[2] a study of British women seeking treatment in Europe found that they resisted the "fertility tourist" label as an inaccurate representation of the difficulties of treatment and their efforts to form a family.[3]

Much of the existing work on cross-border travel comes from experiences in European countries. It is important to recognize that cross-border reproductive travel experiences differ in terms of the linguistic and cultural context, health systems, inconvenience, travel, and costs that travelers encounter. For example, the experience of a French woman traveling across a border to Belgium for treatment is likely to be very different from that of "long haul" cross-border travelers from Australia to Cyprus, Norway to India, or Italy to Thailand. In addition to considerations for the travelers seeking reproductive services, travel between developed and less-developed countries also involves greater concerns about the potential for exploitation among those providing services such as surrogacy.

WHO UNDERTAKES CROSS-BORDER TRAVEL?

No one knows how many people travel for these services as there are no accurate statistics, particularly in developing countries. While individual hospitals and clinics may maintain such statistics, few governments or organizations systematically collect the data. Data also may differ because of definitions. Some hospitals count by patient visits or IVF cycles, rather than by individual patients, for instance, and some may record nationalities, rather than place of residence. However, survey evidence suggests the number of patients traveling for reproductive treatment is large and growing. A 2010 European Society of Human Reproduction and Embryology (ESHRE) survey of 44 clinics in six European countries estimated that 11,000 to 14,000 patients a year seek treatment in other European countries.[4] In 2010, approximately 6 percent of Canadian IVF patients went to the United States for treatment, 80 percent of those for anonymous donor eggs, and 4 percent of all IVF patients in the United States were from other countries.[5] There is evidence of extensive travel from Italy,[6] and data from clinics in Belgium also show a steady growth in patients traveling from nearby France, the Netherlands, Italy, and Germany.[7]

A study of 41 women and 10 men who sought treatment overseas from Britain found them not to differ greatly in demographic characteristics from people who seek fertility treatment in the United Kingdom; they were not substantially older nor wealthier than people using private services in the United Kingdom, although the majority had already undergone one or more treatment cycles in the United Kingdom.[3]

MAJOR HUBS OF REPRODUCTIVE TRAVEL

Certain destination countries have become major hubs for reproductive treatment. In Europe, these include Spain, Belgium, North Cyprus, and the Czech Republic. Jordan, Dubai, Israel, and South Africa are important hubs in Africa and the Middle East. In Asia, India and Thailand are major hubs, although Singapore and Malaysia are increasingly important as destinations. The United States remains an important destination, particularly for commercial ova donation and commercial surrogacy. In South America, Mexico and Argentina have a growing trade. Most of the patients traveling to these destinations come from the surrounding regions; hence familiarity and ease of travel are important considerations in people's choices. But the choice very much depends upon what service is sought.

What these locations tend to have in common is a combination of sophisticated medical infrastructure and expertise; favorable regulatory frameworks (or a lack of regulation); and lower wage structures, which allow for lower costs. Other factors that play important roles in determining the popularity of these sites include the availability of a good tourist infrastructure and visas suitable for longer-term stays, the availability of translators, and religious affiliation (for example, Muslim patients may prefer to travel to Malaysia for care). Different locations have become associated with different services;[2] for example, Spain and the Czech Republic have become known for the plentiful availability of donor eggs, India for affordable commercial surrogacy, and the United States for commercial surrogacy or nonmedical sex selection (choosing the sex of a baby for social rather than medical reasons).

WHY DO PEOPLE TRAVEL?

As Boxes 8.2 and 8.4 illustrate, patients involved in cross-border reproductive care are not a homogenous group.[3] They travel for an array of reasons, as outlined below.[4,8–10]

High Prevalence of Infertility

Approximately 9 percent of couples across the world experience infertility during their reproductive lives.[11] Demographic changes such as later ages of marriage and delayed childbearing and other factors such as obesity and STDs contribute to the demand for access to assisted reproductive technologies.[12]

Regulatory Issues

Regulatory issues also limit the availability or access to particular services in patients' home countries, causing them to travel elsewhere for services.[12] These differences reflect countries' diverse historical, cultural, social, political, and economic and religious traditions. Patients may travel because of legal restrictions on their eligibility for treatment: for example, they may not be eligible because they are unmarried, or in same-sex relationships, or do not fit the age restrictions for publicly funded care. Some people travel because of a desire for donor anonymity that is not possible in their home countries, while others wish to have more information or choice in selecting their donor, options that their countries may not provide or allow. Other restrictions may apply to the types of procedures available. For example, for religious and ethical reasons, countries differ in their responses to IVF technologies, and consequently some may restrict related clinical procedures. Turkey does not allow third party sperm and egg donation, for instance. Other countries have restrictions on cryopreservation of embryos, social sex selection, or preimplantation genetic diagnoses.

A number of countries forbid the commercialization of "third party services" such as surrogacy and commercial ova donation. The availability of commercial surrogacy and commercial ova donation in some locations such as some U.S. states, India, and elsewhere attract couples who may have difficulty obtaining those services in their home countries.

Growing Medical Costs

In many countries, assisted reproductive treatments are expensive, forcing couples to seek more affordable care. This is particularly the case in the United States and other countries where medical insurance may not cover the costs of fertility treatments because they are defined as nonessential. Of 162 countries surveyed by the International Federation of Fertility Societies,[13] 50 of them supplied information on the availability of medical insurance for assisted reproductive services. Even though the responding countries were predominantly developed nations, only 32 reported some form of insurance coverage for reproductive services funded through a national health plan, and the benefits differed markedly depending on the nation.

Lack of Services

Specific reproductive health services may be unavailable due to a lack of expertise, equipment or donor eggs, sperm, or embryos, causing patients to travel across borders to access them. For example, studies of British couples using overseas treatment suggest that the shortage of ova donors in the United Kingdom is the primary motivation for traveling for treatment (7% of 41 cases in the first;[3] 62% of 53 in the second[4]). As the chances of success with IVF technologies decreases with age, and waiting times for treatment in some countries can exceed 12 months, some couples opt to seek timely and affordable services overseas. In other cases, travel may also take place to access higher quality services or expertise. For example, residents of most Pacific nations do not have access to IVF services and may seek them in neighboring countries such as Australia, New Zealand, the United States, and Asia.

Religious and Cultural Compatibilities

Some patients travel to seek culturally and religiously sensitive treatment. For example, countries such as Jordan, Dubai, and Malaysia are attractive destinations for Middle Eastern and Bangladeshi patients due to religious compatibilities such as the perception that fellow Muslim doctors will be more likely to pay due heed to strictly Islamic moral codes and precepts and hence be more scrupulous in the services they provide.[9,14]

Transnational Migrants

Finally, some transnational migrant couples return to their origin countries for treatment in a linguistically and culturally familiar setting close to extended family or for better access to ethnically similar donor gametes.[10]

Growing Knowledge of and Expectations of Access to Reproductive Technologies

The growth in specialist expertise in assisted reproductive medicine and availability of sophisticated laboratory services in countries throughout the world means that more couples are referred to and expect access to these technologies. As more people learn about these technologies through the Internet, media, and social networks, demand for access is growing.

8.2 Access, Quality, and Cost

A study of British patients[15] illustrates the diversity of couples undergoing cross-border treatment. Deborah, a married 36-year-old British woman traveled for IVF treatment in the United States after receiving lengthy and expensive treatment in the United Kingdom with no success. An affluent professional couple, Deborah and her husband were able to access a high-profile clinic in the United States with high success rates: "at the time we thought, oh maybe we should look at [America]. . . . So we went over to [clinic] and we saw them and we were blown away. . . . He [the clinician] just said, 'This isn't a problem. The [UK clinic] shouldn't have been doing this, they should be doing this.' "[15,16]

The first cycle resulted in a successful birth, and they were considering traveling again to undergo further treatment for a second child.

(continued)

In contrast, the study cites an example of Paula, a single woman who traveled from Britain to a clinic in the Czech Republic to undergo a donor insemination cycle because of concerns about cost and poor attitudes in a British clinic: "I think I will probably have change from £1,500 compared to £4,500 for cycles before, it feels like a positive bargain really. And I think the fresh donor cycle is currently about €3,900, which is still quite a lot cheaper than here."

POTENTIAL RISKS AND ETHICAL CONSEQUENCES

Most patients in studies of cross-border treatment in Europe report positively on their experiences.[3,4,7] They tend to make favorable comparisons about the care received and report shorter waiting times, quicker test results, and better access to and choices for gamete donors.[2,3] However, a number of concerns have been raised over quality and safety requirements and standards of care in some countries. Likewise, there are concerns about the conditions under which gamete donations and surrogacy take place.[17–19] Questions have also been raised about the long-term consequences for children conceived from anonymous international donations who will never have access to information on their biological inheritance, or who may struggle with the idea that they were conceived through commercial arrangements.

Quality of Care

Patients in a number of studies report difficulties and negative reactions when attempting to obtain medical advice from medical professionals in their home countries before traveling for treatment.[3] Although in some cases, clinics in the origin country may have affiliations with the destination clinic and are able to swap records and assist with referrals, often such relationships do not exist, or patients are arranging their travel independently. In some cases it may be illegal for clinicians in the sending country to refer for services (for example, in some states of Australia it is illegal to assist in overseas commercial surrogacy arrangements). Consequently, patients undertaking cross-border reproductive services are often left to their own devices to inform themselves about destination clinic protocols and what their treatments may entail, as well as to discern the quality of care provided from one clinic to the next.

In general, people who are traveling for cross-border care tend to have had previous experience with assisted reproductive treatments in their home countries and are familiar with what it entails, including the possible risks.[3] Most also research other individuals' experience in various destination clinics via online community sites. This experience and research can be key, since clinical protocols, expectations, and quality of care may vary from country to country. Very few professional organizations have guidelines for the treatment of foreign patients, although there are some exceptions, such as the European Society for Human Reproduction and Embryology, which has published a "good practice guide" for clinics treating foreign patients.[20]

Differences may exist regarding the medications used and how they are used, the number of embryos transferred in IVF, whether cryopreservation (the freezing of spare embryos) is allowed, and whether counseling or other forms of social support are available for patients. Although English is widely spoken in clinics catering to cross-border patients, miscommunication and misunderstandings are always possible. Patients may find that staff have inadequate language skills to counsel them at times of distress if a cycle fails or if they need to communicate in a language other than English. The quality of translation services provided also may be variable.

Many people contact overseas clinics themselves via the Internet or medical facilitation companies. In doing so, they face difficulties comparing standards of care among clinics and countries because there is no authoritative information source offering such information. Professional organizations have expressed concerns that there is misleading advertising on the Internet and that patients may not fully be informed about the different medical risks involved if they make decisions to pursue treatment overseas without a referring doctor's guidance.[17] Claims of very high IVF success rates need to be treated with caution. Although patients can easily compare costs between clinics, it can be very difficult to compare quality of care and the success of the clinics. There can be large variations in the success rates advertised by clinics depending on whether clinics are reporting their "take home" baby success rates versus pregnancy rates (many of which do not result in a successful birth). Their success will also vary according to the age and complexities of the population of patients treated at that clinic (for example, some clinics refuse older patients and hence report higher success rates).

Not all countries have extensive legal protections for foreign consumers if they experience problems with their medical care, particularly once they have returned to their home country. Medical facilitation companies usually take no responsibility for any problems that may occur as a result of their referrals, and so patients may be left with little means of recompense if problems occur (see chapter 9 for a detailed discussion of these legal considerations). In many cases, the reason that certain procedures are available in a particular country is because of a lack of regulation in that country that also translates into few consumer protections. Overseas patients need to obtain independent legal advice, particularly if they intend to contract surrogacy services and bring a baby home, have an overseas surrogate travel to their country, import frozen embryos following treatment overseas, or import ova or sperm from another country for use. If a patient has medical insurance, she needs to check whether it will cover any medical problems incurred following treatment overseas if she requires follow-up treatment in her home country. Couples obtaining treatment overseas often require follow-up care for their pregnancies back in their home countries. Although it is becoming less common, some clinics have been known to insert multiple embryos to improve chances of successful implantation, a practice that can result in high-risk multiple pregnancies that will require complex care in the sending country.

Ethical Issues

Patients who travel for cross-border care are often concerned about the ethics of such travel, and this may influence where they choose to undertake treatment.[15] The development of a cross-border reproductive care trade raises the general concerns that come with all medical travel, such as the effects on access for local patients in destination countries. More specific concerns relate to balancing the potential for the exploitation of women's bodies as surrogates or ova donors with a patient's right to travel for treatment. The growth of cross-border reproductive travel by patients from wealthy countries to clinics in developing countries raises particular concerns around equity and access. Cross-border trade has arguably benefited destination countries by encouraging the development of labs and clinics with access to the latest assisted reproductive technologies and procedures, and by creating an incentive for IVF specialists to remain in their countries. But it also has encouraged a division between elite clinics oriented to foreigners and the most wealthy local patients and other locally oriented clinics with crowded caseloads and poorer lab facilities. For example, Thailand has reported that its burgeoning medical travel trade is contributing to an internal brain drain of specialists away from its public hospitals, noting that a typical treatment for one foreign patient entails the same number of doctors as treatment for four to five Thai patients.[21,22] Despite claims to the contrary, the growth of a foreign-oriented trade in many countries does not assist in subsidizing access for poorer locals. Patients themselves question the ethics of differential access. As one chat room participant on conceiveonline.com asked in 2008: "Is it, well, ethical to take advantage of another country's health care system? And what about using an egg donor from a country where many people are poor? Is it opportunistic?"[2(p375)]

Little is known about the recruitment and experiences of gamete donors (especially ova donors) or surrogates involved in cross-border services. In many countries, we do not know who they are, how they are recruited, what screening or counseling they receive, how many times they donate or act as surrogates, or whether they are protected from risks.

Those risks include diminished fertility due to surgical procedures or ectopic pregnancies; and excessive ovarian stimulation, which can cause potentially fatal Ovarian Hyperstimulation Syndrome (OHSS). The primary ethical concern is that the growth in cross-border reproductive care is fueling a market for these body products and services, leading to the exploitation of poorer women's bodies and health. Commercial surrogacy and ova donation is banned in most European countries as well as Canada, Japan, and Australia, and a high demand exists for these body products and services. Studies suggest that even in developed countries in Europe and the Middle East, there can be a lack of transparency over the sources and circumstances under which ova are obtained. Patients may not realize that ova may be sourced and traded from clinics in other countries under conditions that may be less than ideal.[23] Unlike sperm donation, ova donation is an arduous and potentially risky medical procedure involving the use of follicle stimulating hormones and the surgical removal of ova. Attracted by the "compensation" payments offered, poorer women, students, and migrants from less-developed regions of Europe are undergoing the rigors of ova donation. Although they technically are not regarded as "commercial" transactions, there are concerns that given the economies in these women's home countries, the "compensation" offered in some cases is in effect a commercial incentive, and some women may not be made fully aware of the risks involved to their health and future fertility.

Likewise, surrogacy arrangements raise a number of issues. Commercial surrogacy is banned in most countries due to ethical concerns over the commodification of women's bodies and procreation. In such countries, surrogacy, if permitted, must be "altruistic"—that is, undertaken as a service with only limited compensation allowed. The difficulty in locating women willing to act as surrogates under these conditions motivates some couples to seek commercial arrangements in other countries. Commercial surrogacy is legal in some states in the United States and also occurs in some countries that have yet to regulate the practice. Commercial surrogacy is the only form of surrogacy permitted in India, where it is believed that a commercial arrangement is more likely to result in a fairer exchange for surrogacy. Even so, Indian surrogacy has become a focal point of concern because of the vast economic disparities in that country (see Box 8.3). In India, the women preferred by clinics for surrogacy tend to be very poor, illiterate women who are portrayed as having clear economic motives for undertaking surrogacy.[24,25] Some feminists question whether in situations of extreme poverty with few economic opportunities or alternate means of employment, women are able to make fully informed free choices to be commercial surrogates. They argue that the trade exploits both impoverished women and their clients.[19]

8.3 Indian Surrogates' Stories

Amrita Pande conducted interviews with 42 Indian surrogates in Anand from 2006 to 2008.[24] The surrogates were usually very poor women living below the poverty line and were encouraged by the clinics to view surrogacy as a gift because it was an opportunity to earn significant income. For example, in her work, she quotes Anjali, a 20-year-old surrogate and mother of two: "I am doing this basically for my daughters; both will be old enough to be sent to school next year. I want them to be educated, maybe become teachers or air hostesses? I don't want them to grow up and be like me—illiterate and desperate."[16]

A disturbing finding from Pande's work was that many of the surrogates interviewed at the time of her study had no formal contract with their contracting parents and were unsure about how much they were to receive. She cites another surrogate, Salma, as explaining: "We don't really have a contract. Will [the intended father] said, 'You make us happy, and we'll make you happy.' He said he would build a house for us—however big we want it to be. I am having twins so perhaps he will build us two rooms instead of one."[16]

The Assisted Reproductive Technologies (Regulation) Bill, introduced in 2010, ensures that formal, enforceable legal contracts exist between surrogates and contracting parents, and provides new protections for surrogates. These include setting the upper age limit for surrogates (who must be married with at least one child) to 35, allowing no more than five live births per woman, limiting the number of times a woman can undergo embryo transfer for the same couple, and forbidding clinics from sending Indian women abroad for surrogacy. Concerns remain, however, that this legislation does not provide enough protection.[26]

Although new legislation now governs surrogacy in India and offers some protections and limits on the number of times women can act as surrogates (see Box 8.3), studies in India have raised concerns about the conditions imposed upon surrogates. In some cases, clinics maintain strict anonymity with no contact between the surrogate and contracting parents (an approach that denies children any future knowledge of the birth mother or donor). Surrogates may be housed in clinic dormitories for the duration of their pregnancy, away from their families and own children, partly to protect them from the stigma attached, and partly to allow the clinic to closely monitor the pregnancy.[25] In a country with a high maternal mortality rate, acting as a surrogate increases a woman's risk of difficulties for her own subsequent pregnancies for which she will not receive the same level of care. In many cases, surrogates use the money they receive to buy a house, support a business, pay off debt, or pay for children's education or daughters' dowries. Although clinics often portray surrogacy as a "life-changing" economic opportunity for surrogates, even a form of development aid, one study of surrogates questions the long-term economic benefits for surrogates and their families[24] (See Box 8.3).

The most vulnerable surrogates and ova donors are those women who themselves travel across borders. These situations can involve two or more countries with conflicting laws and jurisdictional requirements, making it very difficult to regulate or provide any legal protections to those involved. For example, the media reported a case of a woman from the Philippines who traveled to Singapore to undergo intrauterine insemination (IUI) and act as an egg donor and surrogate for a gay Malaysian–Danish couple living in Thailand. A recent case in Thailand involving the trafficking of Vietnamese surrogates is an extreme example of exploitation of women involved in this trade.[27,28] A police raid in Bangkok revealed an alleged trafficking ring involving Vietnamese women used as surrogates in Thailand for Taiwanese couples through a Taiwanese company called Baby 101. Taiwanese law bans the use of surrogates. Thirteen women were arrested during the raid, and 2 more women were arrested later. Of the 15 women, 7 were pregnant. At the time of writing, police were still investigating the case, but media reports suggest that the women were held against their wills. The doctors involved may also face legal and disciplinary action if they are found to have knowledge of or to have benefited from trafficking.

The rights of the children produced from such procedures have been the subject of legal cases in a number of countries where the legal status of children born through international surrogacy arrangements have been questioned. One example was the highly publicized case of a baby girl "Manji," born to a surrogate mother in India who could not be adopted by her Japanese biological father after his wife divorced him. The divorced contracting mother refused to adopt the child, and the surrogate mother also refused to take custody. Under Indian law, a single man cannot adopt children. An Indian court eventually granted custody to the child's paternal grandmother in Japan.[29] Questions have also been raised concerning the rights of children to know about their biological parents and the lack of any information in the case of international anonymous ova donation.[19]

A further ethical question arises when people engage in cross-border reproductive care to avoid legal restrictions or regulations on procedures not allowed in their home countries. A number of countries, particularly in the developing world, have struggled to keep up with developments in assisted reproduction technologies; hence their legislation has left loopholes that form the basis for the services offered in those countries. Whether such "circumvention" travel to access services that are illegal in patients' home countries is ethical, and whether patients have a "right" to undertake such travel is hotly contested.[30] (For further discussion on "circumnavigation tourism," see chapter 10.) An example of this practice is Australians who travel overseas to pursue commercial surrogacy. As noted earlier, commercial surrogacy is banned in Australia. In addition, some states of Australia

(New South Wales and Queensland) have specifically banned residents of those states from arranging, facilitating, or undertaking commercial surrogacy overseas, although it is not clear how such legislation will be enforced. Similarly, Turkish law bans its citizens from pursuing third party donation overseas.[31] Such extraterritorial laws are still rare but point to attempts by some states to regulate cross-border reproductive travel.

Another controversial reproductive technology is sex selection of a child using technologies such as sperm sorting (such as MicroSort) or through the complex intervention of undertaking an IVF cycle and using preimplantation genetic diagnosis (in which cells from embryos are tested to select those embryos with desired sex chromosomes before they are implanted into a woman's uterus). Despite the fact that sex selection for purely social reasons is banned in most countries and is defined as sexist and gender discriminatory under a number of international conventions, it is legal in a limited number of jurisdictions, including some states of the United States, Jordan, and North Cyprus, and its availability heavily promoted on the Internet (see Box 8.4).[32]

8.4 Traveling for Nonmedical Sex Selection

Florence and Joaquim want a son together. They traveled to Thailand to undergo in vitro fertilization (IVF) and preimplantation genetic diagnosis (PGD) for sex selection. Until recently, Thailand had no regulation restricting nonmedical sex selection. They each have a son from previous marriages and have one daughter together. Florence (now 44 years old) dreams of having another one or two children despite her age and said if they had a son together, they will then marry. "I decided I will, everywhere, every year, I will continue to fight until I have one more kid" (Fieldnotes, January 2008).

Both are well-paid and well-traveled professionals (she is a geologist and he a computer engineer) with the resources to pursue their dream. As Florence put it: "it's a high new technology, even expensive, but if you want [it], you must do [it]; we decided to do it." Such treatment is not available in their home country in Africa. They had already traveled twice to South Africa four years ago for treatment, but it was unsuccessful. They wanted to try to undertake treatment in Dubai but found they could only get a visa there for 15 days, insufficient time to complete a cycle.

So they decided to try the clinic in Bangkok, which they found on the Internet. They located hotel accommodation from a list suggested by the clinic. Everything was arranged in advance for them to spend one month to complete one cycle: "we already booked the day to go home on 7th February, and we finish our treatment with everything, PGD, embryo transfer, on 1st of February."

Their two sons, daughter, and a niece came with them for a holiday although their children don't know about their treatment; they just tell them they have gone "shopping." Their treatment will cost them US$7,000, including all testing and drugs. They estimate the total cost is US$27,000 including all their airfares, accommodation, and treatment.

CONCLUSION

Reproductive travel is one of the more controversial forms of medical tourism. The expansion of the market in reproductive services has provided opportunities for many couples to access treatments and produce families, opportunities often denied to them by the inadequacies, costs, or discrimination within their own health systems. No one would deny the joy brought to many families through the children conceived internationally through these technologies. But the growing global circulation of patients, reproductive gametes, embryos, and surrogates poses regulatory challenges and ethical dilemmas. The growth of a global market in ova and surrogacy services presents opportunities for exploitation of disadvantaged women. The promotion of medical care across regulatory boundaries, with the Internet as the source of referrals and little legal protection, carries risks for vulnerable patients. Reproductive travel also may worsen inequalities within destination countries' health services by contributing to a brain drain of specialist medical staff away from public services. Fundamentally, the growth of cross-border reproductive care poses the question of how to balance individual reproductive autonomy with the need for international regulation to prevent undesired consequences. This requires weighing individuals' rights to travel in search of services to form families against the need to protect the rights and health of vulnerable groups also involved in this trade, including women who assist through their ova and gestational services, patients who may not be fully informed of their risks, and the children born of these arrangements. International accreditation standards of clinics involved in the trade might improve quality of care. Better information for prospective patients and greater requirements for transparency around the conditions under which donors and services are recruited would increase the likelihood that patients make informed choices. Countries could also reduce the demand for cross-border reproductive travel by devising strategies to overcome the factors contributing to such travel. For example, countries could consider implementing fair public funding for fertility treatments, improving local recruitment of gamete donors and surrogates, and improving the quality of care within local clinics.

There is still much that is not known about cross-border reproductive travel. Sensational media accounts of "reproductive tourism" do little to inform the public about the realities of treatment and stir up stereotyped and simplistic accounts of what is in reality a complex situation. A lack of data on people traveling for such care and their motivations, experiences, and outcomes as well as a lack of data on the experiences of those who assist them through ova donations or surrogacy limits the ability of policy makers to limit foreseeable harms and protect the reproductive rights and health of all concerned. There is little doubt that traveling to seek reproductive technologies will continue. Understanding cross-border reproductive travel requires understanding both the opportunities it represents as well as the bioethical dilemmas and risks it entails.

ACKNOWLEDGMENTS

This work draws upon research supported by an Australian Research Council Discovery Project funded by the Australian government.

REFERENCES

1. Inhorn M, Pascale P. Rethinking reproductive "tourism" as reproductive "exile." *Fertility and Sterility.* 2009;92(3):904–906.

2. Whittaker A, Speier A. "Cycling overseas": Care, commodification and stratification in cross-border reproductive travel. *Medical Anthropology.* 2010; 29(4):363–383.

3. Culley L, Hudson N, Blyth E, Norton W, et al. *Transnational reproduction: An exploratory study of UK residents who travel abroad for fertility treatment. Summary report.* Leicester: De Montfort University; June 2011.

4. Shenfield F, de Mouzon J, Pennings G, et al. Cross-border reproductive care in six European countries. *Human Reproduction.* 2010;25(6):1361–1368.

5. Hughes EG, Dejean D. Cross-border fertility services in North America: A survey of Canadian and American providers. *Fertility and Sterility* 2010;1 (June): e16–e19.

6. Bartolucci R. Cross-border reproductive care: Italy, a case example. *Human reproduction* 2008;23 (Supplement1; i88).

7. Pennings G, Autin C, Decleer W, Delbaere A, et al. Cross-border reproductive care in Belgium. *Human Reproduction.* 2009;24:3108–3118.

8. Blyth E, Farrand A. Reproductive tourism—a price worth paying for reproductive autonomy? *Critical Social Policy.* 2005;25(1):91–114.

9. Inhorn M, Shrivastav P. Globalization and reproductive tourism in the United Arab Emirates. *Asia-Pacific Journal of Public Health.* 2010;22:86S-74S.

10. Whittaker A. Global technologies and transnational reproduction in Thailand. *Asian Studies Review.* 2009;33:319–332.

11. Boivin J, Bunting L, Collins JA, Nygren KG. International estimates of infertility prevalence and treatment seeking: Potential need and demand for infertility medical care. *Human Reproduction.* 2007;22(6):1506–1512.

12. Sorenson C, Mladovsky, P. *Assisted reproduction technologies in Europe: An overview, research note. European Commission Directorate-General Employment, Social Affairs and Equal Opportunities, social and demographic analysis.* London: London School of Economics and Political Science; 2006.

13. International Federation of Fertility Societies (IFFS). *IFFS surveillance 2010:* International Federation of Fertility Societies; September 2010.

14. Inhorn M. *Local babies, global science: Gender, religion and in-vitro fertilization in Egypt.* New York: Routledge; 2003.

15. Hudson N, Culley L, Assisted reproductive travel: UK patient trajectories. *Reproductive. Biomedicine Online.* 2011;23:573–581.

16. Pande A. Transnational commercial surrogacy in India: Gifts for global sisters? *Reproductive Biomedicine Online.* 2011;23:618–625.

17. Collins J, Cook J. Cross-border reproductive care: Now and into the future. *Fertility & Sterility.* 2010;94(1):e25–e26.

18. Deech R. Reproductive tourism in Europe: Infertility and human rights. *Global Governance.* 2003;9(4):425.

19. Donchin A. Reproductive tourism and the quest for global gender justice *Bioethics.* 2010;24(7):323–332.

20. Shenfield F, Pennings G, de Mouzon J, Ferraretti A.P, Goossens V. ESHRE's good practice guide for cross-border reproductive care for centres and practitioners. *Human Reproduction.* 2011;26(7):1625–1627.

21. Na Ranong A, Na Ranong V. The effects of medical tourism: Thailand's experience. *Bulletin of the World Health Organization.* 2011;89:336–344.

22. Kanchanachitra C, Lindelow M, Johnston T, et al. Human resources for health in southeast Asia: Shortages, distributional challenges, and international trade in health services. *The Lancet.* 2011;377(9767):769–781.

23. Nahman M, "Reverse traffic": Intersecting inequalities in human egg "donation." *Reproductive Biomedicine Online.* 2011;23:626–633.

24. Pande A. *Commercial surrogate mothering in India: Nine months of labor?* PhD Thesis, Amherst, University of Massachusetts; 2009.

25. Vora K. Selling Potential: Surplus fertility and biocapital in the production of transnational Indian surrogacy. Paper presented at the American Anthropological Association 107th Annual meeting, November 19–23. San Francisco, 2008.

26. Qadeer I. Benefits and threats of international trade in health: A case of surrogacy in India. *Global Social Policy.* 2010;10:303–305.

27. Inthaket M. Police bust Taiwanese gang for "ensnaring" 13 women. *The Nation.* February 5, 2011.

28. Anon. Two surrogate mothers decide to keep their babies. *The Nation.* March 1, 2011.

29. Wade M. Warning to couples on Indian surrogacy laws. *The Age.* January 26, 2009.

30. Pennings G. Reproductive tourism as moral pluralism in motion. *Journal of Medical Ethics.* 2002;28(6):337.

31. Gürtin Z, Banning reproductive travel? Turkey's ART legislation and third-party assisted reproduction. *Reproductive Biomedicine Online.* 2011:23:555–564.

32. Whittaker A. Reproductive opportunists in the new global sex trade: PGD and non-medical sex selection. *Reproductive Biomedicine Online.* 2011;23:609–617.

Part III

Legal and Regulatory Questions

Chapter 9

Into the Void: The Legal Ambiguities of an Unregulated Medical Tourism Market

Nathan Cortez

An irony surrounds medical tourism. In the United States, health care is perhaps our most heavily regulated industry. We spend a great deal of time and energy calibrating (and recalibrating) the laws that govern hospitals, medical professionals, and health insurance, among many other things. We periodically agonize over health reform and wring our hands over new advances in the biosciences. In the United States, we use overlapping layers of federal, state, and local laws; agency regulations; court decisions; and even voluntary private codes of conduct that, together, govern virtually everyone and everything concerned with health care.

Yet medical tourism presently escapes most if not all of this oversight. When a patient travels to a foreign hospital—whether at the behest of an insurer, with the help of a facilitator, or simply on his or her own—the transaction largely occurs in a legal void. Swirling around in this void are vapors of various legal duties and standards that might apply, and one goal of this chapter is to examine these possibilities. But no one really knows which laws apply and when. These possibilities have not been tested by courts or explored by regulators.

As such, the medical tourism industry is characterized by pervasive legal uncertainty for all those involved. Given its cross-border dimensions, with transactions consummated in foreign jurisdictions, it is fair to say that medical tourism operates beyond our traditional regulatory system in the United States and even punctures our understanding of how to regulate health care.[1]

This chapter considers the legal ambiguities that medical tourism presents by addressing some of the most intriguing legal questions surrounding it. For example, could it be illegal for patients to leave the United States for health care? Can patients injured overseas sue in the United States if something goes wrong? If they cannot sue in the United States, can patients sue overseas? How might governments regulate medical tourism? If the U.S. government cannot regulate foreign hospitals and physicians, who can? Is it legal for insurers to ask patients to leave the country for care? And how will the U.S. health reform law affect the medical tourism market?

The unifying theme is that very few laws and regulations govern medical tourism, and this uncertainty creates legal risks for all the parties involved. Unfortunately, these risks are being shifted to perhaps the least sophisticated parties in these transactions—patients.

IS IT ILLEGAL FOR PATIENTS TO LEAVE THE UNITED STATES FOR HEALTH CARE?

Federal and state laws neither explicitly permit nor prohibit U.S. patients from leaving the country for medical care. Although medical tourism might trigger certain laws in unique situations, it is not immediately clear how these laws would apply. Moreover, whether a particular trip is illegal depends on a number of subsidiary questions, such as why the patient is traveling, to which country, and for which treatment.

Research on medical tourists shows they are far from monolithic.[2] Patients can have very different motivations for leaving the United States. For decades, patients have left the country for medical care without prohibition, mostly to seek treatments that are not accessible, for one reason or another, where they live. Today, patients leave for treatments that are banned by law, that are not approved by regulators, that are not offered by domestic hospitals or physicians, or that are not paid for by insurers.[3]

Legal scholars have not identified any laws that would prohibit price shoppers from seeking care elsewhere if they cannot afford it domestically. And it is hard to imagine policymakers objecting to such travel, assuming the treatments are lawful here in the United States. But it becomes murky when patients travel for treatments that are banned by law, or are not approved by U.S. regulators—what I. Glenn Cohen calls "circumvention tourism" (see chapter 10). For example, women in some countries travel for abortions when they are banned domestically, the classic cases being women from Ireland and other predominantly Catholic countries traveling to more permissive jurisdictions.[3]

There are other well-known permutations, such as cancer patients leaving the United States to take Laetrile in Mexico, as well as other examples of patients traveling for drugs not approved by the U.S. Food and Drug Administration (FDA).[4,5] Medical products and technologies used in the United States must be approved by the FDA, and some patients have left the country for treatments that the FDA either has delayed approving or rejected outright.[3] For example, when the FDA lagged behind its counterparts in Europe and Asia in approving a new hip resurfacing technology, U.S. patients traveled to those regions for it.[3] And when the FDA began prohibiting certain fertility treatments, patients simply found them elsewhere.[3] The FDA was virtually powerless to intervene because its jurisdiction is limited to medical products and the companies that produce them, not patients. (Contrast this to Congress, which is not powerless to intervene, and could probably ban such travel, per chapter 10.)

One could imagine a public health crisis—like a more dangerous, more transmissible version of SARS or the Swine Flu—prompting the U.S. Centers for Disease Control and Prevention (CDC) and the State Department to prohibit patients from traveling to certain countries. For example, the FDA has long been concerned about xenotransplantation—the practice of using animal parts and cells in humans therapeutically—based on the risk of transferring animal diseases to humans.[6] If such fears came to fruition outside the United States, these agencies could probably invoke their emergency powers to prevent such travel, even if it would be difficult to enforce. But aside from these nightmare scenarios, it is difficult to imagine price shoppers or even "forum shoppers" in search of more permissive regulatory environments being prohibited from seeking care overseas. As chapter 10 explains, it would take an act of Congress to ban such activities, and no such laws currently exist in the medical context.

CAN INJURED PATIENTS SUE IN THE UNITED STATES?

Another important but unanswered legal question is whether patients injured overseas can sue in U.S. courts. Medical errors are an unfortunate but persistent reality in all health care systems, including the United States. The medical and legal professions generally accept that despite best efforts, at least some minimum quantum of errors is an unavoidable consequence of modern medicine. Even the best hospitals staffed with the best medical professionals and the best technologies will make mistakes—a truth that holds equally for U.S and non-U.S. hospitals. Thus, even assuming that magnet hospitals in countries like India and Thailand can achieve outcomes that are equal to or better than U.S. hospitals—a disputed assertion, to be sure—there will still be errors that injure patients. Medical malpractice is a matter of *when*, not *if*. In such cases, can U.S. patients sue in U.S. courts for medical errors committed overseas?

Although current research has yet to identify any publicly reported court cases involving U.S. medical tourists, word-of-mouth reports have percolated among industry insiders, most of which suggest that the parties have settled out of court. Thus, we have yet to test whether U.S. medical tourists can successfully sue for medical negligence occurring in a foreign country. But many in the industry assume the answer is a qualified *no* and often urge patients to reconsider medical tourism if they are worried about their legal remedies. At least one government body, the United Kingdom's National Health Service (NHS), has advised outgoing British medical tourists that they must rely on the legal system of the host country to redress any grievances against foreign providers.[1, 7] In contrast, California specifically designed its state law that regulates cross-border insurance plans to avoid situations in which California residents would have to rely on Mexican courts.[7]

Ultimately, it remains entirely unclear whether U.S. patients can sue in U.S. courts for malpractice committed abroad. The most logical targets for lawsuits would be the foreign hospital or physician that caused the injury. But various procedural rules make it difficult to sue foreign providers here. These three sets of rules, deriving from the U.S. Constitution, the Federal Rules of Civil Procedure, and various judicial decisions interpreting them, require that U.S. courts (1) assert proper jurisdiction over the parties, (2) serve as an appropriate venue to resolve each dispute, and (3) select either domestic or foreign law to govern the conduct that gave rise to the lawsuit.

First, to be subject to the jurisdiction of a U.S. court, our laws require that the defendant have at least some minimum contacts with the state in which the court sits. This requires that the defendant either had some purposeful contacts with the state, or some substantial and ongoing connection with the state, such as a business license, regular visits, or some property ownership there. Most foreign hospitals and physicians would not satisfy either standard unless systematically targeted U.S. patients as customers—such as through a website interacting with U.S. customers via contracts with insurers or facilitators in that particular state, or possibly via other activities. State "long-arm" statutes also allow courts to reach out and assert jurisdiction over a party that transacts or sometimes even solicits business in that state.

One of the core principles animating these jurisdictional requirements is that out-of-state residents must have at least some minimum contacts with the state to be hauled into court there. A related notion is that foreign parties that purposefully avail themselves of the rights and benefits given to them by U.S. law also ought to be accountable in U.S. courts—a sort of symmetry between rights and obligations that attach to each state. Given these policies, U.S. courts might be reluctant to breach this symmetry and assert jurisdiction over foreign hospitals or physicians. Defendants must have some genuine contacts with the state in which the lawsuit is filed, which would make it difficult to sue most foreign providers in U.S. courts. Even foreign hospitals that are affiliated with U.S. institutions, like Harvard or Johns Hopkins, for example, structure their relationship in such a way to minimize potential liability for the U.S. affiliate.

A second procedural requirement for suing foreign parties in U.S. courts is that the court must be the proper "venue" for deciding that dispute. Courts can dismiss a case if it would excessively burden the defendant to appear in that court, and if there is an alternative court that can hear the case. In deciding whether to dismiss, courts typically balance the burdens to plaintiffs and defendants, as well as the public's interest in hearing such disputes in that state. For example, if the conduct giving rise to the suit occurred overseas and is thus governed by the law of that country, a U.S. court might dismiss the case. Courts have also dismissed cases when the defendant, the witnesses, and the evidence are located overseas.[7] In such cases, the law calls this an inconvenient forum (*forum non conveniens*). An important caveat for medical tourism lawsuits is that courts will dismiss cases even when the foreign jurisdiction provides very weak remedies by U.S. standards. It can be relatively easy for defendants to demonstrate that a foreign jurisdiction is an "adequate" alternative to U.S. courts, even if U.S. plaintiffs would scoff at the damage awards. This a real hurdle for medical tourists.

A third procedural hurdle for suing foreign providers in U.S. courts is winning the battle over which country's laws apply. Even if a U.S. court can properly assert jurisdiction and venue, the court might have to apply foreign law. If a Thai surgeon commits malpractice against a U.S. patient in a Thai hospital, will Thai or U.S. medical malpractice law govern? In deciding this "choice of law" question, courts will consider several factors, including where the injury occurred, where the actions that caused the injury occurred, where the parties reside and do business, and where the parties interacted with each other.[4] In medical tourism cases, courts are likely to apply the law of the country where the procedure took place. This makes a certain amount of sense: why should a Thai physician be held to U.S. legal standards when performing surgeries in Thailand? At the same time, if a Thai hospital markets itself to U.S. patients claiming that it meets U.S. quality standards, and patients therefore expect the hospital to meet those standards, a court might apply U.S. law. Also, if the Thai hospital contracts with U.S. insurers and facilitators, this might tempt a court to apply U.S. law, particularly if the contract stipulates that U.S. law applies.

This "choice of law" question can be paramount, because the laws governing personal injuries and medical malpractice in host countries can be much less friendly to patients than U.S. laws.[7]

In summary, it could be difficult—although certainly not impossible—for U.S. patients to resolve the jurisdiction, venue, and choice of law questions in their favor when trying to sue foreign providers in U.S. courts.

As an alternative, U.S. patients might try to sue a U.S.-based party, such as a medical tourism broker, or an employer or insurer that arranged the trip. Any U.S.-based parties in the so-called supply chain might be sued, because these defendants do not present the same problems with jurisdiction, venue, or choice of law as foreign defendants. Still, it might be difficult for patients to convince a court that these parties should be held responsible for injuries caused not by the parties themselves but by a foreign hospital or physician.

Lawyers and academics have sketched out possible legal claims that patients could assert against U.S.-based parties.[3,4,8,9] For example, a medical tourism facilitator might be liable for corporate negligence if it sent patients to foreign providers that it knew were unfit or incompetent. A facilitator might be liable if it misrepresented or exaggerated the quality of foreign providers—and anyone that has browsed facilitator websites knows this happens.[10] Facilitators and insurers might be liable for malpractice by a foreign provider if they worked closely enough with and exerted some control over the provider, although that would be unusual in medical tourism arrangements.

Health insurers could be liable to patients under some of these same legal theories, and might also be liable under laws that require certain types of insurers to make benefit decisions that protect their beneficiaries' interests without ulterior motives like saving money by outsourcing.[11] Each of these theories might be difficult for plaintiffs to sell convincingly. But they continue to float around in the legal fog that surrounds medical tourism.

Another layer of legal uncertainty for patients derives from the prophylactic measures that facilitators, employers, and insurers have taken to shield themselves from liability. Companies routinely ask medical tourists to sign or acknowledge legal waivers, disclaimers, and liability releases. These documents are often dense and intimidating for patients to understand, and most patients will not push back. These contracts often also require patients to limit the damages they can claim, resolve their disputes out of court, or resolve their disputes in a more hostile foreign jurisdiction.

In some respects this is fitting. If we are going to outsource health care, then it seems logical that we would also outsource any legal disputes that it generates.[7] On the other hand, even though it is not clear whether a court would enforce these contractual devices against patients, they shift much of the legal risk from employers, insurers, and medical tourism facilitators—all of whom profit or at least save money by outsourcing care—to patients, perhaps the least sophisticated and least knowledgeable parties in these transactions.

CAN INJURED PATIENTS SUE OVERSEAS?

If suing in the United States is not realistic, can patients seek recourse overseas? The medical tourism industry greatly prefers that patients resolve disputes outside the United States—and for good reason. Many host countries tend to be less hospitable, if not downright hostile, to medical malpractice suits. To date, the medical tourism literature has evaluated the legal systems of only four destinations: India, Thailand, Singapore, and Mexico.[7] This research finds that it is highly unlikely that U.S. patients will recover satisfactory compensation by our (admittedly high) domestic standards. The average medical malpractice payout in the United States, through both court judgments and settlements, is around $312,000.[7] In contrast, the average payout is only $2,500 in Thailand and $4,800 in Mexico. And anecdotal reports from India and Singapore show amounts that are also dwarfed by the U.S. payouts.[7]

There are many complicated reasons for such large discrepancies, including foreign laws not granting noneconomic damages like pain and suffering, and not awarding punitive damages, both of which can amplify U.S. recoveries in comparison. Thus, as purely a bottom-line calculus, medical tourists should understand what the industry already firmly grasps—damage awards in host countries will be paltry compared to those in U.S. courts.

Aside from these very different endgames, there are various practical obstacles to suing overseas. Patients will have to navigate a foreign legal system, most often in a foreign language. They may have to travel back periodically for court hearings and other proceedings. And they will have to overcome other home field advantages that domestic defendants may enjoy over foreign plaintiffs. In aggregate, these obstacles may make suing overseas not particularly worthwhile.

In addition to these general obstacles, each host country presents its own problems. For example, in India it can take upwards of 15, 20, or even 25 years to resolve a lawsuit.[7] For that reason, most malpractice plaintiffs prefer to sue in India's consumer dispute forums, or Consumer Dispute Redressal Agencies (CDRAs). But even these consumer forums, which were designed to be a quicker alternative to courts, can be difficult to navigate. There can be delays even with their truncated procedures. The forums are not well equipped to handle cases involving complex medical evidence, and sometimes transfer such cases to civil courts, where they can languish for years. Hospitals and physicians often refuse to provide patients with copies of their medical records, which makes it difficult for patients to prove what happened. And many patients cannot find a physician willing to testify on their behalf, which makes it extraordinarily difficult to prove that the treating physician did not provide reasonable care. For all these reasons, very few malpractice lawsuits are successful in India.

In Thailand, patients face some of the same problems, in addition to others.[7] Thai civil courts are not hospitable to medical malpractice claims, and patients do not achieve much when they file complaints with the Thai Medical Council, the Ministry of Public Health, or Thailand's Consumer Protection Agency.[7] The laws governing medical malpractice in Thailand are underdeveloped, with very few publications that lawyers, judges, and doctors might use for guidance. And as in India, Thai patients struggle to access their medical records, which makes it difficult to prove in court what happened. Thus, it is not surprising that very few patients in Thailand file formal complaints of any sort when injured.

Unlike India and Thailand, Singapore has both the resources and capacity to closely regulate its health care facilities and professionals. But patients suing for medical malpractice there face very similar obstacles to patients in India and Thailand. Patients in Singapore rarely sue their doctors, for a variety of reasons—damage awards are modest; finding a medical expert to testify is difficult; plaintiffs who lose their cases must pay the litigating expenses of the defendant; and Singapore does not allow lawyers to charge contingency fees, which means plaintiffs must be able to afford lawyers out of pocket, without waiting for an award or settlement.[7] And as in India, Singaporean courts can be overly deferential to medical experts. This often means that defendant physicians will not be held liable if they can muster even one expert who testifies that he or she was not negligent, despite convincing evidence to the contrary.[12] Putting all these together, Singapore can be just as hostile to medical malpractice suits as India or Thailand.

Mexico, the fourth legal system evaluated in the literature, paints just as bleak a picture for plaintiffs.[7] Its civil courts are inhospitable to medical malpractice complaints in many ways, and its legal system will be alien to U.S. patients. Mexican courts do not use juries and are not really bound by judicial precedents[13,14] (previous court decisions that establish legal principles or rules that courts must follow in similar cases, a hallmark of U.S. law). Thus, medical malpractice lawsuits are exceedingly rare in Mexico. Mexico does use a relatively workable system for arbitrating medical disputes, the National Commission for Medical Arbitration, known as "Conamed."[7,15] But the average recovery is only $4,800, largely because damages are calculated according to Mexico's outdated worker's compensation formula.[7,13] Very few U.S. patients would find this adequate.

Other host countries not yet explored are likely to present similar challenges to plaintiffs. In evaluating these countries, it is important to appreciate some of the deeper cultural contributors that make foreign jurisdictions so much different from our own. In the four jurisdictions above, there seems to be both a general reluctance to challenge medical authority and an aversion to using U.S.-style adversarial litigation to resolve disputes. In fact, in each of the four jurisdictions above, there have been concerns that there is a looming malpractice litigation crisis that will drive away doctors and threaten to close hospitals. The evidence does not really support these doomsday concerns, which in some cases are based on U.S. statistics rather than on statistics from the countries that are allegedly facing these crises. The evidence also suggests that patients treated in these countries are often deterred from filing legitimate complaints.

For all these reasons, medical tourists should understand what the industry already does—host countries will not provide remotely adequate forums for resolving malpractice disputes.

HOW MIGHT GOVERNMENTS REGULATE MEDICAL TOURISM?

Short of banning medical tourism (see chapter 10), is there a way to regulate it? Federal and state governments in the United States have largely ignored medical tourism to date. At the federal level, Congress has not considered a single bill that would address it. In 2006, a U.S. Senate committee held hearings on medical tourism, featuring testimony from various interests.[16] But the hearings were not associated with any bills and did not generate any legislative action.

At the state level, only two states have passed laws addressing a narrow aspect of medical tourism—cross-border health insurance that covers at least some care abroad. California passed a law in 1998 legalizing cross-border health insurance plans with Mexican providers. The law was designed to introduce legal standards to the underground market for cross-border plans in Southern California.[17] In the following years, other border states considered similar frameworks, including Texas. But in 2007, the Texas state legislature changed course and banned insurance plans that require or encourage patients to leave the country for medical care.[18] The legislative history to the law cited concerns with hospitals in Thailand and other faraway locales, but the law is widely understood to be a protectionist effort to shield Texas physicians from competition from less expensive Mexican providers. Two other states—West Virginia and Colorado—have considered bills that would have given state public employees financial incentives to have high-cost surgeries overseas, but none have passed. Thus, in every state aside from California and Texas, and for every other type of medical tourism arrangement, there are no laws and regulations that clearly govern these transactions.

Of course, our state and federal governments certainly are not novices at regulating health care. And there is an endless variety of legal tools and techniques they might use to regulate medical tourism. Legal academics have identified several possibilities here, including mechanisms that:

- generate more and better information about foreign providers;
- steer patients to higher-quality providers;
- reallocate the legal risks between parties, or alter the legal rules that apply;
- require prescreening and postoperative care domestically;
- ban unfair practices and arrangements;
- harmonize quality standards across countries;
- leverage insurance reimbursement for meeting quality goals;
- use free trade agreements to impose standards; and
- provide comprehensive regulatory oversight by an administrative agency.[1,3,4,7,8,9]

None of these proposals has come to pass, but they all remain possibilities if the government does intervene.

Meanwhile, various nongovernmental groups have tried to fill the regulatory void and introduce standards to the industry. Several groups have created international hospital accreditation schemes, which in theory can help assure that foreign hospitals meet at least some minimum quality standards. Trade groups like the Medical Tourism Association (MTA) have created a program to certify medical tourism facilitators based on various criteria. Even the American Medical Association (AMA), which represents U.S. physicians and has no direct involvement with the medical tourism industry, introduced its own guidelines that ask companies to observe nine principles.[19]

Aside from these pseudo-regulatory stopgaps, legal academics have also identified analogues that might serve as models for regulating medical tourism. For example, the U.S. Department of Defense's health insurance program for overseas military personnel (TRICARE Overseas) shows how regulators can identify high-quality foreign providers, encourage contractors to meet various standards, and even monitor fraud and abuse.[3] TRICARE certifies foreign providers into its provider network and uses regional networks to locate specialty care.

The European Union's experience with what it calls "patient mobility" is both instructive and inapposite. Various EU laws and opinions by the European Court of Justice require member states to allow their citizens to travel to other member states for medical care, subject to certain limitations. The EU's experience is instructive because after struggling with patient mobility for several years, European legislators in February 2011 passed a comprehensive law addressing it, including various provisions that protect patients.[20] But the EU experience is also inapposite because the United States cannot similarly rely on supranational institutions like the European Union to pass laws beyond its territorial jurisdiction.

CAN ANYONE REGULATE FOREIGN HOSPITALS AND PHYSICIANS?

If U.S. regulators cannot reach foreign hospitals and physicians, who can? Regulators in host countries obviously have jurisdiction over their domestic providers, but they have little incentive to spend their scarce resources imposing additional regulatory burdens on them, particularly for the benefit of foreign patients. Is there a way for U.S.-based institutions to impose standards or exert any regulatory pressures on foreign providers?

Fortunately, there is. Nongovernment groups can leverage access to U.S. markets to require foreign providers to meet U.S.-based standards. The best example is international hospital accreditation. Accreditors in the United States, the United Kingdom, and Australia, among others, offer international accreditation to foreign hospitals, which can signal that the hospitals meet internationally recognized quality standards. For example, Joint Commission International (JCI) is the international division of the Joint Commission, which itself accredits U.S. hospitals on behalf of Medicare.[21] JCI has accredited hundreds of foreign hospitals, most of which have aspirations of attracting foreign patients. Accreditation is based on a JCI investigation that determines whether the hospital meets six broad "International Patient Safety Goals" and dozens of corresponding standards and criteria. Once accredited, hospitals readily advertise their JCI status to foreign patients. Because of the Joint Commission's official responsibilities with Medicare, JCI accreditation can carry with it the imprimatur of the U.S. government, via a sort of misplaced transitive theory of accreditation.

Although accreditation is entirely voluntary, it has become a de facto industry standard, which has made it an avenue of private regulation. Hospitals that attract medical tourists have significant reputational incentives to comply with these standards. A loss of accreditation could be catastrophic to the hospital's efforts to attract foreign clients, possibly even jeopardizing contracts that require accreditation as a condition of doing business. Thus, hundreds of foreign hospitals now meet international quality standards, not because they are required to by "hard" law that is enforced through legal sanctions, but because competitive pressures have made it a sort of de facto requirement or "soft" law. For further discussion of accreditation, see chapter 11.

A second but far less successful example of filling the regulatory void is the certification program by the MTA. The MTA is the major trade association for the medical tourism industry, claiming as its members hospitals, clinics, facilitators, insurers, and other businesses. It claims to operate five different certification programs: one each for facilitators, international patient departments, hotel and hospitality organizations, travel and tour operators, and global spas.[22] Like international hospital accreditation, the MTA's certification program tries to introduce some standards in an otherwise unregulated market. The MTA's goal is to create "best practices" for facilitators and ensure that they meet basic standards, although it is unclear precisely what these standards are or how the certification program will enforce them.[7] Still, by introducing standards, the program ostensibly tries to protect patient interests, as well as generate credibility (and presumably a competitive advantage) for facilitators. It is not clear how many entities have been certified in each of the five programs, but the MTA's website lists only four facilitators that have been certified and one in progress.[22] Dozens if not hundreds of facilitators seem to have chosen to forego voluntary certification, which means the certification program remains more a theoretical possibility for providing standards than a reality.

A third example of nonbinding standards trying to fill the regulatory void is the guidelines published by the AMA, the largest physicians' organization in the United States. In 2008, the AMA published guidelines that call for "employers, insurance companies, and other entities that facilitate or incentivize medical care outside the U.S." to adhere to various standards, most of which revolve around patient rights and safety.[7,19] For example, the guidelines say that patients should be informed about the risks of traveling for surgery and the legal recourse available to them. The AMA also says that patients should have access to information about the physicians and hospitals that treat them. Again, no one is bound by these guidelines, and they are not enforceable in any legal sense, except to the extent they are adopted voluntarily by contract.

Each of these quasi-regulatory standards has its shortcomings. As "soft" law standards and best practices, none are legally enforceable. All suffer from potential conflicts of interest, or at least self-interest by the standard setters. JCI is paid significant fees by the hospitals it accredits, many of whom also pay JCI consultants additional fees to help them pass inspections. JCI's parent organization has been criticized in the United States for similar problems, including its track record of accrediting virtually every applicant and revoking virtually no accreditations once granted.[23] The MTA's certification program is susceptible to similar criticisms. And the AMA's guidelines could be interpreted by the skeptic as nothing more than protectionist interference from a domestic physician lobby that wants to discourage foreign competition.

Thus, in the absence of robust regulation by host countries, various voluntary standards, best practices, and guidelines have emerged. Though these can be poor alternatives to more traditional, legally enforceable requirements, they are probably better than nothing. For patients, there is some assurance that standards might govern these transactions. For foreign providers, these standards also reduce the legal uncertainty.

Treating foreign patients presents unique challenges. Physicians cannot physically examine patients until they arrive. Postoperative, follow-up care is possible only for a short time. Foreign patients can underestimate how long it will take to recover from surgery when making travel arrangements. Departing patients make it difficult to track outcomes more than superficially. Providers cannot always be certain that patients will get the necessary follow-up care after they leave.[3] Foreign providers should welcome these private standards, as they help legitimize the industry and differentiate credible providers from noncredible ones.

IS IT LEGAL FOR INSURERS TO ASK PATIENTS TO LEAVE THE COUNTRY FOR CARE?

Like others in the medical tourism industry, health insurers have ventured into the legal void. Nearly every species of insurer—including HMOs, PPOs, and self-insured employer plans—has experimented with medical tourism. Some plans give beneficiaries financial incentives to have expensive surgeries overseas. Some have added select foreign hospitals to their provider networks. And some have created genuine cross-border plans with more extensive medical tourism components. There are seemingly endless permutations.[4,24] Plans can use positive incentives (like lowering premiums or waiving deductibles for overseas care) or negative incentives (like charging higher premiums or higher deductibles for domestic care). As I. Glenn Cohen astutely observes, it can be hard to distinguish positive from negative incentives if there is enough money at stake, and both forms can be coercive.[4]

Some insurers have been more adventurous than others. Indeed, some have yet to send a single patient overseas, instead using the plans as leverage to negotiate lower prices domestically. Either way, these experiments buck the long-standing tradition that health insurance is generally nonportable—meaning it does not cover care outside the country except perhaps in emergencies, when a traveler needs unplanned care.[25] For that reason, very few state or federal laws that govern health insurance even contemplate portable plans.

Between public and private insurers in the United States, public insurers have been much less inclined to experiment with portable insurance. Among the public insurers, Medicare will pay for treatment outside the United States only if it is an emergency, or only if a non-U.S. hospital is more accessible to a U.S. resident, circumstances that very rarely apply.[3] For federal programs like Medicare and Medicaid, any experiments with overseas coverage beyond these narrow parameters would probably require Congress to pass a law specifically allowing it. David Warner has argued convincingly that Medicare should extend coverage to Mexico for American retirees, but acknowledges the legal and practical impediments to doing so.[26] Politically, it is hard to imagine a proposal that would better galvanize U.S. providers than the threat of using public funds to pay for overseas competitors. As such, it remains highly unlikely that federal programs will experiment with medical tourism.

States have been slightly less reluctant. Two states have considered bills that would encourage state public employees to go overseas for surgery. A well-publicized bill that died in the West Virginia legislature would have given public employees various financial incentives to have surgery overseas, at hospitals accredited by JCI.[27] The Colorado legislature contemplated a similar proposal,[28] which also was not seriously considered. In West Virginia's case, the bill's sponsor was trying to make a political point that U.S. hospitals and physicians, by far the world's most expensive, should have to compete with low-cost foreign providers. So as with federal programs, it seems highly unlikely that states would experiment with medical tourism.

Private insurers have been much more adventurous. And as I note above, only Texas and California have laws that directly address private, cross-border plans. Texas bans HMOs and other state-regulated insurers from requiring beneficiaries to go overseas, or from offering financial incentives to do so; California allows cross-border plans that contract with providers in Mexico, subject to various requirements.[17,18]

Other than these two laws, no state laws directly address cross-border insurance plans or even medical tourism more broadly. And it is unclear whether *existing* state laws focused on traditional domestic plans might clash incidentally with cross-border plans. For example, state regulations sometimes require that HMOs and other insurers that use provider networks to contract with providers that are accessible within certain geographic distances, which would functionally bar cross-border plans. Given the volume and variety of state insurance regulation, it is possible that cross-border plans could be barred incidentally in several states. This does not mean that state regulators would necessarily enforce these laws against cross-border plans. But anyone wishing to challenge cross-border plans being offered in their state might be able to find ammunition in existing laws that do not even contemplate medical tourism.

Another breed of health insurance is largely immune from state laws, and it is these plans that have experimented the most with medical tourism. Plans offered under the Employee Retirement Income Security Act (ERISA) are self-funded plans that are typically offered by larger employers or industrial or professional organizations. So-called ERISA plans are subject to very little state regulation (pursuant to ERISA provisions that preempt state requirements), which gives them flexibility to experiment with medical tourism. For example, the Western Growers Association (WGA) offers self-funded ERISA plans to immigrant agricultural workers, largely in California and the Southwest. The WGA allows beneficiaries to add "riders" to their plans that allow them to seek care in Mexico. The WGA offers several types of cross-border plans, relying on its contracts with primary care and specialty providers in both Mexico and the United States. Thus, if cross-border plans are attacked via state laws, they are largely immune to such attacks if structured as self-funded ERISA plans.

Thus, it is unclear whether it is unlawful for insurers to ask patients to travel overseas for care. There are virtually no federal laws that confront this question directly and only two state laws that do. Although many state regulations might bar cross-border plans by implication, without even contemplating medical tourism, self-insured plans structured under ERISA are not similarly constrained. Nevertheless, if cross-border plans become more prominent, it would not be surprising to see domestic providers unite to ban such plans, as they did in Texas.

HOW WILL U.S. HEALTH REFORM AFFECT MEDICAL TOURISM?

This last question might be the most intriguing and the most important for the industry's long-term prospects: How will landmark health reform in the United States affect medical tourism? In 2010, Congress passed the Patient Protection and Affordable Care Act,[29] the most important new health law since the Social Security Act Amendments created Medicare and Medicaid in 1965. This new law (which was being challenged on constitutional grounds at the time of this writing; see endnote) will affect the entire health care industry, including its cross-border elements.

Like other laws, the Affordable Care Act does not address medical tourism directly. But it includes many provisions that might affect the medical tourism market incidentally. If the law survives the current constitutional challenges, by far its most significant impact on medical tourism will be reducing the number of uninsured. The Congressional Budget Office predicted that the Act would reduce the number of uninsured by 31 million over the next decade, from 54 million to 23 million.[30] An obvious concern for the industry is whether reducing the number of uninsured would also reduce the number of patients who would consider leaving the country for care. Will there indeed be 31 million fewer potential customers for the medical tourism industry?

It is difficult to make any firm predictions here for a few reasons. The medical tourism market is notoriously opaque—we have no firm sense of how many patients leave the United States, where they go, or for what procedures. Many popular estimates are not particularly reliable. More-over, we are still in the initial phases of implementing the Affordable Care Act. Its many pilot programs, demonstration projects, and other experiments may make much more or much less of a difference than we expect—if the law survives.

That said, we do have a good sense of the following. Roughly 50 million U.S. residents will remain uninsured until 2014, when several major provisions in the Affordable Care Act are scheduled to be implemented. In 2014, the number of uninsured should drop from 50 million to roughly 31 million, largely due to expanding Medicaid enrollment and the availability of individual and small group insurance plans through new state exchanges. After 2014, the number of uninsured is expected to drop at a slower pace, until it settles at around 21–23 million over the next several years. So the medical tourism industry might be comforted to know that the Affordable Care Act is not expected to shrink the number of uninsured by half overnight.

At the same time, not everyone who is uninsured is a candidate for medical tourism. A report for the Robert Wood Johnson Foundation evaluated the different populations that would remain uninsured after the Act was fully implemented,[31] and this shows with more granularity who might travel post-reform. Of the 23 million who are expected to remain uninsured, around 4 million are children or elderly and thus less likely to travel, leaving 19 million. Of this 19 million, roughly 7 million will be eligible for Medicaid but not enrolled. This population is also unlikely to travel, because to be eligible for Medicaid, you must earn less than 138 percent of the Federal Poverty Line. The report found the average annual income to be only $3,000 for this group, which is not enough to afford even low-cost foreign care.

The remaining 12 million uninsured can be divided into four groups. The first is a group of 3 million that will be exempt from the Act's individual mandate to maintain health coverage, because there are no affordable plans where they live. The average age for this group is 51, and the average family income is $31,000—which still may not be enough to afford overseas care, unless border state residents travel to Mexico and thus spend less on travel.

The second group consists of 1.4 million uninsured who will also be exempt from the mandate but who qualify for federal subsidies to buy insurance in the new state insurance exchanges. It is not clear if this group would be more or less likely to travel for care. The average income is slightly higher, roughly $36,000, and the average age much lower, at 33. Their younger age and slightly higher income might make them more likely to travel, but they could probably purchase subsidized plans in the new state exchanges more cheaply than overseas care.

The third group seems markedly more likely to travel. It consists of 2.8 million who are not exempt from the individual mandate but who are expected to elect to remain uninsured and thus pay a modest tax penalty. The average age in this group is 43, and the average income is significantly higher, at roughly $66,000. This population may be the most likely to travel.

The fourth group is probably the largest group likely to leave the United States for care. It consists of 4.5 million undocumented immigrants, who by design will remain uninsured despite the Affordable Care Act, which expressly limits insurance coverage and subsidies to those lawfully present. Undocumented immigrants probably have the biggest motivations to travel but face two obstacles—first, they might be reluctant to leave the United States and risk problems at reentry, and second, their average income is only $18,000. However, if this population traveled to Mexico and Central America rather than Asia, it might not be cost prohibitive.

Thus, although it is hard to predict precisely how the Affordable Care Act might affect the pool of medical tourism candidates, it is safe to say that it is likely to shrink the number of uninsured who might travel.

But will *insured* patients travel post-reform? This depends on two questions—whether cross-border insurance will satisfy the individual mandate (again, assuming the mandate survives constitutional challenge) and whether such plans will be allowed to be sold in the state exchanges. On the first question, the Act requires almost all U.S. residents to maintain "minimum essential coverage" or pay a tax penalty. The Act does not define what minimum coverage entails, except by referencing existing public and private plans. So although it is possible that cross-border plans would not qualify as "minimum essential coverage" as government agencies further define it through regulation, nothing in the bill presently disqualifies such plans.

On the second question, there is also nothing in the Affordable Care Act that would prohibit insurers from selling cross-border plans in the state insurance exchanges. Congress created the state exchanges so individuals and small groups could purchase insurance in an open, competitive market. Plans offered in the exchanges must meet various requirements, some of which would not conflict with cross-border plans but some of which might.

Thus, insurers might still find it worthwhile to offer low-cost cross-border insurance after health reform, and U.S. residents might be able to use these plans to satisfy the new individual mandate. Again, nothing in the Act contemplates cross-border plans or medical tourism. There are several other provisions in the Act that might conflict with cross-border plans, but there are at least as many provisions that encourage flexibility and innovation, which might pave the way for medical tourism experiments by private insurers. For example, states like California, Arizona, and New Mexico could use these provisions to authorize private cross-border plans targeted at border residents. The Affordable Care Act includes numerous pilot programs, demonstrations, and waivers that encourage insurers to experiment with insurance coverage. But again, at the time of publication, the Act's constitutionality was very much in question.

All of this makes it difficult to say with much confidence what the medical tourism market will look like in 10 years. The legal void may very well remain.

CONCLUSION

Medical tourism was incubated in a legal and regulatory void, where it largely remains. Very few laws address or even contemplate medical tourism, and lawyers and academics are uncertain how laws that target other activities might incidentally affect it. This creates legal uncertainty for the medical tourism industry, which has tried to shift most of these risks to patients through contractual waivers, disclaimers, and other legal devices. This chapter discusses some the most intriguing legal ambiguities in the medical tourism market, each of which has generated significant articles or books on its own.

And there are many other legal ambiguities that this chapter does not address. For example, is the industry susceptible to laws that prohibit unfair and deceptive trade practices, given its aggressive promotion?[3] Do medical tourism facilitators violate anti-kickback laws by accepting referral fees from foreign hospitals?[32] Will medical tourism insurance fill the legal void and protect patients from the risks of overseas surgery?[33] What are the legal implications of outsourcing ancillary medical services?[34] Do free trade agreements create legal obligations for countries that send or receive patients?[35] And how should host countries that spend resources attracting foreign patients and perhaps subsidizing private hospitals address the concerns of local patients?[36] A growing body of scholarship is evaluating these questions, trying to identify possible sources of law that might govern. But in the meantime, medical tourism will continue to operate in a legal void.

NOTE

At the time of publication, the U.S. Supreme Court was considering constitutional challenges to the Affordable Care Act. The court heard oral arguments in a very rare three-day session in March 2012, during which it contemplated the constitutionality of several key reforms in the Act. An opinion by the court is expected in June 2012. The three related cases being decided by the court are *National Federation of Independent Business, et al. v. Sebelius* (11-393), *Department of Health and Human Services, et al. v. Florida* (11-398), and *Florida v. Department of Health and Human Services* (11-400).

REFERENCES

1. Terry NP. Under-regulated health care phenomena in a flat world: Medical tourism and outsourcing. *Western New England Law Review.* 2007; 29: 415–463.

2. Glinos I, Baeten R, Helbe M, Maarse H. A typology of cross-border patient mobility. *Health & Place.* 2010; 16: 1145–1155.

3. Cortez N. Patients without borders: The emerging global market for patients and the evolution of modern health care. *Indiana Law Journal.* 2008; 83: 71–132.

4. Cohen IG. Protecting patients with passports: Medical tourism and the patient-protective argument. *Iowa Law Review.* 2010; 95: 1467–1567.

5. Cohen IG. Medical tourism: The view from ten thousand feet. *The Hastings Center Report.* March–April 2010: 11–12.

6. Food & Drug Administration. Guidance for industry: Source animal, product, preclinical, and clinical issues concerning the use of xenotransplantation products in humans. http://www.fda.gov/BiologicsBloodVaccines/GuidanceComplianceRegulatoryInformation/Guidances/Xenotransplantation/ucm074354.htm. Accessed July 14, 2011.

7. Cortez N. Recalibrating the legal risks of cross-border health care. *Yale Journal of Health Policy, Law, & Ethics.* 2010; 10: 1–89.

8. Mirrer-Singer P. Medical malpractice overseas: The legal uncertainty surrounding medical tourism. *Law and Contemporary Problems.* 2007; 70: 211–232.

9. Howze K. Medical tourism: Symptom or cure? *Georgia Law Review.* 2007; 41: 1013–1052.

10. Lunt N., Carrera P. Systematic review of web sites for prospective medical tourists. *Tourism Review.* 2011; 66: 57–67.

11. Brady CJ. Offshore gambling: Medical outsourcing versus ERISA's fiduciary duty requirement. *Washington & Lee Law Review.* 2007; 64: 1073–1114.

12. Amirthalingam K. Judging doctors and diagnosing the law: *Bolam* rules in Singapore and Malaysia. *Singapore Journal of Legal Studies.* 2003: 125–146.

13. Vargas JA. Mexican law and personal injury cases: An increasingly prominent area for U.S. legal practitioners and judges. *San Diego International Law Journal.* 2007; 8: 475–522.

14. Vargas JA. Tort law in Mexico. In Vargas JA, ed. *Mexican Law: A Treatise for Legal Practitioners and International Investors.* Eagan, MN: West Group; 1998: § 21.5.

15. Comisión Nacional de Arbitraje Médico (Conamed). http://www.conamed.gob.mx/index.php. Accessed July 14, 2011.

16. U.S. Senate. The globalization of health care: Can medical tourism reduce health care costs?, Hearing 109–659 before the Special Committee on Aging. 109th Congress. June 27, 2006.

17. California Health & Safety Code, §§ 1345, 1351.2.

18. Texas Insurance Code Annotated, article 1216.004.

19. American Medical Association. New AMA guidelines on medical tourism. http://www.ama-assn.org/ama1/pub/upload/mm/31/medicaltourism.pdf. Accessed July 14, 2011.

20. European Union. Directive of the European Parliament and of the Council on the Application of Patients' Rights in Cross-Border Healthcare. February 21, 2011.

21. Joint Commission International. About Joint Commission International. http://www.jointcommissioninternational.org/about-jci/. Accessed July 14, 2011.

22. Medical Tourism Association. Certification programs. http://www.medi caltourismassociation.com/en/certification.html. Accessed July 14, 2011.

23. Jost TS, Medicare and the Joint Commission on Accreditation of Health-care Organizations: A healthy relationship? *Law & Contemporary Problems.* 1994; 57: 39–40.

24. Cortez N. Embracing the new geography of health care: A novel way to cover those left out of health reform. *Southern California Law Review.* 2011; 84: 857–929.

25. Mattoo A, Rathindran R. How health insurance inhibits trade in health care. *Health Affairs.* 2006; 25: 358–368.

26. Warner DC. Medicare in Mexico: Innovating for fairness and cost savings. *A Report by Policy Research Project on Medicare in Mexico,* Lyndon B. Johnson School of Public Affairs, University of Texas, Policy Research Project Report No. 156; 2007.

27. H.B. 4359, 77th Leg., 2d Sess. (West Virginia, 2006).

28. H.B. 07–1143, 66th General Assembly, 1st Regular Session (Colorado, 2007).

29. Patient Protection and Affordable Care Act, Public Law No. 111–148, as amended by the Health Care and Education Reconciliation Act, Public Law No. 111–152 (2010).

30. Letter from Douglas W. Elmendorf, Director of Congressional Budget Of-fice, to Nancy Pelosi, Speaker of the U.S. House of Representatives, March 20, 2010.

31. Buettgens M, Hall MA. Who will be uninsured after health insurance re-form? Robert Wood Johnson Foundation, March 2011.

32. Spece RG. Medical tourism: Protecting patients from conflicts of interest in broker's fees paid by foreign providers. *Journal of Health & Biomedical Law.* 2010; 6: 1–36.

33. International Medical Travel Journal, Medical Tourism Insurance. http:// www.imtj.com/marketplace/medical-tourism-insurance/. Accessed July 14, 2011.

34. McLean TR. The offshoring of American medicine: Scope, economic issues, and legal liabilities. *Annals of Health Law.* 2005; 14: 205–266.

35. World Health Organization. Summary Report, Workshop on the Movement of Patients Across International Borders: Emerging Challenges and Opportunities for Health Care Systems. February 24–25, 2009.

36. Pasquale F. Access to medicine in an era of fractal inequality. *Annals of Health Law.* 2010; 19: 269–310.

Chapter 10

Medical Outlaws or Medical Refugees?: An Examination of Circumvention Tourism

I. Glenn Cohen

While many medical tourists are motivated to travel by the price of service, the ability to jump queues, or greater expertise of a foreign provider, there is also a very different kind of medical tourism afoot in the world today that I call "circumvention tourism"—travel to access services that are *legal* in the receiving country but *illegal* in the patient's sending country, thereby circumventing a domestic prohibition on the service.

Consider the following four examples of circumvention medical tourism:

- Susan is a 50-year-old-woman diagnosed with Lou Gehrig's disease, which typically results in death within three years of diagnosis due to the wasting of respiratory muscles. Before death ensues, patients with the disease face difficulty with speech, chewing, and swallowing. Susan is unable to end her own life. Because assisted suicide is illegal in her home state of Connecticut, her brother Jon helps her travel to Switzerland where a clinic assists her in ending her life. Upon his return to Connecticut, can the state prosecute Jon for assisting Susan's suicide? Should it be able to do so? Does the answer change if the federal government was the one to undertake the prosecution?

- Andrea, a 21-year-old Irish woman, experiences an unwanted pregnancy. Abortion is illegal in Ireland. She therefore travels by boat to Women on Waves, a floating abortion clinic anchored in international waters off the coast of Ireland. Ships in international waters are governed by the law of the country whose flag they fly, and this ship flies the flag of the Netherlands, where abortion is legal. Nevertheless, on Andrea's return to Dublin, the Irish government initiates criminal process against her. Can the Irish government do so? Should it be able to do so?[1]

- Jason and his partner Jonathan are frustrated by the difficulty of securing a surrogate in their sending country of Canada, where paid surrogacy is criminalized. They turn to a clinic in the village of Anand, in India, where the practice is legal. Can Canada prosecute the couple? Should Canada be able to do so?[2]

- Nawal is a two-year-old U.S. citizen whose parents, both now U.S. citizens, emigrated from the Sudan 20 years earlier and gave up their Sudanese citizenship. The family now lives in a largely Sudanese American community in Baltimore, Maryland. Nawal's grandparents have pressured her parents to have female genital cutting (FGC) performed on Nawal. Performing the procedure is illegal in the United States,[3] so Nawal's parents take her to Sudan, where a local doctor legally performs the surgery. Could the United States close this loophole by applying the criminal prohibition to her parents for their acts abroad? Should it do so?

This chapter examines these and other questions pertaining to circumvention tourism. Part One further describes these four case studies of circumvention tourism: abortion, assisted suicide, female genital cutting of minors, and reproductive technology. Part Two describes sending countries' powers under international law to criminalize the activities of their citizens abroad to prevent circumvention tourism. Part Three examines the question of when home countries should try to do this.

PART ONE: FOUR CASE STUDIES

Abortion

Medical tourism can be used to circumvent domestic criminal prohibitions on abortion, an issue that West Germany wrestled with before reunification and that Ireland, Poland, and Portugal face even today.[4]

The West German law, paragraph 218 of the Criminal Code, made abortion a criminal offense unless the mother's health was in danger, or in cases involving "(1) pregnancies which result from criminal activity, (2) an 'incurable defect' in the unborn child and (3) overall poor social conditions which would adversely affect pregnancy," although "incurable defect" and "overall poor social conditions" were not defined.[1] The paragraph 218 criminal prohibition extended extraterritorially to reach abortions by citizens done abroad unless women received a *Beratungsschein,* or a certificate from a West German doctor, in advance.[5] In order to enforce the law against circumvention abroad, German customs officials performed gynecological examinations on women reentering West Germany (in one case prompted by a nightgown and a brochure for a Dutch abortion clinic spotted in the woman's car) that could result in penalties of up to three years of imprisonment if the authorities detected an illegal abortion.[5,6] Since reunification, with a more liberal set of abortion laws currently in place, German abortion tourism appears to have decreased.[7]

Ireland's difficulties with abortion tourism stem from its electorate's September 1983 adoption of the Eighth Amendment to the Irish Constitution, now codified in Article 40.3.3, which provides that "[t]he State acknowledges the right to life of the unborn and, with due regard to the equal right to life of the mother, guarantees in its laws to respect, and, as far as practicable, by its laws to defend and vindicate that right."[1(p394),8]

In *Attorney General v. X* (the "X Case"), a 14-year-old rape victim sought to travel to England to obtain an abortion, but when the victim's family contacted the Irish police to ask about how to properly collect DNA evidence during the procedure to assist with the rape prosecution, the attorney general petitioned for an injunction to prevent the travel. The patient argued that her life was at stake because the prospect of giving birth under the circumstances made her suicidal, and thus abortion was permissible under Article 40.3.3's provision for "due regard to the equal right to life of the mother." However, the High Court found that the prospect of suicide did not qualify as a threat to the mother's life and so enjoined the trip. The Supreme Court ultimately reversed on the grounds that suicide was a threat to the mother's life but did not say that the trip would have been permissible in the absence of a life-threatening condition.[1,9]

In response to the X Case and the fear that the European Court of Justice and European Court of Human Rights would rule against the Irish abortion law, the Irish people passed the Thirteenth Amendment (often called the "Travel Amendment"), which provides that Article 40.3.3 "shall not limit freedom to travel between the State and another state."[1(p412),8] However, subsequent case law and commentary leave unclear whether the state has the power to enjoin travel of Irish citizens seeking abortion outside the narrow case of threat to the mother's life (including suicide risk).[1,10] Ireland also has tried to control counselor and physician speech regarding the possibility of abortion outside of the country, which has given rise to a separate line of cases.

Before *Roe v. Wade*,[11] at least one U.S. case considered the application of domestic criminal law prohibitions to abortions performed outside of the United States.[12] *People v. Buffum* involved a Long Beach, California, doctor who arranged for an associate to transport pregnant women to Tijuana, Mexico, where an abortion was performed by another individual.[13] The court ultimately reversed a conviction under California criminal law on the ground that the "statute makes no reference to the place of performance of an abortion, and we must assume that the Legislature did not intend to regulate conduct taking place outside the borders of the state," while noting that the prosecution had not advanced a theory that the defendant conspired *in California* to violate *Mexican* abortion law.[13(p320)]

Assisted Suicide

Medical travel for assisted suicide, including physician-assisted suicide, has consisted mainly of travel to Switzerland. While other countries permit assisted suicide, only Switzerland permits it without requiring the user to be a resident. The most well-known legal cases involving assisted suicide tourism emanate from the United Kingdom in the 2000s. Among those is the case of Diane Pretty, who suffered from motor neuron disease, a degenerative illness that rendered her increasingly debilitated. She sought confirmation from the Director of Public Prosecution (DPP) that her husband would not face prosecution were he to assist her to commit suicide by accompanying her to a Swiss suicide clinic.[14,15] The relevant criminal offense fell under the Suicide Act of 1961, which stated that "[a] person who aids, abets, counsels or procures the suicide of another, or an attempt by another to commit suicide, shall be liable on conviction on indictment to imprisonment for a term not exceeding fourteen years."[16]

When the DPP refused the confirmation, Pretty argued before the House of Lords and then before the European Court of Human Rights (ECHR) that her rights under Article 8 of the European Convention of respect for private and family life were being infringed.[17] Both courts rejected her claim.[17] The Lords held that Article 8 did not include the right to control one's own death, while the ECHR found that any infringement of Article 8 could be justified as necessary to protect the interests of the state in preventing terminally ill people from being taken advantage of by those with an interest in encouraging their suicide. The ECHR also found that a blanket ban was not disproportionate to the aim of public protection because the DPP retained considerable flexibility in his prosecutorial decisions.

The most recent case involved Deborah Purdy, a multiple sclerosis sufferer who anticipated a time when she would want to end her life. She applied to the High Court seeking an order that the DPP issue a guidance clarifying that her husband would not face charges under the Suicide Act if he assisted her to travel to Switzerland to die.[18] The High Court refused to make the order, noting the prior decision in *Pretty*, at which point Purdy took her case to the House of Lords. The Lords upheld the criminal prohibition on assisted suicide, but found a problem of fair warning and consistency of application under Article 8 of the European Convention in the inadequacy of the Code for Crown Prosecutors, which outlines the principles under which prosecutors exercise their discretion. They found it problematic that an individual assisting a loved one with his or her suicide could not adequately determine from the Code before acting whether prosecutorial discretion would be exercised in favor or against the individual's prosecution. In response to the decision, in 2010 the DPP issued final guidelines listing 16 factors in favor of and 6 against prosecution.[15] Irish authorities have also recently indicated an intention to crack down on their citizens' use of assisted suicide in Switzerland.[19]

Female Genital Cutting

Female genital cutting (FGC), also referred to as female genital mutilation or female circumcision, is a surgical procedure involving the "partial or total removal of the external female genitalia or other injury to the female genital organs for non-medical reasons."[20] The World Health Organization (WHO) estimates that between 100 million and 140 million currently living women and girls worldwide have undergone FGC. The WHO divides FGC into four types from most to least invasive. These include "[t]ype 2 Excision: partial or total removal of the clitoris and the labia minora, with or without excision of the labia majora" and "[t]ype 3: Infibulation: narrowing of the vaginal opening through the creation of a covering seal . . . formed by cutting and repositioning the inner, or outer, labia, with or without removal of the clitoris."[20]

The WHO notes that FGC "has no health benefits" and states that its immediate complications include "severe pain, shock, hemorrhage (bleeding), tetanus or sepsis (bacterial infection), urine retention, open sores in the genital region and injury to nearby genital tissue," and long-term consequences include "recurrent bladder and urinary tract infections; cysts; infertility; . . . increased risk of childbirth complications and newborn deaths" and the need for later surgeries, for example the "procedure that seals or narrows a vaginal opening (type 3 above) needs to be cut open later to allow for sexual intercourse and childbirth."[20]

Motivations for performing FGC have been described as social pressure to conform to community norms about cleanliness, beauty, femininity, virginity, and constraining premarital female libido, along with some disputed claims that it is required by some variants of Islam. For the purposes of this chapter, I will take the facts as stated by the WHO as given, but I note that even in the medical community there are dissenting voices about whether FGC has long-term reproductive health consequences[21] or interferes with sexual activity.[22] A study by Nawal Nour and her associates at the Brigham and Women's Hospital in Boston, based on 2000 U.S. Census data, suggested that 44,500 women under age 18 and 165,000 women over age 18 living in the United States were "at risk" for FGC, with California, New York, and Maryland having the most female immigrants and refugees from countries where FGC is prevalent.[23]

In 1996, the United States criminalized the action of anyone who "knowingly circumcises, excises, or infibulates the whole or any part of the labia majora or labia minora or clitoris of another person who has not attained the age of 18 years," with a punishment of up to five years in prison.[24] The statute exempts cases where FGC is medically necessary.[25] The statute also makes clear that in applying the health exception, "no account shall be taken of the effect on the person on whom the operation is to be performed of any belief on the part of that person, or any other person, that the operation is required as a matter of custom or ritual."[26] Although the statute has been in place for 15 years, it has apparently given rise to only one prosecution: in 2006, 30-year-old Ethiopian immigrant Khalid Adem was successfully prosecuted for performing genital cutting on his 2-year-old daughter in Georgia and sentenced to 10 years in prison.[27,28] Because it has not been interpreted to apply extraterritorially (i.e., outside the territorial borders of the sending country), the statute allows citizen parents to take their daughter to another country for FGC and then return to the United States. I am not aware of any reliable statistics regarding how many U.S. parents use medical tourism to circumvent the FGC prohibition, although those in the field have suggested the problem is not insignificant among some communities.[29]

In contrast to the U.S. law, the United Kingdom's Female Genital Mutilation Act of 2003 makes it an offense for UK nationals or permanent residents to carry out female genital mutilation abroad, or to aid, abet, counsel, or procure the carrying out of female genital mutilation abroad, even in countries where the practice is legal, with penalties ranging from 5 to 14 years imprisonment.[30,31] Sweden also criminalizes the activity extraterritorially, and Canada, New Zealand, and the Australian state of Victoria make it a crime to arrange for a child to be taken out of the sending country in order to procure FGC.[32]

In April 2010, Congressman Dennis Crowley and Congresswoman Mary Bono Mack introduced the "Girls Protection Act of 2010" seeking to extend the existing U.S. prohibition of FGC extraterritorially.[33] It has yet to become law.

Reproductive Technologies

Many countries (or their states or provinces) limit or ban certain Assisted Reproductive Technologies (ARTs). Italy's Law 40 confines use of reproductive technologies to infertile women of "potentially fertile age" who are married or part of a "stable" heterosexual couple and prohibits the use of donated sperm or egg.[34] The Australian states of Western Australia, South Australia, and Victoria have all enacted similar legislation forbidding access to ARTs by lesbian, gay, bisexual, transgender, and single individuals and permitting use only where "the reason for infertility is not age."[34] Greece and Japan also restrict access to ARTs to women 50 or younger. Egypt, Iran, Kuwait, Jordan, Lebanon, Morocco, Qatar, Turkey, Indonesia, Malaysia, and Pakistan ban all forms of sperm or egg donation.[35] Austria, Germany, Switzerland, the Australian States of Victoria and Western Australia, the Netherlands, Norway, and most recently New Zealand and the United Kingdom prohibit anonymous sperm donation. Britain, Canada, and the Australian states of Victoria and New South Wales have banned or limited compensation for egg and sperm donation beyond expenses incurred. Canada, the Australian states of Victoria, New South, Wales, and Western Australia have made commercial surrogacy a crime, as have the U.S. states of New York, Michigan, Washington, and the District of Columbia, with Louisiana, Maryland, Nebraska, New Mexico, and Oregon rendering commercial surrogacy contracts unenforceable. Britain de facto prohibits commercial surrogacy by forbidding the transfer of parentage rights absent a showing of "no financial or other beneficial consideration in exchange."[34] The French Civil Code states "all agreements relating to procreation or gestation on account of a third party are void," imposes a penalty of up to 10 years and a fine of €150,000 (US$201,150) for violating that law, and grants the surrogate automatic parental rights over the resulting child.[36] This list is far from exhaustive.

These restrictions have prompted significant amounts of medical tourism. Major destinations for these services include Australia, Canada, Germany, India, Israel, South Africa, and the United States. There are also "niche markets": Romania, Ukraine, and the United States are common destinations to obtain ethnically Caucasian sperm or eggs, while Jewish couples often travel to Israel to access procedures that comply with Jewish law.[37]

Efforts to circumvent domestic prohibitions also influence receiving country choice. Denmark, which permits anonymous sperm provision, attracts patients from nearby Sweden, Finland, Norway, and the Netherlands, which prohibit the practice. Because they permit payment for sperm and egg donors, Spain and Romania attract patients from many Western European countries where compensation is banned or limited, and Taiwan attracts patients from China and Japan for the same reason.

Some patients will go to Belgium, Finland, Greece, India, or the United States: destination countries where sex selection is not illegal.[34] India and California have become popular destinations for surrogacy because they permit commercial surrogacy and enforce surrogacy contracts.[38] Over all of this, price hangs as an additional consideration.[39]

The Akanksha Infertility Clinic, centered in the village of Anand, India, run by Doctor Nanya Patel and featured on the *Oprah Winfrey Show,* gives a good sense of surrogacy tourism today.[2,40] The clinic only employs women who have been married and have had at least one child. In 2008, there were 45 surrogates on the payroll, who lived away from their families in a compound, which one author described as "a classroom-size space . . . dominated by a maze of iron cots that spills out into a hallway." Surrogates receive $50 a month, plus $500 at the end of each trimester, and the balance upon delivery. A successful Akanksha surrogate makes between $5,000 and $6,000 (slightly more if she bears twins), an amount that exceeds a typical salary for several years of ordinary labor in India. If a woman miscarries, she keeps what she has been paid up to that point. If she chooses to abort—an option the contract allows—she must reimburse the clinic and the client for all expenses. The clinic charged American medical tourists $15,000 to $20,000 for the entire process, including in vitro fertilization (IVF), somewhere between a third and a fifth of what clients would pay for a similar service in the United States. As in the United States, the surrogate receives roughly a quarter of the total fees the couple pays to the provider. There have been reports that the Ankansha clinic routinely implants five or more embryos at a time, considerably more than the one or two implanted embryos recommended by the American Society for Reproductive Medicine. Under guidelines issued by the Indian Council of Medical Research, surrogate mothers sign away their rights to any children, and the surrogate's name is not even put on the birth certificate. (For further discussion of reproductive travel and surrogate mothers, see chapter 8.)

Despite the rampant circumvention of domestic prohibitions on reproductive technology through medical tourism, the vast majority of countries have not taken steps to deter it. The exceptions are notable. In March 2010, Turkey extended its domestic criminal prohibition on reproducing with donor sperm or egg (other than from a spouse) to apply to activities by its citizens abroad, such that a Turkish woman inseminated with donor sperm in the United States could face up to three years in prison.[41] In 2004, Italy announced that it would prosecute doctors who referred patients abroad for prohibited reproductive technology services.[42] Two Australian states have also made it a crime for their citizens to undertake commercial surrogacy overseas, with penalties of up to two years of imprisonment and fines of $275,000.[43]

France has also extended its criminal prohibition to citizens who travel abroad to use surrogacy services, and has used its family law provisions declaring who is the legal parent in children born through surrogacy as a further deterrent.[34] French courts have nullified U.S. declarations of parenthood and refused to recognize adoption orders in cases arising out of circumvention tourism for commercial surrogacy in California and Minnesota; in one case, a court denied the commissioning parents any possibility of ever adopting the children.[34,44] Japan and the United Kingdom have also had controversial cases where immigration was initially denied to children born to surrogates abroad.[45,46]

PART TWO: SENDING COUNTRIES' POWER TO CRIMINALIZE CIRCUMVENTION MEDICAL TOURISM UNDER INTERNATIONAL LAW

In this section, I show that international law will permit sending countries to criminalize the circumvention tourism of their citizens in these cases but does not require them to do so. That said, it is worth emphasizing that even if international law forbade it, the United States or other countries could simply violate international law in this respect.[47] There is also a separate question of whether, independent of international law, domestic (and, in the case of the European Union, supranational) law obligates, forbids, or gives the sending country discretion to criminalize the circumvention tourism of its citizens. This analysis can only be done on a country-by-country basis, a task I will not undertake in this short space.

Before I set out this analysis, I should be a bit more specific about the question I am seeking to answer. First, my focus is on the extraterritorial application of *criminal* law and not, for example, tort or contract law or even administrative regulatory requirements that are not administered by the criminal justice system. As I explain in greater depth in the next section, on both communitarian and social contractarian political theories, there is a special role accorded to criminal law as the judgment of the community, making extraterritorial application more justified.

Second, although I will speak of "citizens" going forward, I intend to restrict my analysis to cases where the citizen against whom the sending country seeks to apply its criminal law is also its domiciliary, and not living in the receiving country (or another country)—thus excluding the case of an expatriate. I will thus put to one side less clear cases that do not seem like true circumvention tourism—for example, a country that continues to claim an individual as its citizen by her blood relation to prior "full" citizens, even though the individual has never lived there or had other significant ties.

Third, I am only interested in cases where the activity is prohibited by criminal law in the citizen's sending country but *not* in the receiving country, such that circumvention is possible. Thus, I leave for other work cases of medical tourism for services illegal in both the sending and receiving country but with lax enforcement regimes in the receiving country, most notably organ sale tourism.

Fourth, my focus is on "jurisdiction to prescribe" or "prescriptive jurisdiction," which involves the power to render a particular offense criminal, for example, to make it a crime in Ireland for an Irish citizen to engage in an abortion in the Netherlands.[48,49] It is to be contrasted with "enforcement jurisdiction," for example, the ability of Ireland in that circumstance to violate Dutch sovereignty and march in to the Netherlands to arrest the citizen for a crime made illegal by Irish criminal law. Even when a country has and exercises its power to prescribe, it typically does not have jurisdiction to enforce and instead relies on extradition processes to get the offender back into its sovereign territory and custody. Sometimes, these two jurisdictions are further contrasted with "jurisdiction to adjudicate" or "curial jurisdiction," involving the right of courts to try and receive cases referred to them.[48]

It is commonplace under existing international law doctrines for a country to have prescriptive jurisdiction to declare an extraterritorial activity of its citizen a crime under its domestic law but not jurisdiction to enforce the law by arresting its citizen *in the foreign country*. Because many patients intend to return to their sending countries after engaging in prohibited activities, prescriptive jurisdiction unaccompanied by enforcement jurisdiction remains an important tool for deterring and punishing circumvention medical tourism. While detection of and the ability to prove extraterritorial circumvention will be imperfect, as the historical cases that I discussed above show, many countries have been able to detect, deter, and punish these violations. The difficulties are not uniform across all my case studies. Detecting and proving abortion tourism seems the most difficult, whereas the other cases seem easier: family and immigration law involving the return of new children from abroad will more likely ferret out circumvention reproductive technology. The fact that a frail individual never returns from a trip abroad may alert the sending country to assisted suicide in the receiving country. Later visits to sending country physicians will reveal that FGC has been performed on a minor, and physician reporting requirements for child abuse can alert authorities that the law has been violated either at home or abroad. In any event, through the so-called expressive function of law, criminalizing these acts may have additional force in discouraging them notwithstanding these difficulties.

While, for reasons I will discuss, the sending country is likely to have the power to criminalize the circumvention tourism of its citizens in the case studies I have been discussing, its power to criminalize the activity of receiving country citizens—for example, the doctors who perform abortions—is much less certain.

Bases for Prescriptive Jurisdiction

Under customary international law, prescriptive jurisdiction may be premised on several possible bases. For some sending countries under some interpretations of some existing human rights treaties, the FGC case may be different in that there may be some obligation to criminalize FGC abroad, though I think the weight of authority is to the contrary.[50] Because I limit this chapter to cases where the "perpetrator" is a sending country citizen who has engaged in medical tourism to skirt the domestic prohibition, all my case studies fall comfortably within the "National Principle" basis for prescriptive jurisdiction—permitting a state to assert jurisdiction over the acts of its citizens wherever they take place.[48,51,52] Citizenship or nationality of a person might be the result of birth in the country or to a parent who is a citizen, or the result of naturalization.[48,49] As a leading treatise observes, "[f]or practical purposes . . . States remain free to decide who their nationals are," while flagging potential exceptions that prove the rule such as "[t]he mass imposition of nationality upon unwilling people, or nationality obtained by fraud or corruption."[49(p347)] While for my cases the National Principle would be enough, there are other possible bases of jurisdiction, some of which would be needed if the country criminalized the activities of its citizens—the topic of this chapter—*and* sought to criminalize the activities of receiving country citizen providers.

"Subjective territorial jurisdiction" comprehends crimes that are initiated in one's home territory but completed in another territory, such as loading a bomb in the United States onto a plane that will explode in Israel.[49,51,52] This basis may apply in our cases when referrals to foreign physicians are involved; or when much of the planning and arrangements are done on home soil; or when some of the activity begins in the sending country, such as hormone treatments for in vitro fertilization that will ultimately be performed abroad.[54]

"Objective territorial jurisdiction" refers to the opposite case, a crime initiated abroad but completed in one's home territory.[49,51,52] Some countries, most notably the United States, have sought to extend this jurisdiction through an "effects doctrine," especially asserting antitrust jurisdiction against non-U.S. companies based on acts done entirely outside the United States that had economic repercussions for the price of a commodity in the United States.[49,55,56] Perhaps prescriptive jurisdiction could be premised on this basis in some of our cases as well—for example, the children born through prohibited reproductive technology usage will return to the sending country to be reared, or girls on whom FGC is performed may incur medical or psychological expenses in the sending country, etc.

A third basis, "passive personality," represents the flipside of the National Principle, in that jurisdiction is asserted based on the fact that the *victim* (rather than perpetrator) is a national of the sending country. The principle is controversial, and a leading treatise suggests that its increased acceptance is category specific: while it is "widely tolerated when used to prosecute terrorists" it is far from clear that it would be found "acceptable if used to prosecute, for example, adulterers and defamers."[49] Passive personality may be used to justify extending extraterritorially sanctions on assisting suicide or FGC, based on the theory that it protects the sending country citizen whose life is ended or minor whose genitals are cut. Relying on passive personality in the abortion case would be more controversial and depend on treating the fetus as a citizen, a matter on which there is no established precedent. I return to a parallel issue on the normative side in Part Three.

While there are other bases of prescriptive jurisdiction, such as "universal jurisdiction" and the "protective principle," neither seems likely to apply to medical circumvention tourism.

Limitations on Jurisdiction to Prescribe

Notwithstanding the presence of a basis for prescriptive jurisdiction, as the *Restatement (Third) of Foreign Relations Law* cautions, "a state may not exercise jurisdiction to prescribe law with respect to a person or activity having connections with another state when the exercise of such jurisdiction is unreasonable."[51(s403)] The Restatement then suggests that whether jurisdiction is unreasonable should be determined by "evaluating all relevant factors, including," (thus not exhaustively) "where appropriate" a set of eight factors.[51(s403)]

Although the outcome of any multifactor highly standard-like test is hard to predict, in each of my case studies there is a strong argument that jurisdiction is reasonable. I explain factor by factor:

1. "The link of the activity to the territory of the regulating state, i.e., the extent to which the activity takes place within the territory, or has substantial, direct, and foreseeable effect upon or in the territory": While the health care activity takes place out of the United States, abortions and assisted suicide result in one fewer member of society being born or staying alive. Reproductive technology access will result in an additional citizen being born, and certain practices such as allowing multiple gestation or older mothers may produce children that are severely premature, or suffer from genetic abnormalities that cause externalities upon the family's return to the sending country. In a case from Canada, 60-year-old Canadian Ranjit Hayer traveled to her native India when Canadian doctors refused to provide her access to IVF. She returned to Canada and delivered twins seven weeks premature who required intensive neonatal care, and

she needed to have her uterus removed, with all costs incurred by the provincial health care system.[57] All these seem like "substantial, direct, and foreseeable" effects on the sending country. The same is true of the medical and psychological needs of girls who have FGC performed on them as minors.

2. "The connections, such as nationality, residence, or economic activity, between the regulating state and the person principally responsible for the activity to be regulated, or between that state and those whom the regulation is designed to protect": In all these cases, the "perpetrator" is a citizen, and for most (the abortion case is more controversial) at least one "victim" is a sending country citizen.

3. "The character of the activity to be regulated, the importance of regulation to the regulating state, the extent to which other states regulate such activities, and the degree to which the desirability of such regulation is generally accepted": Creating and ending life are activities that are highly important to and heavily regulated by most countries, as suggested by the case studies above. How "desirabl[e]" such regulation would be is, of course, in the eyes of the beholding country, but even regimes that are relatively permissive with regard to abortion or assisted suicide typically regulate things like timing, information provision, age of consent, mental competency evaluation, waiting periods, etc. Similarly, the U.S. approach to FGC invokes the deeply imbued tradition of U.S. family law and child protection law that "[t]he state appropriately steps in, as parens patriae protector of the welfare of these non-autonomous persons, to act in their behalf, choosing for them."[58(p411)] Moreover, through S-CHIP, Medicaid, or other means, the state may bear some of the future medical costs associated with FGC.

4. "The existence of justified expectations that might be protected or hurt by the regulation": Given that the activity is illegal at home, the circumventing patient is unlikely to have justified expectations in accessing the service. Perhaps the receiving country medical tourism sector might claim its expectations in patient flow from that country were justified, but with the possible exception of the reproductive technology industry in destination countries, it seems unlikely that circumvention medical tourism is a significant share of that sector's total business. I discuss a related point on the normative side in the next section.

5. "The importance of the regulation to the international political, legal, or economic system": It is unclear what this means in our cases, but for FGC, the fact that many international treaties condemn it may suggest regulating it is important to the international legal system.

6. "The extent to which the regulation is consistent with the traditions of the international system": The application of this factor to our cases is also not obvious. There certainly have been other instances where the international system has allowed sending countries to criminalize the activities of their citizens in destination countries where the practice is legal. Jeffrey Meyer has provided an illustrative list of the numerous instances where the United States has criminalized extra-territorial conduct on the basis of its citizens' activity as well as lists of crimes that are "geoambiguous" in their scope.[59] For example, the U.S. PROTECT Act levies either a fine or 30 years in prison or both for any U.S. citizen or permanent resident "who travels in foreign commerce, and engages in any illicit sexual conduct" including "any commercial sex act . . . with a person under 18 years of age."[60]

7. "The extent to which another state may have an interest in regulating the activity," and

8. "The likelihood of conflict with regulation by another state": Of all the factors, these two seem the most likely basis for arguing against reasonableness, but the argument does not seem strong. This chapter is only about criminalization of the conduct of the sending country citizen, not a receiving country doctor or other provider, which somewhat dilutes the interest of the receiving country. Moreover, these conflicts can largely be avoided by adopting the solution that countries other than Switzerland have used regarding assisted suicide: a requirement that the person seeking to use the service be a resident of the receiving country. (To be more precise, it is possible that a U.S. citizen becomes a resident of Switzerland and thus qualifies under the Swiss rule. This would involve a case of split domicile of the kind that I am bracketing for the purpose of my discussion here.) Unlike the extraterritorial extension of a country's antitrust or fair labor standards, these cases entail minimal interference with the existing practice in the receiving country—one need not remake competition policy or wage and hour regulation in the receiving country; the industry can persist as is; it merely becomes inaccessible to foreigners.

The reproductive technology case seems slightly harder in this regard, in that it is plausible that the receiving country receives significant economic benefit from circumvention tourism and that foreign patients secure higher wages for the doctors in the industry, which some contend helps counteract physician brain drain.[61] Still, given the extent to which the other factors favor reasonableness, this contrary fact seems insufficient even with regard to reproductive technologies. One useful point of comparison is the PROTECT Act covering child sex tourism, which has been upheld as consonant with both U.S. and international law by several U.S. Circuit Courts.[62]

Thus, I conclude that criminalizing circumvention tourism will not run afoul of the balancing approach of the Restatement. That conclusion follows still more easily under U.S. Supreme Court jurisprudence, which has, at times, suggested a move away from the balancing approach to comity toward an even more permissive test.[63] In sum, this analysis shows that existing doctrinal international law will *permit* sending countries to apply extraterritorially the criminalization of abortion, assisted suicide, FDC, reproductive technology use, and similar prohibitions should they so decide. It neither forbids nor mandates sending countries from doing so.

PART THREE: WHEN SHOULD SENDING COUNTRIES CRIMINALIZE CIRCUMVENTION MEDICAL TOURISM?

Having established that under international law, sending countries have discretion to criminalize many forms of circumvention tourism, the question is whether they should do so. This is complicated terrain, which I have written about more in depth elsewhere,[50] and here I can only briefly scratch the surface.

Let us bracket for present purposes the question of whether the sending country's own domestic prohibition is itself justified—for example, whether Ireland is justified in banning abortion within its territory. If we assume for the sake of argument that it is justified, what do we need to consider in determining whether the sending country ought to apply that same prohibition extraterritorially to its citizens engaged in circumvention tourism? Deciding whether states should criminalize circumvention tourism requires taking a position on two very large questions.

The first question is the meaning of citizenship and whether, on either communitarian or social contractarian theories of the state's power to punish, the territorial location of the conduct and the fact that the conduct is not prohibited under the law of the foreign sovereign matters. One way of putting the point is whether we see the sovereignty of the sending country and its power to make people answer to it through criminal law as extending primarily based on territoriality (the presence in the territorial boundaries of the sending country), or citizenship (the ties of being a citizen of the sending country), or both. The more citizenship is thought of as a justifiable basis for the sovereign to exercise its criminal jurisdiction, the less problematic criminalizing circumvention tourism becomes. Additionally, in analogy to the "effects test" under international law discussed above, the more the sending country will face significant externalized costs from the activity (for example in the case of multiple embryo transfer), the stronger its interest in applying its law abroad.

On the other side of the ledger, one needs to develop a way of weighing the receiving country's interest in enabling the circumvention tourist to engage in the domestically prohibited activity within its territory. This interest might be economic, as in fertility tourism where the commerce of circumvention tourism could be a substantial boon to the economy. The receiving country's interest might also be more moralistic—the desire to serve as a refuge for those governed by what the receiving country views as unjust laws at home. Because a sending country's criminalization of the conduct of its own citizens abroad is minimally disruptive to the receiving country—the provision of services by receiving country citizen doctors and the design of its health care system is otherwise unaffected—it is easier to justify on this score than, for example, criminalizing the activity of receiving citizen physicians who provide the service.

Second, one must examine a constellation of questions that might go under the heading of "cost of Exit," "accommodation," and "cultural defense." Circumvention tourism offers the citizen a middle ground between the political theoretical diptych of being bound by the domestic law, or Exit—the renunciation of one's citizenship and presence in the sending country. We can think of it as a kind of "Exit Light," where the Citizen need only temporarily leave the territorial boundaries of the country in order to avoid its criminal laws. Guido Pennings has been the most staunch proponent of this approach in relation to abortion or assisted suicide, claiming that "a certain norm is applicable and applied in society as wanted by the majority while simultaneously the members of the minority can still act according to their moral views by going abroad," and suggests that "[a]llowing people to look abroad demonstrates the absolute minimum of respect for their moral autonomy."[64(p340)] Circumvention tourism thus becomes a kind of modus vivendi, which "prevents a frontal clash of opinions, which may jeopardise social peace."[64 (p340)] In the case of something like FGC with strong religious or cultural origins, we can also see this as a kind of accommodation to "cultural defender" claims by minority groups within the society.[65]

At the same time, this position is not without its problems. First, it would result in a kind of masking of what some might think of as an instance of murder or child abuse, where we allow ourselves to avoid confronting it by making sure it happens outside our view. Second, the accommodation privilege seems to be distributed in a morally arbitrary way in that it tracks whether the individual can afford to travel to the receiving country at the right time. If we were serious about accommodation, the argument might go, we in theory should instead hold a lottery for all those who wanted to receive the service in the sending country and grant them a fixed number of "permits," or at least pay for the expense of traveling abroad for those who want to circumvent. If we are uncomfortable with such suggestions, this may suggest there is also something wrong with this form of accommodation. Finally, when the interest is preventing harm to someone who has not meaningfully consented (e.g., a fetus, a child), it seems irrelevant to the "victim" that the actual injury took place outside of the territory; it is still a sending country citizen who has been harmed by another sending country citizen, and in most of these cases this is a "victim" that is not in the receiving country voluntarily.

The push and pull of these considerations cannot be resolved in a domain-general way. Instead, as I have suggested in other work,[50] it should be evaluated in light of the reasons that underlie the sending country's domestic prohibition along with a determination of who the "victim" is. On communitarian and social contractarian grounds, the permissibility (and indeed perhaps obligation) of the sending country to criminalize the activities of its citizens engaged in circumvention tourism is at its zenith when there is what I call a "double coincidence of citizenship"—when both the "perpetrator" and "victim" are citizens of the same sending country that has a domestic prohibition in place that would criminalize the act. In such cases, the sending country can only excuse the perpetrator–citizen from criminal liability if it forces the victim–citizen to forego the protection of its criminal law. Extraterritorial criminalization is particularly appropriate when the "victim's" presence in the receiving country is not voluntary in a meaningful sense: this is certainly the case with abortion and, given the infancy of the "victim," FGC. For reproductive technology, it depends on a specification of who the "victim" is, and for assisted suicide on whether the sending country is willing to accept consent to the act as negating its criminality. Putting these two criteria together—type of justification and victim citizenship—can help us sort through the four case studies above.

Where the justification for the domestic prohibition is preventing serious bodily harm, and the "victim" is also a sending country citizen—fetuses in abortion, or children in FGC, for example, and on some accounts some reproductive technology use (although I am somewhat skeptical about this claim[34]), the state has very good reasons to extend its prohibition extraterritorially, and the claim for accommodation is at its weakest. This is because under criminal law theory, the sovereign is most justified in criminalizing in order to prevent serious bodily injury by one citizen against the other, the core of the Harm Principle. FGC fits comfortably into this analysis. In the case of abortion it raises the additional and difficult question of whether a fetus should be considered a "citizen" of the sending country when its parents are, and whether doing so requires taking a stance on the personhood of the fetus. In other words, must citizenship-type interests on the sending country's part follow recognition of legal or moral personhood, or may it also precede that recognition? I have argued in depth elsewhere[50] that the better view is that fetuses are, for political theory purposes, best seen as citizens of the sending country when it comes to harm-prevention justifications, and that this does not require ascribing them personhood. I have also argued that even if I am wrong about this, they should at least be viewed as stateless individuals, in which case the sending country still has a strong (albeit slightly weaker) interest in punishing its citizens who have engaged in abortion.

A second set of justifications for acting is based on "corruption" or "attitude-modification" concerns. This type of justification frequently underlies prohibitions on commercial surrogacy (that women's sexuality will be devalued by commodification), slippery slope concerns with allowing assisted suicide, and less often reasons for criminalizing abortions (that it is not harm to fetuses but the devaluation of the personhood of those already born who are very young or mentally impaired that justifies a ban on abortion). The "victims" in this category are other sending country citizens whose attitudes will be corrupted by these practices.

For these types of justifications it is important to distinguish what I have elsewhere called "consequentialist" and "intrinsic" corruption. Consequentialist corruption justifies intervention to prevent changes to our attitudes or sensibilities that *will* occur if the practice is allowed: for example, that we will regard each other as objects with prices rather than as persons. Intrinsic corruption is a more metaphysical objection—that something wrong has been done through the act of value denigration at the moment sperm or eggs or surrogacy services are sold irrespective of what follows thereafter.[66]

For consequentialist corruption, the sending country may be less justified in criminalizing the activity abroad if the geographical distance between the receiving and sending country will reduce the norm-modifying effect as to its citizens. This is a quasi-empirical question, whether "out-of-sight, out-of-mind" really obtains. The same claim does not apply to intrinsic corruption, where wrong has been done at the moment the act is done (whatever its consequence); and the act of criminal condemnation is needed both to deter that act and, on retributivist or corrective justice-type grounds, to re-right the balance. Because the wrong is free floating, the sending country's "standing" to punish it does not depend on its effects on its citizens, though given the detection difficulties discussed above, perhaps it has less good reason to police these activities abroad.

A different set of justifications focuses on concerns that receiving country citizens have been exploited; commercial surrogacy is an excellent example. This differs from the first set of justifications in two key ways: the focus is not on harm prevention but more on relational/distributive justice concerns, and the victim is now a receiving rather than sending country victim. The question is whether the sending country ought to intercede because it views the receiving country surrogate as exploited even though her own sovereign disagrees. I would argue that for a number of reasons (including available alternatives, whether redistribution is possible, etc.), a sending country's conclusion that paying a gestational surrogate in the sending country $20,000 wrongfully exploits her does not necessarily entail a conclusion that paying an Indian surrogate the same amount wrongfully exploits her. Further, to the extent that exploitation is thought of as a relational/distributive justice violation, under several theories of Global Justice, a sending country citizen or government may have quite different obligations to fellow citizens than those abroad.[61] All this has led me to conclude that *if* the justification for the domestic prohibition relates to matters of distributive justice and not physical harm, *and* the exploited party's country of citizenship (the receiving country) has determined that it is not exploitation, *and* the exploited party's participation is voluntary (in the sense of lacking immediate coercion though perhaps not in a deeper sense of freedom), *and* the exploited party is adequately represented in the governance of the country, *and* the activity takes place in the receiving country's territorial sovereignty, *then* the sending country does not have good reason to criminalize extraterritorially.

Finally, when the concern is paternalism, there are countervailing dynamics at play, as is evident in the assisted suicide case. On the one hand, there are reasons to be more concerned about the circumvention tourism than its domestic equivalent because the state cannot use its existing laws relating to the supervision of its physicians (including licensure and disciplinary rules) as a bulwark against undue influence by family or doctors. On the other hand, perhaps the sending country thinks that the very activity of traveling abroad and the planning that goes into it evidences more self-reflection and fixedness of will than the equivalent activity undertaken domestically, such that the consent of the patient—which is irrelevant under the sending country's domestic prohibition—deserves more weight in this setting. While this latter force may persuade the sending country, especially when combined with a desire to accommodate minority beliefs within its polity, since assisted suicide tourism involves serious bodily harm by one citizen against another citizen, it is also a case where the sending country's criminal law interests in intervening are at their zenith.

CONCLUSION

In this chapter I have explained a sending country's power under international law to criminalize circumvention tourism, and the normative considerations that go to whether they ought to do so, and applied them to a series of case studies that are typical instances of circumvention tourism going on today. I have shown that home countries have strong reasons to criminalize the activity of their citizens abroad for abortion and FGC, and fairly strong reasons in the case of assisted suicide. For reproductive technology, much will turn on the underlying justification for the domestic prohibition, but on the basis of many of those justifications, the home country does *not* have a strong reason to criminalize the activities of its citizens abroad.

The globalization of health care, the ease of international travel, and the divergences between countries as to whether to criminalize certain procedures within their territory has given rise to circumvention tourism, which is likely to grow only more pronounced as the medical tourism industry expands and becomes more institutionalized. While I have focused on unilateral criminalization by the home country, it is my hope that we will move to more multilateral approaches, such as treaties. That said, I do not see this happening in the short or middle term.

ACKNOWLEDGMENTS

I thank Bill Alford, Betsy Bartholet, Gabriella Blum, Rachel Brewster, Grainne De Burca, Einer Elhauge, Nita Farahany, Dov Fox, Charles Fried, Jesse Fried, John Goldberg, Jim Greiner, Janet Halley, Adriaan Lanni, Martha Minow, Gerald Neuman, Vijay Padmanabhan, Ben Roin, Bill Rubenstein Ben Sachs, Jed Shugerman, Joseph Singer, Robert Sitkoff, Carol Steiker, Matthew Stephenson, Jeannie Suk, Mark Wu, Detlev Vagts, Carlos Vasquez, and Jonathan Zittrain for comments on earlier drafts. I also thank participants at the Harvard Law School Petrie-Flom Health Law Workshop on April 18, 2011, the Harvard Law School Petrie-Flom Center Globalization of Health Care Conference on May 21, 2011, and the ASLME Health Law Professors Conference on June 11, 2011. I also thank in advance audiences at the NYU/Brooklyn Law School Criminal Law Theory Workshop on September 15, 2011, and the University of Texas at Austin Faculty Workshop on October 28, 2011 for comments. Mollie Bracewell, Joseph Brothers, Sean Driscoll, Cormac Early, Mischa Feldstein, Katherine Hicks, Russell Kornblith, Katherine Kraschel, Rebecca Livengood, Lisa Sullivan, and Desta Tedros provided excellent research assistance. Material in this chapter is adapted from a much longer discussion in Cohen IG. Circumvention tourism. *Cornell L. Rev.* 2012; 97 (forthcoming).

REFERENCES

1. Clifford AM. Comment, Abortion in international waters off the coast of Ireland: Avoiding a collision between Irish moral sovereignty and the European Community. *Pace Int'l L. Rev.* 2002;14:385–433.

2. Gentleman A. India nurtures business of surrogate motherhood. *New York Times.* March 10, 2008:A9.

3. 18 U.S.C. § 116(a) (2006).

4. Dixon R, Posner EA. The limits of constitutional convergence. *Chi. J. Int'l L.* 2011;11:399–423.

5. Crabbs KY. The German abortion debate: Stumbling block to unity. *Fla. J. Int'l L.* 1991;6:213–231, 220.

6. Jones T. Wall still divides Germany on the abortion question. *Los Angeles Times.* October 19, 1991:A3. http://articles.latimes.com/1991–10–19/news/mn-515_1_legal-abortions. Accessed August 28, 2011.

7. Davis MF. Abortion access in the global marketplace. *N.C. L. Rev.* 2010;88:1657–1685.

8. Art. 40.3.3., Constitution of Ireland, 1937. http://www.taoiseach.gov.ie/at tached_files/Pdf%20files/Constitution%20of%20Ireland.pdf. Accessed August 28, 2011.

9. [1992] 1 I.R. 1 (Ir. S. C.).

10. *A and B v. E. Health Bd.*, 1 I.L.RM. 460 (Ir. H. Ct.) (1998).

11. 410 U.S. 113 (1973).

12. Bradford CS. What happens if *Roe* is overruled? Extraterritorial regulation of abortion by the states. *Ariz. L. Rev.* 1993;35:87–171.

13. *People v. Buffum,* 256 P.2d 317, 319 (Cal. 1953).

14. *Pretty v. UK* (App no 2346/02) (2002) 35 EHRR 1.

15. Mullock A. Overlooking the criminally compassionate: What are the implications of prosecutorial policy on encouraging or assisting suicide? *Med. L. Rev.* 2010;18:442–470.

16. Suicide Act 1961, 50 Eliz. c. 60, § 2 (Eng.)

17. Greasley K. *R(Purdy) v. DPP* and the case for willful blindness. *Oxford J. Legal Stud.* 2010;30:301–326.

18. *R(Purdy) v. DPP* [2009] EWCA Civ 92, [2009] 1 Cr App R 32.

19. Irish woman prevented [from] going to Switzerland for assisted suicide. *Newstalk.* May 5, 2011. http://www.newstalk.ie/2011/uncategorized/6irish-woman-prevented-going-to-switzerland-for-assisted-suicide70/. Accessed August 28, 2011.

20. World Health Organization. Fact sheet no. 241 on female genital mutilation. http://www.who.int/mediacentre/factsheets/fs241/en. Accessed August 28, 2011.

21. Morrison L, Scherf C, Ekpo G, et al. The long-term reproductive health consequences of female genital cutting in rural Gambia: A community-based survey. *Tropical Med. & Int'l Health.* 2001;6:643–653.

22. Obermeyer CM. The consequence of female circumcision for health and sexuality: An update on evidence. *Culture, Health, and Sexuality.* 2005;7:443–461.

23. Brigham and Women's Hospital. Female genital cutting research: Number of women and girls with or at risk for female genital cutting is on the rise in the United States. http://www.brighamandwomens.org/Departments_and_Ser vices/obgyn/services/africanwomenscenter/research.aspx. Accessed August 28, 2011.

24. 18 U.S.C. § 116(a) (2006).

25. 18 U.S.C. § 116(b) (2006).

26. 18 U.S.C. § 116(c) (2006).

27. McKinley MA. Cultural culprits. *Berkeley J. Gender L. & Just.* 2009;24:91–165 (discussing *State v. Adem,* No. 04-B-1291–5 (Gwinnett County Super. Ct. Nov. 2, 2006)).

28. Associated Press. Georgia: Man convicted in daughter's mutilation. *New York Times.* November 2, 2006.

29. Nour N. Female circumcision: Ethics and human rights considerations. Presentation, Harvard Law School, March 3, 2011.

30. The Female Genital Mutilation Act, 2003, c. 31 (Eng.).

31. Malik M. Feminism and its "other": Female autonomy in an age of "difference." *Cardozo L. Rev.* 2009;30:2613–2628.

32. New Zealand: Crimes Act 1961 No. 43, § 204B; Canadian Criminal Code, § 273.3; Sweden: Act (1982:316) on Prohibiting the Genital Mutilation ("Circumcision") of Women, § 3; Victoria, Australia: Crimes Act 1958, § 33.

33. H.R. 5137, 111th Cong. (2d Sess. 2010).

34. Cohen IG. Regulating reproduction: The problem with best interests. *Minn. L. Rev.* 2011;96:423–519.

35. Inhorn MC. Fatwas and ARTs: IVF and gamete donation in *Sunni v. Shi'a Islam. J. Gender Race & Just.* 2005;9:291–317.

36. Hunter-Henin M. Surrogacy: Is there room for a new liberty between the French prohibitive position and the English ambivalence? In: Freeman M, ed. *Law and Bioethics: Current Legal Issues* 2008;11:334–336.

37. Ikemoto LC. Reproductive tourism: Equality concerns in the global market for fertility services. *Law & Ineq.* 2009;27:277–309.

38. *Johnson v. Calvert,* 851 P.2d 776 (Cal. 1993).

39. Cohen IG. Protecting patients with passports: Medical tourism and the patient-protective argument. *Iowa L. Rev.* 2010;95:1467–1567.

40. Carney S. Inside India's rent-a-womb business. *Mother Jones.* March/April 2010. http://motherjones.com/politics/2010/02/surrogacy-tourism-india-nayna-patel. Accessed August 28, 2011.

41. Turks barred from receiving sperm or egg donations abroad. *Hurriyet Daily News and Econ. Rev.* March 15, 2010. http://www.hurriyetdailynews.com/n.php?n=turks-are-banned-to-receive-sperm-or-egg-donations-abroad-2010–03–15. Accessed August 28, 2011.

42. Robertson J. Protecting embryos and burdening women: Assisted reproduction in Italy. *Hum. Reprod.* 2004;19:1693–1696.

43. Surrogacy Bill 2010. http://www.parliament.nsw.gov.au/prod/parlment/NSWBills.nsf/0/71c024816771a264ca2577c100195683?OpenDocument. Accessed August 28, 2011.

44. Cuniberti G. French court denies recognition to American surrogacy judgment. *Conflict of Laws.Net.* June 30, 2009. http://conflictoflaws.net/2009/french-court-denies-recognition-to-american-surrogacy-judgement/. Accessed August 28, 2011.

45. Parks JA. Care ethics and the global practice of commercial surrogacy. *Bioethics.* 2010;24:333–340.

46. Smerdon UR. Crossing bodies, crossing borders: International surrogacy between the United States and India. *Cumb. L. Rev.* 2008–2009;39:15–85.

47. Knox JH. A presumption against extrajurisdictionality. *Am. J. Int'l L.* 2010;104:351–396.

48. Council of Europe Res (68) 17 pf 28 June 1968.

49. Lowe V. Jurisdiction. In: Evans MD. *International Law.* 2006;335(2d ed.):335–360.

50. Cohen IG. Circumvention tourism. *Cornell L. Rev.* 2012;97 (forthcoming).

51. Restatement (Third) of the Foreign Relations Law of the United States § 402 (1987).

52. *United States v. Yousef*, 327 F.3d 56, 91 n.24 (2d Cir. 2003).

53. Watson GR. Offenders abroad: The case for nationality-based criminal jurisdiction. *Yale J. Int'l L.* 1992;17:41–84.

54. Cohen IG, Chen DL. Trading-off reproductive technology and adoption: Does subsidizing IVF decrease adoption rates and should it matter? *Minn. L. Rev.* 2010;95:485–577.

55. *United States v. Aluminum Co. of Am.*, 148 F.2d 416 (2d Cir. 1945).

56. *Rio Tinto Zinc Corp. v. Westinghouse Elec. Corp.* [1978] 1 All ER 434 (HL).

57. Coutts M. Ethical concerns raised as woman, 60, gives birth to twins. *National Post.* February 5, 2009. http://www.nationalpost.com/most_popular/story.html?id=1256913. Accessed August 28, 2011.

58. Dwyer JG. The child protection pretense: States' continued consignment of newborn babies to unfit parents. *Minn. L. Rev.* 2008;93:407–492.

59. Meyer JA. Dual illegality and geoambiguous law: A new rule for extraterritorial application of U.S. law. *Minn. L. Rev.* 2010;95:110–186.

60. 18 U.S.C. §2423 (b), (c), (f).

61. Cohen IG. Medical tourism, global justice, and access to health care. *Va. J. Int'l L.* 2011;51:1.

62. *United States v. Tykarsky*, 446 F.3d 458, 470 (3d Cir. 2006); *United States v. Clark*, 435 F.3d 1100, 1103–04 (9th Cir. 2006); *United States v. Bredimus*, 352 F.3d 200, 205–07 (5th Cir. 2003); *United States v. Han*, 230 F.3d 560, 563–64 (2d Cir. 2000).

63. *Hartford Fire Ins. Co. v. California*, 509 U.S. 764, 769–770 (1993).

64. Pennings G. Reproductive tourism as moral pluralism in motion. *J. Med. Ethics.* 2008;28:337–341.

65. Minow M. About women, about culture: about them, about us. In: Shweder RA, Minow M, Markus HR, eds. *Engaging cultural differences: The multicultural challenges in liberal democracies.* 2008:252.

66. Cohen IG. Note, The price of everything, the value of nothing: Reframing the commodification debate. *Harv. L. Rev.* 2003;117:689–710, 691–692.

Chapter 11

Independent Health Care Accreditation: Medical Tourism and Other International Aspects

Stephen T. Green and Hannah King

People traveling outside of their countries to access health care services put a great deal of faith in the hospitals, clinics, and health care professionals they are visiting, as well as the authorities and the legal services of the countries where the health care providers are located. Medical tourists are in effect trusting that the health care they receive will meet or exceed a certain level of quality and safety. In all likelihood, they are seeking a similar or improved level of quality to what they would receive at home. Few reasonable people would dispute that health care providers should always consider themselves bound by an ethical duty to provide the safest achievable health care of the highest possible quality for all of their patients, wherever they happen to be from.[1] Nonetheless, it certainly cannot be taken for granted that the standard of services on offer for medical tourists will always be adequate. Even in the wealthiest countries, such as the United States, health care providers struggle with quality problems.[2]

Consequently, as a growing number of countries seek to develop and improve their credentials as providers of health care services for

Disclosure: Stephen T. Green is a Director of QHA Trent Accreditation Scheme.

overseas populations, one vital question that has to be asked is: just how safe and fit for purpose are the medical tourism services on offer? Most governments and their agencies have some form of compulsory process in place for regulating and licensing health care providers. While these processes are clearly valuable, they essentially serve to set baseline standards and do not constitute rigorous, holistic assessments of quality and safety. In addition, in some cases, the agencies responsible for setting and enforcing these standards are controlled by governments that are promoting medical tourism as part of a national economic strategy. Ultimately, the medical tourism industry remains largely unregulated.[3] The extent to which quality and safety issues in medical tourism can, or should be, a matter for regulation, either nationally or internationally, and whether the response should remain voluntary, is the subject of ongoing debate.

In the meantime, if hospitals and clinics anywhere in the world are simply left to their own devices, can they be trusted to be of high quality? The principal reason that most health providers, facilitators, and governments target medical tourists is profit. Depending on a hospital's perspective, investing resources to elevate quality and safety may or may not contribute to that profit. Patients typically struggle with a similar calculus; as medical tourists they look to acquire the best possible health care for the lowest possible personal expenditure. Although the commercial nature of medical tourism may engender a focus on the volume of patients seen and procedures delivered, ultimately it is obvious that quality must also be an integral part of any successful business strategy. Patients want, need, and deserve the best and the safest health care services possible. True professionals will wish to do the best they can for their patients, and financial managers recognize the importance of creating the best image possible for the services they provide.

So how do hospitals and clinics maximize quality and minimize risk? Similarly, how does a patient determine if a hospital or clinic is genuinely safe and fit for purpose? One option gaining currency in the global market for health care services is accreditation, or a third-party evaluation of the safeguards and systems in place to promote quality and safety at hospitals and clinics. This chapter will examine the strengths and limitations of accreditation, as well as the challenges that arise in the context of medical tourism, including assessing the full spectrum of care, from pre to postoperative services. It also explores issues around setting global standards for health care quality.

ACCREDITATION IN HEALTH CARE

The implication of a free market within a capitalist system is, in theory, that businesses can introduce any product to the market, and the public then can examine and purchase if it appears to have merit. But the system only works efficiently and safely if the public is able to accurately assess the quality, efficacy, and safety of these products, and if competition is allowed to flourish. However, due to the complexities entailed in genuinely assessing the efficacy of a health care provider (and the vast amount of data that would need to be collected to realistically assess risk), individuals are unable to accurately determine the quality of the providers and the safety of their activities. There is a need, therefore, for some kind of "honest broker"—an independent system of external quality assessment to help guide health care consumers.

Accreditation is a very particular form of external quality assessment carried out by a third-party assessment body known as an accreditation scheme. The process generally applies to organizations rather than individuals, although it can be as readily applied to a small dental clinic as a full hospital. If the accreditation process applies to the whole hospital or clinic, it is referred to as "holistic accreditation."

The route to becoming accredited combines self-assessment and external peer review by a team of surveyors. The survey will often come after preparatory work and other initial visits to the hospital and should involve all those who are involved in making the hospital function. This formalized assessment by the surveyors from an independent external body is a vital element of effective accreditation, and if it is done properly, it is this independent hands-on survey that gives accreditation its robustness and credibility. Without this externally led step in place, there exists no unbiased verification, or refutation, of what may be being claimed by a health care–providing organization. Independent external assessment is what gives accreditation its power and value within medical tourism.

Accreditation has come to be thought of as a "stamp of approval" verifying the authenticity and quality of the services provided, and as such has been adopted as a marketing tool for health care providers targeting medical tourists.

Assessing Quality

For an organization to be considered genuinely high quality, it should be constantly seeking to maintain and improve its standards. In health care, this will be achieved through (a) maximizing safety by identifying and minimizing risks and (b) continually pushing up quality. To best manage risk in the context of a hospital, it is important to recognize that a hospital's structures and processes interact in such a way that poor functioning in one component will resonate throughout the organization, and the final result will be dysfunctional. To ensure effective multidisciplinary working, it is essential that all of a hospital's services, from the kitchens to the intensive care unit, attain at least the minimal standards that will enable that hospital to function. Ideally, the hospital should be performing better than this by actively maintaining and improving the quality of health care it provides, but this cannot happen until risks are first recognized and minimized.

A risk-management culture that puts the patient first should be a fundamental aspect of the day-to-day running of all hospitals and incorporated into any ongoing developments.[4] This can only be accomplished by establishing an organizational framework designed to assess quality, identify risk, and deal with all relevant issues; and by promoting a culture of remaining vigilant, of being prepared to listen, and of maintaining an open mind. These are among the features that a good accreditation process will encompass and address.

It is beyond the scope of this chapter to look at every small facet of how all the major international health care accreditation schemes operate, but there are a number of principal components that are common to all schemes:

- The accreditation process should be grounded upon the application of predetermined published standards for assessing and benchmarking organizations' performance.
- Standards should be based upon the best available evidence, and where evidence is not available, opinion generated by an expert peer group.
- Professional peers with appropriate training should conduct surveys and reviews.
- A reputable, genuinely independent body should administer the accreditation process.
- The process should encourage organizational development and aim to improve quality and reduce risk to patients, staff, and the wider society.
- Processes should be put into place to prospectively identify and correct problems.
- The accreditation process should include a mechanism to ensure that recommendations are acted upon and that problems identified by the measurement process are corrected.
- The assessment process should be repeated periodically, usually every two to four years.

"Benchmarking," the process of comparing quality, safety, cost, or time measurements among organizations, can also be incorporated into the process.

Establishing Standards

The standards that accreditation schemes use in their surveys vary. Whatever standards they employ, accreditation schemes must develop them in consultation with relevant professional organizations, and they must be based on best available evidence, reflect currently accepted best practice, be widely accepted by all relevant parties, and have a sound footing in ethics and probity. They should reflect the patient care process, be patient focused, and emphasize multidisciplinary collaboration. Accreditation standards encompass not only clinical governance and care, but also a wide range of other factors, including buildings, grounds and equipment, staff credentialing, ethics, customer service, informed consent, and infection control.

ISO, the Europe-based International Organization for Standardization, is often mentioned in the same breath as accreditation. The ISO process is similar to accreditation in that it focuses on the application of certain established standards, but its emphasis is more technical than clinical. ISO standards focus on adhering to a particular process of quality management and are designed to consistently produce a product (or service) that meets preestablished specifications. While ISO 9000 quality management systems in the health care sector are considered a valuable way of improving quality in health care delivery,[5] they assess only whether the quality management system and the buildings and business systems are fit for purpose, and whether they have embraced a culture of continuous self-improvement and efficiency.[6] Some clinical accreditation schemes also have the capacity to offer ISO certification or work with ISO provider organizations as a complement to their services.

Accreditation Schemes

Accreditation schemes for health care services have grown up in many countries throughout all continents. Some are independent companies, and others are government-supported "Quasi-Autonomous Non-Governmental Organizations" (quangos). Some schemes are holistic, while others have a specialized focus, such as primary care; rehabilitation; or services designed to meet specific needs, such as autism or ambulatory health care.

In some countries, such as France, Malaysia, and South Africa, only one main accreditation program has developed to date. In others, including the United States, United Kingdom, and Australia, several accrediting organizations operate in parallel. Some schemes (often quangos) only operate within their own national borders, while others have gone on to assess hospitals outside of their base country and thus become international

Table 11.1
Holistic international accreditation schemes

Name/Country	Ownership	Works only in health care	Offers ISO certification
JCI (Joint Commission International), United States http://www.jointcommissioninternational.org/	Independent US 501(c) corporation (nonprofit & tax-exempt).	Yes	No
DNV (Det Norske Veritas) & NIAHO, United States & Norway http://www.dnv.com/industry/healthcare/services_solutions/accreditation/niaho_dnv_international_accreditation/	Multinational company, with multiple business interests.	No	Yes
QHA Trent Accreditation UK (Quality Healthcare Advice Ltd.), United Kingdom http://www.qha-international.co.uk	Independent private limited company (PLC).	Yes	Yes
CHKS (Caspe Healthcare Knowledge Systems), United Kingdom http://www.chks.co.uk/	Part of Capita PLC, a large business process outsourcing and professional services company with multiple business interests.	No	Yes
Accreditation Canada International, Canada http://www.accreditation.ca/en/default.aspx	Nongovernment organization (quango) with Canadian Government Observers on the Board.	Yes	No
ACHSI (Australian Council for Accreditation of Health Standards International), Australia http://www.achs.org.au/ACHSI/	Company limited by guarantee in Australia, with representation on Council from Departments of Health of Australian States.	Yes	No

(continued)

Table 11.1 (continued)

Name/Country	Ownership	Works only in health care	Offers ISO certification
NABH (National Accreditation Board for Hospitals & Healthcare Providers), India http://www.nabh.co/	A constituent board of the "Quality Council of India" (QCI), itself a government-supported quango with a Chairman appointed by the Indian Prime Minister's office on recommendation of the Government and industry. QCI works in multiple areas.	No	No
ISO (International Organization for Standardisation), Multinational http://www.iso.org	Multiplicity of PLCs around the world (NB. ISO is not a clinical accreditation scheme). Works in multiple areas outside and inside health care.	No	Yes

Note: The major holistic international accreditation schemes for hospitals and clinics are primarily private and nongovernmental organizations, some of which focus exclusively on health care. This information is current as of December 2011.

accreditation schemes. Many, but not all, of the accreditation schemes operating internationally are private companies or corporations independent of governmental-level interference, an important factor in medical tourism. Table 11.1 presents details of some of the major holistic schemes involved in international accreditation.

Confidential Feedback

While hospitals are happy to publicize the results of a successful bid for accreditation on their walls and websites, the results of the actual survey—the feedback the hospital receives from surveyors—are generally private. There is debate regarding whether the results of surveys should be publicly available. In general, transparency in health care is considered of great value as it provides consumers with the necessary information to choose health care providers based on quality and value. The U.S. Department of Health and Human Services, for example, champions such transparency in its value-driven health care agenda.[7] However, to date, hospitals' final accreditation reports typically have not been made available in the public domain. Clearly, publicizing the results has the potential to be of value in improving safety and quality in medical tourism.

Does Accreditation Work?

Based on the foregoing discussion, one might assume that accreditation would always be of value. However, as Brent James has suggested, "accreditation is not a guarantee of high quality."[8] In their proposed study design for investigating health sector accreditation, Jeffrey Braithwaite and colleagues concluded that "empirical evidence to sustain many claims about the benefits of accreditation is currently lacking."[9] In a later systematic review of health sector accreditation research, Braithwaite and colleagues stated that "while the anecdotal literature contains arguments about the value and merits of accreditation, the evidence has not been assembled and reviewed."[10]

So, while in some quarters there is considerable enthusiasm for accreditation and indeed for accrediting the accreditors as well, it is not entirely certain that it has genuine value in health care.[11] In view of the paucity of firm evidence unequivocally supporting the value of the accreditation model itself, it may be prudent to maintain a degree of healthy skepticism in many aspects of this field. In particular, no one model of health care accreditation and no single set of standards have been proven unequivocally to be the correct one, or even the best one, so an open mind should be maintained and the differing options kept in mind. We examine some of the potential limitations of accreditation below.

Accreditation and Medical Tourism

Medical tourism highlights both the potential benefits and limitations of accreditation and raises additional issues for consideration. Theoretically, accreditation provides medical tourists with the ability to assess the quality of far-flung facilities and to select caregivers that meet a certain standard of quality. Likewise, accreditation can serve as a marketing tool for providers seeking to signal the quality of the care they provide. However, the universal standards and pricing structures that define accreditation can make for an awkward fit for some medical tourism providers and destinations. Moreover, from a patient perspective, accreditation fails to cover the full spectrum of health considerations that arise as the patient's journey unfolds. The following sections will examine how accreditation does and does not work in the diverse global health care market.

POTENTIAL BENEFITS OF INTERNATIONAL ACCREDITATION

Accreditation has the potential to improve the quality—and image—of care provided to medical tourists, and as a result attract business. As the preceding sections outline, a competent, independent accreditation process can help a hospital or clinic identify risks and take steps to minimize them, and put into place a system for ongoing quality improvement. In the assessment of the World Health Organization (WHO), "accreditation can be the single most important approach for improving the quality of health care structures."[12] This potential for quality improvement has related business benefits that can help persuade health care providers to make the substantial investments required to pursue accreditation. There are two important caveats regarding the business benefits of accreditation. The first, which is discussed in further detail below, is that the cost of acquiring accreditation may limit its accessibility for some hospitals. The second is that if an accreditation scheme loses its reputation for independence or integrity, its value as an assessor of quality will, at the very least, be seriously impaired.

Business Benefits

From a business standpoint, accreditation offers a variety of potential benefits for health care providers. It may:

- Help guide consumer choices. For example, the UK National Travel Health Network and Centre (NaTHNaC) has identified accreditation as a way for medical tourists to establish whether a hospital is safe.[13]
- Reduce hospitals' insurance and legal liability.

- Minimize hospitals' risk of bad publicity.
- Attract business through third-party payers. Insurance companies are increasingly looking at whether or not a hospital has accreditation.
- Facilitate access to overseas markets. For example, in the United States, accreditation schemes such as the Joint Commission on Accreditation of Healthcare Organizations (JCAHO) and the American Osteopathic Association are a means to access Medicare-financed business.

Marketing Quality

Among the factors influencing a hospital's decision whether to seek accreditation, or a medical tourism facilitator's or insurance company's inclination to insist upon it, is its marketing and advertising potential. Many of the medical tourism facilitators that cater to this market will tout the fact that the hospitals that they make use of are accredited. Indeed, accreditation is now common practice in many provider countries, and some regard it as a competitive necessity. It may be important for access to health insurance or access to capital markets and, should negative news emerge about a particular hospital, one of the first queries that may arise from the media may be regarding the organization's accreditation status.

Hard evidence of the value of accreditation in this arena is difficult to come by. In recent years there have been two major reports by business consultants dealing with medical tourism, *Mapping the market for medical travel*[14] by Tilman Ehrbeck and colleagues and *Medical Tourism: Consumers in search of value*[15] by Deloitte LLP. Both reports contain some observations regarding accreditation. The latter states that accreditation "helps consumers select a provider based on maintenance of certain standards, medical ethics and quality,"[15(p8)] while the former asks more probing questions and notes that, "the providers themselves . . . are divided about whether the JCI accreditation process made their patients more confident about the quality of their services."[14(p6)]

The private sector in the United Kingdom represents an interesting case. UK health care retains a strong brand image, and the UK private sector currently remains a significant provider of incoming medical tourism services. Yet as of 2012, few UK private sector hospitals or clinics had voluntarily undergone comprehensive holistic accreditation. UK hospitals tend to rely instead on credentials such as possession of the compulsory registration given by the Care Quality Commission (CQC), the regulator for health and social care services in England, even though this process does not provide the same assurances as independent accreditation. It will be interesting to see if over time the absence of holistic accreditation will affect the United Kingdom's standing in the medical tourism market.

Currently, accreditation is most often used as a marketing tool by wealthier provider hospitals, medical tourism facilitators, and the governments of provider countries seeking to grow their share of the medical tourism business. In some cases, governments have directly supported the process by actively encouraging their hospitals to acquire accreditation. This has been the case in not only wealthy countries, but also in some countries where resources are relatively scarce and accreditation is difficult for hospitals to afford. Accreditation by reputable agencies can serve as an indication of the quality of care patients can expect to receive and facilitate relations with foreign insurance companies.[16] There are many examples of hospitals and individual clinics (and even entire countries) advertising that they have passed international accreditation or are in the process of trying for it. The growing appeal of the marketing aspect of accreditation appears to have led to cost inflation and served as an incentive for the suppliers of accreditation to, in turn, market their schemes to the growing band of countries who wish to participate in the medical tourism industry.

Some health care providers have employed other alternatives to accreditation for improving image and visibility. For example, in the U.S. private sector, formalized partnerships between hospitals and universities are used to oversee foreign providers. Affiliation with a recognized medical provider or educator, such as Partners Harvard Medical International, the Mayo Clinic, or the Cleveland Clinic can increase brand recognition and trust among potential medical tourists.

Some providers may incorrectly portray other forms of assessment, such as an individual country's statutory registration, for instance the United Kingdom's CQC, as genuine accreditation. While these entities certainly have intrinsic value, being assessed and certified by them does not mean that the organization has been subjected to and passed rigorous holistic accreditation.

Encouraging Medical Tourism

Does accreditation actually induce people to undertake medical travel? This is an extremely difficult question to answer, in part because of the lack of accurate data on the number of medical tourists and a lack of understanding of their decision-making processes. Countries themselves are often unsure as to precisely how many people are traveling in or out for medical services.

Even in the absence of international accreditation, patients would and do find reasons to engage in medical tourism, including cost, quality, and access to services not available in their local communities. Despite this, it is possible that accreditation status may influence the distribution and destinations of medical tourists, if not the absolute numbers traveling.

For example, after achieving international accreditation from a U.S.-based scheme in 2009, a hospital in Mexico arranged a deal with U.S.-based insurance group Blue Cross Blue Shield that enabled the plan's members to use that hospital's services.[17]

However, even if accreditation leads to an increase in foreign patients, it does not necessarily result in additional foreign revenue if, for example, the destination facilities were owned by foreign companies. In addition, accreditation schemes themselves charge hospitals and governments for their services, and this may also remove capital from the country. Finally, it is important to note that the interactions between medical tourism and accreditation are functioning within shifting paradigms, such as the major worldwide economic downturn in late 2008 that could alter prospects for medical tourism providers, and as a result, accreditation schemes.

POTENTIAL LIMITATIONS AND PROBLEMS OF INTERNATIONAL ACCREDITATION

Accreditation in general is not without its critics, and there are some particular problems with accreditation in the context of medical tourism:

- Accreditation of individual hospitals or clinics does not cover the full spectrum of health care services for medical tourists.
- Accreditation may be cost prohibitive for countries and hospitals with limited resources.
- Having a variety of different accreditation schemes and standards around the world makes it difficult to compare quality across hospitals. However, efforts to standardize approaches to accreditation across the globe may stifle the development and innovation necessary to ensure that the standards used by accreditation schemes reflect the latest evidence.
- As discussed above, the link between accreditation and quality improvement remain in question.
- Improving quality may increase the costs to hospitals without a corresponding increase in revenue if, for example, a scheme requires hospitals to make large investments in hardware and real estate.
- The commercial image, needs, and aspirations of the accreditation schemes themselves can come to dominate the picture and the accreditation market may become overshadowed by marketing hype and manipulation.[18]
- There is potentially a conflict of interest in situations in which the accreditation schemes that are assessing are also involved in

preparing organizations for the assessment. Therefore, a robust accreditation scheme must be willing to fail health care providers, or require them to do further work to be deemed of an adequate standard to pass.

- Universal standards themselves raise difficulties, given that health care is delivered locally where there may be varying cultural expectations.

The following sections will discuss the first three points in greater detail.

Quality and Safety of Pre- and Post-Care Support Systems in Medical Tourism

There is more to the medical tourism process than just the surgical or medical procedure itself. Patients should receive appropriate advice and input at all stages of the caring process. Risk minimization in the stages before and after the period of hospital care, wherever that care might be located, should not be an optional extra. All parts of the system are closely interconnected, and one part breaking down can endanger the integrity of the rest.

A variety of risks and needs must be addressed at different stages of the medical tourism process. Prior to travel, there may be a need for pre-counseling and informed consent for whatever procedure is being contemplated. Intending medical tourists may have a preexisting illness, such as diabetes mellitus, cardiovascular deficiency, or renal failure, or be taking medication that will need to be considered at the earliest possible opportunity. In addition, if the patient is traveling to a country with a tropical or subtropical climate, such as Thailand or India, where the disease ecosystem differs from the home country, then this should be considered and addressed. Problems can develop in transit during the flights there and back, such as deep venous thrombosis and pulmonary thromboembolism, or a myocardial infarct.

While abroad, the medical tourist may become ill, perhaps in a way quite unrelated to their primary reason for becoming a medical tourist (e.g., dengue or malaria); they might develop complications or side effects related to their treatment and stay in the hospital (e.g., drug-resistant wound infections, *Clostridium difficile* colitis); or worse, may die. They may have problems paying or may dispute the bill, and medicolegal issues may develop.

On arriving home, complications, side effects, and postoperative care generally become the responsibility of the domestic medical care system, and patients may encounter problems accessing adequate care. For example, physicians in the United States may be uncomfortable dealing with patients who have traveled overseas to another country and undergone an operation to implant a purchased kidney.

These wider issues around receiving care abroad clearly merit attention. Accordingly, apart from hospital accreditation, if patients are to benefit maximally, there is a need to consider and address the whole medical tourism process. It is therefore appropriate to consider some form of external quality assessment, which could possibly be accreditation based. To date, there are a number of international examples of organizations responding to this challenge, although individually their validity and value may be variable. Groups such as Temos (German), Treatment Abroad (British), and Medical Tourism Association (U.S.) have all developed their own codes of practice or programs of certification. For some schemes, there are no specific standards to reach for these programs, and thus the certification means very little and is not quality assured.

Accreditation Costs

There is only limited data regarding the true cost of international accreditation in the scientific literature and even in the marketing literature. Program costs typically cover clinical time, which includes travel, accommodation, etc.; preparation; accreditation itself; and follow-up visits. A 2003 study estimated the annual costs for a typical, medium-sized U.S.-based organization to participate in the National Committee for Quality Assurance (NCQA) accreditation process to be around $US630,000 a year.[19] NCQA is a domestic U.S.-based accreditor that accredits behavioral health providers. A 1989 study (published in 1993) found that preparation and first-year costs for an initial survey by JCAHO was on the order of $US327,000.[20]

At the time of writing, very few accreditation schemes were openly publishing any data about the charges and incidental expenses of accreditation on their websites. The USA's JCI publishes an average accreditation survey cost of $US46,000, and an explanation of additional costs, including onsite costs for the team (travel, accommodation, food), preparation, and other consultation.[21] QHA Trent also publishes their charges and a breakdown of the way costs are assessed, including fees and on-site costs for presurvey and survey visits, as well as optional training seminars, and a resurvey two years later. Depending on the size and type of the organization, the minimum total price ranges from £5,300 (approximately $US8,200) for a GP clinic to £52,000 (approximately $US80,450) for a hospital outside of the European Union with more than 600 beds.[22] With respect to costs on the ground, in 2008, as part of the preparation for a WHO report, one of the authors of this chapter, Stephen T. Green, contacted the major international accreditation schemes and ISO and asked for approximate costs for a 500-bed hospital, but the results were extremely difficult to interpret. An objective study of the true costs of preparing for and achieving accreditation would be of value.

These examples indicate that the overall cost incurred by an organization to enable them to pass an accreditation may extend well beyond the cost of the survey itself. Such costs can render accreditation prohibitively expensive for hospitals in low-resource countries that cannot afford the preparation, let alone the survey itself. Moreover, the costs noted above are for just a single health care organization; the extrapolated, whole-of-system financial commitments for several organizations within a particular country would likely be very substantial.

MAKING ACCREDITATION MORE WIDELY AVAILABLE WORLDWIDE

In light of the expenses incurred, hospitals typically pursue international accreditation in an effort to attract lucrative patients from overseas rather than to improve services for the local population. Accordingly, if their products could be rendered more affordable, accreditation schemes could significantly contribute to the wider quest for good health in the world.

The core principles and standards offered by the majority of the main holistic accreditation schemes are very similar, with the main differences generally related to style and cost rather than content. However, the intensive competition and marketing among accreditation schemes can obscure this reality and unnecessarily hike up costs. Therefore, for the development of a worldwide accreditation service to be possible, effective, and affordable, existing accreditation providers would have to work together instead of competing for individual business. The implications for medical tourism would be to level the playing field as more hospitals and clinics would be able to access the accreditation process.

Taking International Standards in Accreditation Forward

At the present time, consideration of a unifying approach or standards for international hospital accreditation is at a relatively early stage. Health care delivery around the world is heterogeneous and in many countries involves both the public and private sectors. Full involvement of both sectors would be necessary to create a universally useful accreditation process.

A number of organizations have attempted to address this issue, such as the International Society for Quality in Health Care Ltd. (ISQua),[23] which has created the "ISQua ALPHA standards," a template for standardizing and harmonizing accreditation approaches. This has considerable value as a starting point, along with other possible sources for developing a uniform scheme. Other possibilities that may serve as a foundation for these efforts include the well-established ISO standards for health care

Table 11.2
Creating common standards

Scheme	ISQua Institutional Member	ISQua Alpha Standards	UKAF Member	Offers ISO certification
JCI (Joint Commission International), United States	Yes	Yes	No	No
DNV (Det Norske Veritas) & NIAHO, United States & Norway	Yes	No	No	Yes
QHA Trent Accreditation UK (Quality Healthcare Advice Ltd.), United Kingdom	Yes	No	Yes	Yes
CHKS (Caspe Healthcare Knowledge Systems), United Kingdom	Yes	Yes	Yes	Yes
Accreditation Canada International, Canada	Yes	Yes	No	No
ACHSI (Australian Council for Accreditation of Health Standards International), Australia	Yes	Yes	No	No
NABH (National Accreditation Board for Hospitals & Healthcare Providers), India	Yes	Yes	No	No

Note: Work to harmonize accreditation activity could tap standards and early efforts by ISO, ISQua, and the UKAF.

and the clinical governance standards established by major public sector services, such as the UK's National Health Service (NHS) and CQC. The United Kingdom Accreditation Forum (UKAF) has also undertaken work to harmonize and standardize accreditation activity.[24] Some of the major international accreditation schemes already are connected to these sources and efforts (see Table 11.2).

Would it be possible to develop a credible universal system within which an umbrella accreditation scheme could function, improving health care for both domestic and international patients? One solution may lie with basing such a system on the existing representative organizations, such as the WHO, the UN World Tourism Organization, and possibly the World Trade Organization (WTO). The WHO has attempted in the past to create viable regional accreditation schemes. The Eastern Mediterranean Regional Office of WHO (EMRO) developed a model for hospital accreditation that would have been appropriate for that region and was flexible enough to allow for adaptation at country level,[11] however, the model was never fully developed due to an apparent lack of interest by potential participating nations. There have also been moves toward similar regional schemes in Latin America.[25]

The World Tourism Organization (UNWTO/OMT), a specialized agency of the United Nations and the leading international organization operating in the field of tourism, plays a central and decisive role in promoting the development of responsible, sustainable, and accessible tourism and pays particular attention to the interests of developing countries, some of which are, or plan to be, provider countries for medical tourists. The WTO could also play a useful role, as it "provides a forum for negotiating agreements aimed at reducing obstacles to international trade and ensuring a level playing field for all, thus contributing to economic growth and development."[26] Economic expertise of this quality could have value in ensuring both that medical tourism and international accreditation are placed on a sound trade footing with an appropriate degree of nonpartisan oversight and with due regard to the needs of less wealthy economies.

The formation of a truly effective overall advisory body, or bodies, for accreditation would require wide representation and hence ownership. The input of not only national governments and bodies like the United Nations, UNICEF, the European Union, the Association of Southeast Asian Nations (ASEAN), and the British Commonwealth, but also of relevant independent international and regional societies and other stakeholders, would be of the greatest value. The views of specialist representative groups, such as ISQua and UKAF, as well as the ISO-related organizations such as the United Kingdom Accreditation Service (UKAS), would certainly be essential.

In addition, at the present time patients have only a limited voice within the worlds of medical tourism and hospital accreditation. Involvement of bodies such as the International Alliance of Patients' Organizations (IAPO) would help empower patients and bring great benefit.

Out of such a conglomeration of expertise, and with an appropriate measure of effort, it would not be too difficult to envisage a credible and inclusive international accreditation scheme for hospitals emerging along the lines outlined earlier. Such a scheme might help provide a more affordable alternative for hospitals catering to medical tourists and domestic populations alike. Entities such as the WHO Patient Safety and the Alliance for Health Policy and Systems Research provide clear examples of how the basis for an accreditation initiative of this type might be established.

To take things forward, leadership of the right caliber would need to be identified and procured, covering not only health care but also, as already argued, the tourism and business aspects of medical tourism. An affordable and pragmatic accreditation scheme based on realistically attainable standards and undertaken by a range of trained surveyors with appropriate skills and experience drawn both locally and from overseas could be developed. An example of such a system as this is the Royal College of Physicians in the United Kingdom, which conducts high-quality postgraduate examinations for doctors in many countries outside of the United Kingdom using volunteer medically qualified examiners drawn from all over the world. Whether a single accreditation scheme could be developed to suit the whole world is debatable, as one size does not fit all; and regional variants may be appropriate, provided there were accepted basic universal standards underpinning the accreditation activities.

CONCLUSION

Entrepreneurism is fundamental to global economies, but when it comes to health care it has to be balanced against the needs for ethics, equity, and professionalism. It must be kept in mind that medical tourism is largely a private sector business and, as such, entails potential clashes between business and health care priorities and the potential for harm. Relying on trust, goodwill, and slick adverts may not be enough to protect medical tourists, and may not guard health care providers against publicly visible complaints and legal action by disgruntled customers. Accordingly, there is a need for some form of externally sourced monitoring or accreditation, and indeed perhaps regulation.

Accreditation is one of the various options that exist for conducting external quality assessments of those hospitals and clinics working in medical tourism. While accreditation has often been used as a marketing tool, and its effectiveness as a quality improvement tool remains in question in some quarters, in much of the world there remains a general acceptance that the process of accreditation can be a valuable tool for quality improvement. However, at the present time it can be very expensive for a hospital to become involved in accreditation, especially if there is a wish to make use of those schemes that offer services internationally. In less well-resourced parts of the world, these costs can be prohibitive. Meanwhile, commercial incentives exist among the accreditation schemes themselves to denigrate less costly options.

Work should be undertaken to develop and improve the current system for international oversight of accreditation schemes, so as to best ensure their genuine independence, maximum immunity from all relevant stakeholder-related conflicts of interest (e.g., agendas of governments, insurance, health care providers, and accreditation schemes themselves), ability to respond to challenges, and affordability.

There is virtually no incentive at the present time for good quality accreditation to be made available to hospitals and clinics in less well-resourced parts of the world at reasonable and affordable prices. This is regrettable, as an inability of hospitals and clinics located in lower- and middle-income countries to access good-quality accreditation because of cost constraints denies them the opportunity to improve their clinical governance. It could be argued that WHO initiatives such as WHO Patient Safety would benefit from successful accreditation-type initiatives becoming a more common feature of the landscape, but to achieve this, an effort will be required.

In the growing medical tourism market, at the present time the safety of patients traveling from the developed world to less well-resourced parts of the world depends to a considerable extent upon the private sector being "policed" by international holistic accreditation schemes. It is worth keeping in mind that while populations from the United States and some other parts of the world are accustomed to having the vast majority of their health care provided by the private sector and consequently may have a degree of aversion to regulation, this is not the case for much of the rest of the developed world.

Increased collaboration at the international level may help eliminate or minimize problems that might adversely affect medical tourism and accreditation, such as restrictive business practices, failure of probity, and conflicts of interest. However, at the present time, the relevant official international bodies associated with health care (WHO), cross-border human travel (UNWTO), and trade (WTO) are playing no significant role in this process, either in an advisory or regulatory capacity. To best assure a healthy future, new models may need to be developed.

To date, much of the available research into this field has been undertaken as a result of commercial drive rather than scientific interest. There is an important need for a program of well-thought-out, nonbiased, nonjudgmental, epidemiological, clinical and socially oriented research in the field of accreditation. Richard D. Smith provides good advice, recommending that "the academic sector, international organisations and individual countries undertake to give priority to such research."[27]

Accordingly, if things are to be taken forward in a rational way, good quality research in this field must be encouraged: "The necessity for an empirically grounded, comprehensive evidence base for accreditation has long been recognized. Without this, the varying positive and negative views about accreditation will remain anecdotal, influenced by ideology or preferences, and driven by such biases."[9(p181)]

REFERENCES

1. Gaston M. Primary obligations and managed care. *J Dent Hyg*. 1998;72(2):3–4.

2. Gaynor M. What do we know about competition and quality in health care markets? Working Paper No. 06/51. Bristol: Centre for Market and Public Organisation; 2006.

3. Patsner B. Medical tourism: A serious business undergoing serious change. *Health Law Perspectives*. University of Houston Law Center; January 2008.

4. Pattinson R. *Audit and feedback: Effects on professional practice and health-care outcomes*. Geneva: World Health Organization; 2006.

5. British Standards Institute (BSI) Australia. *ISO 9001 health service accreditation*. http://www.bsigroup.com.au/en-au/Assessment-and-Certification-servi ces/Management-systems/Standards-and-schemes/ISO-9001-Health/. Accessed January 17, 2012.

6. International Organization for Standardization. *ISO 9001:2000 quality management systems—requirements*. http://www.iso.org/iso/catalogue_detail?csnumber= 21823. Accessed December 28, 2011.

7. Leavitt M. Building a value-based health care system. *The Prologue Series*. Washington, DC: U.S. Department of Health and Human Services; 2008.

8. James B. *Minimising harm to patients in hospital*. Australian Broadcasting Corporation Radio National Health Report. October 1, 2001. http://www.abc.net. au/radionational/programs/healthreport/minimising-harm-to-patients-in-hos pital/3488594. Accessed December 28, 2011.

9. Braithwaite J, Westbrook J, Pawsey M, et al. A prospective, multi-method, multi-disciplinary, multi-level, collaborative, social-organizational design for researching health sector accreditation. *BMC Health Serv Res*. 2006;6:113.

10. Greenfield D, Braithwaite J. Health sector accreditation research: A systematic review. *Int J Qual Health Care*. 2008;20(3):172.

11. Greenfield D, Braithwaite J. Developing the evidence base for accreditation of healthcare organisations: A call for transparency and innovation. *Qual Saf Health Care*. 2009;18(3):162–163.

12. WHO Regional Office for the Eastern Mediterranean. *Technical discussions: Accreditation of hospitals and medical education institutions—challenges and future directions*. Paper EM/RC50/Tech.Disc.1. Regional Committee for the Eastern Mediterranean. Agenda item 7; 2003.

13. National Travel Health Network and Centre. Britons travelling abroad for treatment. *Travel Health Information Sheets*. http://www.nathnac.org/travel/misc/ medicaltourism_010911.htm#facilities. Accessed December 28, 2011.

14. Ehrbeck T, Guevara C, Mango P. Mapping the market for medical travel. *The McKinsey Quarterly*. McKinsey & Company. 2008. https://www.mcki nseyquarterly.com/Mapping_the_market_for_travel_2134. Accessed April 12, 2012.

15. Deloitte Center for Health Solutions. *Medical tourism: Update and implications*. Deloitte LLP. 2009.

16. United Nations Economic and Social Commission for Asia and the Pacific. *Medical travel in Asia and the Pacific—challenges and opportunities*. Bangkok: United Nations Economic and Social Commission for Asia and the Pacific. 2007.

17. Kim H, Anderson B, Gaitz C, et al. *Medical tourism from U.S. to border region of Mexico: Current status and future prospects.* Tucson: University of Arizona. 2009.

18. Berg R, Barnes J, Segall M. *The elephant in the room: Integrating the private sector in quality improvement mechanisms.* Abt Associates. 2006. http://www.icohere-presentations.com/presentations/MiniU/2006/31ElephantRoom-PrivateSector.pdf. Accessed December 28, 2011.

19. Mihalik G, Scherer M, Schreter R. The high price of quality: A cost analysis of NCQA accreditation. *J Health Care Finance.* 2003;29(3):38–47.

20. Rockwell D, Pelletier L, Donnelly W. The cost of accreditation: One hospital's experience. *Hosp Community Psych.* 1993;44(2):151–155.

21. Joint Commission International. *Costs of accreditation.* http://www.jointcommissioninternational.org/Cost-of-Accreditation/. Accessed December 28, 2011.

22. QHA Trent, *How much does QHA Trent charge for accreditation services?* http://www.qha-international.co.uk/what-charges-do-qha-trent-make-for-accreditation-services. Accessed December 28, 2011.

23. ISQua. *Accreditation.* http://www.isqua.org/accreditations.htm. Accessed December 28, 2011.

24. United Kingdom Accreditation Forum. http://www.ukaf.org.uk/. Accessed December 28, 2011.

25. Zeribi K, Marquez L. *Approaches to Healthcare Quality Regulation in Latin America and the Caribbean: Regional Experiences and Challenges.* LACHSR Report No. 63. Bethesda: Latin America and Caribbean Health Sector Reform Initiative—Quality Assurance Project. 2005.

26. World Trade Organization. *About the WTO—a statement by the director general.* http://www.wto.org/english/thewto_e/whatis_e/wto_dg_stat_e.htm. Accessed December 28, 2011.

27. Smith R. Foreign direct investment and trade in health services: A review of the literature. *Soc Sci Med.* 2004;59:2320.

Part IV

Ethical Considerations

Chapter 12

Medical Travel and the Global Health Services Marketplace: Identifying Risks to Patients, Public Health, and Health Systems

Leigh Turner

Whether prospective medical travelers seek orthopedic procedures, dental care, ophthalmologic surgery, stem cell injections, in vitro fertilization, kidney transplantation, or other medical interventions, if they can afford to pay out of pocket for medical care, they have access to a global health services marketplace. While this market enables patients to access medical services that might otherwise be unavailable to them, it also exposes individuals to risks they would not necessarily encounter in domestic health care facilities. This chapter provides an overview of different types of risks related to increased medical travel and globalization of health care. In addition to considering risks to individual medical travelers, the chapter considers risks to public health and health systems.

The development of transcontinental transportation networks, the emergence of the Internet as a global communication medium, and the establishment of reputable hospitals and clinics around the world make it feasible for citizens of such countries as Australia, Canada, England, and the United States to obtain medical care in countries within Asia, Eastern Europe, Latin America, South America, the Caribbean, and elsewhere. Of course, medical travel is multidirectional and does not simply flow from "West" to "East" and "North" to "South." Just as travel for business and pleasure has increased, a growing number of individuals leave their local communities and receive treatment at international medical facilities.

Various factors prompt individuals to travel abroad for medical care. Cost of care; wait times; unavailability of particular treatments in nearby medical facilities; the desire to access treatments that are available abroad but have not been approved by domestic regulatory bodies; interest in accessing illegal treatments such as organ transplants and commercial surrogacy; and the possibility of receiving high-quality, "VIP treatment" in modern, well-staffed, technologically advanced facilities all contribute to increased medical travel. Many "push" factors prompt medical travelers to seek treatment outside their local communities. Likewise, various "pull" factors draw patients to particular international health care facilities.

PARTICIPANTS IN THE GLOBAL HEALTH SERVICES MARKETPLACE

Numerous businesses and medical facilities promote medical travel and the global health services marketplace. In some countries, individual medical facilities such as Bumrungrad International in Thailand and Mayo Clinic in the United States have developed reputations for excellence or special services that attract international patients. In other countries, hospital chains in the private sector and government ministries in the public sector work together and support national medical tourism initiatives. In countries such as India and Singapore, for example, both private sector and government agencies support national efforts to promote medical tourism. National and regional governments promote medical tourism initiatives because they see an opportunity to attract foreign direct investment, increase tourism revenues, and expand employment opportunities in the health care sector and hospitality industry. Governments support medical tourism initiatives by eliminating tariffs on imported medical devices and providing financial assistance and infrastructure support to hospitals and clinics seeking to attract international patients. In addition, they sponsor international trade shows, exhibitions, trade missions, marketing campaigns, and other initiatives designed to showcase medical travel destinations. Destination hospitals and clinics typically participate in these initiatives by sending marketing executives and senior managers to conferences and trade shows.

International accreditation bodies play an important role in promoting medical travel.[1] Joint Commission International, or JCI as it is often called, is the international branch of the U.S.-based Joint Commission. The Joint Commission, formerly known as the Joint Commission on Accreditation of Healthcare Organizations, accredits hospitals in the United States. JCI offers accreditation to health care facilities around the world.[2] Destination hospitals and clinics use JCI accreditation to signal that they provide an "international" level of care. Though JCI does not directly promote particular medical facilities, the "gold seal of approval" provided by JCI plays a significant part in hospital marketing campaigns. Visitors to JCI-accredited medical facilities can find the JCI gold seal prominently displayed on promotional brochures, in elevators and hotel lobbies, and in the offices of health care providers. JCI is the most visible organization providing international hospital accreditation, but it is not the only body providing this service. Accreditation Canada, the Australian Council on Healthcare Standards, and other organizations also provide international accreditation of hospitals and clinics. International hospital accreditation has a powerful marketing function. Obtaining international accreditation enables medical facilities to advertise themselves as offering high-quality, independently assessed medical care.

Individual hospitals and clinics, large hospital chains, government agencies, and international accreditation bodies all contribute to promotion of medical travel and construction of a global marketplace for selling and purchasing health services. In addition, medical tourism companies play a key role in marketing health services available at international facilities. These businesses use company websites, print media advertisements, and Internet-based advertisements to promote medical travel.[3,4] Though some companies specialize in particular domains such as dental care, cosmetic surgery, bariatric surgery, or reproductive medicine, most medical tourism agencies offer comprehensive lists of medical procedures. In addition to advertising medical procedures, medical tourism companies commonly offer airline reservations, concierge services, tours before or after surgery, and postoperative stays in resorts and luxury hotels.

Businesses, government agencies, and public–private partnerships populate the medical travel marketplace.[5] Destination hospitals and clinics market and provide health services. Medical tourism companies and international patient centers at destination medical facilities advertise medical procedures, coordinate patient travel and treatment, and book accommodations. International accreditation bodies help legitimate destination health care facilities. In summary, numerous participants in the global health services marketplace are deeply invested in efforts to promote medical travel and expand the global health services marketplace.[6] Though there are many organizations invested in promoting medical travel and convincing prospective clients to leave their local communities and travel abroad for health care, many risks accompany medical travel. Proponents of increasing trade in health services claim that the benefits of medical travel outweigh whatever risks accompany globalization of health services. Acknowledging that access to a global healthcare marketplace aids some patients and has potential for generating social and economic benefits if adequate regulatory structures are in place, medical travel, absent suitable safeguards, poses risks to patients, public health, and health systems.

MARKETING MEDICAL PROCEDURES AND RISKS TO INFORMED DECISION MAKING

Medical tourism companies and destination medical facilities have a financial interest in selling health services. Websites of medical tourism companies and destination hospitals and clinics are designed to promote medical procedures and make international medical travel seem safe and appealing.[7,8] Some medical tourism companies and destination hospitals offer package deals and special offers if customers purchase multiple procedures. Other medical tourism companies offer financial incentives when clients refer friends or family members and generate additional business. In an article describing how medical tourism companies can convert calls into sales, marketing consultant Rob Passmore describes the many different conversational techniques and incentives medical tourism companies can use.[9] Passmore recommends that medical tourism companies use procedure discounts, hotel upgrades, free limousine service, complimentary flight upgrades, and other "high perceived value, low actual cost" offers to turn callers into customers. Standard marketing techniques are used to attract customers and emphasize the benefits of traveling abroad for medical care. Both medical tourism companies and destination hospitals employ customer sales representatives or "facilitators" ready to speak with prospective clients and promote "all-inclusive" health care packages.

Ethical tensions, coupled with professional norms intended to promote ethical behavior and prohibit unethical conduct, are built into the practice of medicine. One example of an ethical tension found in the practice of medicine is the fee-for-service model common in the United States and a number of other settings. With the fee-for-service model, on the basis of pure financial self-interest, physicians benefit from performing as many procedures as possible. However, medical interventions are not always in the best interest of patients. In medical training, codes of conduct, and professional guidelines, physicians are reminded that they are to perform medical procedures only when they are clinically warranted. Physicians are supposed to "first, do no harm" and act in the best interests of patients even if what is best for patients conflicts with what is most profitable for clinicians and the health care facilities where they work. In the global health services marketplace, it is unclear whether physicians' moral imperative to do no harm, serve their patients, and act as fiduciaries supersedes commercial interests. The manner in which medical tourism company websites are designed, marketing efforts at trade shows and exhibitions, and the promotional material of destination hospitals and clinics reveal hospitals' and medical tourism companies' interest in selling medical procedures. The various ways in which medical tourism companies are paid—receiving a percentage of the total price of health services sold, payments for referring clients to destination facilities, or a set fee from customers—suggest that these companies, in many cases, have more incentive to sell medical procedures than to dissuade prospective clients from purchasing medical care they might not need.

Financial interests also appear to influence how information about the risks and benefits of medical care is communicated to prospective medical travelers. Medical parentalism, a hierarchical relationship in which physicians relate to their patients as parents relate to their children, was once regarded as the primary obstacle to providing information to patients and helping them make informed, voluntary, autonomous choices. Medical parentalism assumes that doctors know what is best for their patients, that patients cannot adequately understand the complexities of medical treatment, and that doctors rather than patients should make decisions about whether to proceed with particular medical interventions. Contemporary efforts to provide information about the risks and benefits to patients and help them make choices about medical interventions are intended to reduce the power and authority of physicians and ensure that patients are able to make considered decisions about whether or not to undergo particular medical procedures.

In countries around the world, introduction of legislation concerning informed consent has resulted in a shift away from medical parentalism and toward increased information disclosure and informed patient choice. Informed consent requires that patients have access to information, comprehend that information, and have decision-making capacity. Embedded in the concept of informed consent is the understanding that health care providers have a moral obligation to be honest with patients, disclose risks and benefits of treatment options and consequences of nontreatment, and help patients understand immediate and long-term implications of making particular decisions. However, what informed consent means in the context of a highly competitive medical tourism industry is unclear. There is considerable risk that commercial interests, rather than medical parentalism, play a significant role in shaping how information is provided to patients.

The commercial objective of selling medical procedures is very different from the goal of helping patients develop an informed understanding of the risks and benefits of medical interventions, risks and benefits of alternative treatments, and risks and benefits of declining treatment. Full disclosure of the risks and benefits of treatment is a vital component of promoting informed patient choice. However, several recent analyses of medical tourism company websites reveal that much of the information provided to prospective medical travelers emphasizes the benefits of purchasing treatment and provides little information concerning the risks associated with undergoing particular medical procedures, postoperative complications, and legal recourse in the event that medical travelers are harmed while receiving care at international medical facilities.[10,11] One study of 100 websites marketing plastic surgery abroad found that 37 percent of those websites provided no information concerning advertised procedures, 10 percent contained information about the possibility of complications, and 4 percent mentioned details concerning aftercare and follow-up procedures in the event of postoperative complications.[12] Another study of 66 medical tourism websites found that risk of procedures was noted by 11.9 percent of the websites, the possibility of complications was mentioned by 21.5 percent, postoperative complications were mentioned by 35 percent, and legal recourse was mentioned by 9.8 percent of the websites.[13] These studies, along with other content analyses of websites of medical tourism companies, raise serious questions about the quality of information provided medical travelers.[14] Chapter 13 provides additional insight into the role of medical tourism facilitators in providing information to prospective clients.

The absence of transnational regulatory authorities in the global health services marketplace and lack of regulations governing how information about medical procedures is provided puts patients at risk of receiving interventions that are profitable for destination hospitals, clinicians, and medical tourism companies but not necessarily beneficial for medical travelers. At present, customer service representatives at medical tourism companies and destination hospitals play key roles in providing health-related information to clients. The patient–physician relationship is displaced by interactions between prospective clients and medical tourism company facilitators. Some medical travelers agree to medical procedures, sign contracts and waiver of liability documents, purchase treatment, and fly to destination health care facilities without having meaningful discussions with health care providers about risks and benefits of treatment.

Traditional models of informed consent assume that physicians are key figures in sharing information with patients. Sales agents are not part of this model. The involvement of sales agents employed by medical tourism companies and international patient centers at destination hospitals in communicating information to patients prompts concerns that medical travelers are at risk of making decisions on the basis of information provided by parties with direct financial interests in encouraging medical travelers to purchase health services and go abroad for treatment. Content analysis of websites of medical tourism companies raises questions about the quality of information provided to medical travelers. These studies suggest the need for better oversight of the medical tourism industry and more stringent regulation of how health care packages are advertised to prospective medical travelers.[15]

QUALITY OF CARE, PATIENT SAFETY, AND RISKS TO HEALTH

Medical tourism companies and destination health care facilities emphasize the high-quality care medical travelers receive. Marketing material often highlights high ratios of doctors and nurses to patients, health care professionals' qualifications, and low infection rates at destination hospitals and clinics. Notwithstanding these claims about the outstanding quality of care provided at medical tourism destinations, some patients travel to international medical centers and return home with surgical complications, infections, and other significant medical problems requiring postoperative treatment.[16,17]

Given the absence of large-scale studies addressing how many individuals travel abroad for care and what percentage of these individuals experience postoperative infections and other complications related to treatment, it is not possible to compare morbidity and mortality rates in medical travelers with morbidity and mortality rates in comparable patient cohorts treated at domestic health care facilities. At present, there is no way to benchmark care provided at international medical facilities against quality of care provided within the local communities of medical travelers. Caution is therefore necessary when examining the subject of quality of care and patient safety at destination health care facilities. Noting the need for better quantitative data, there are many case reports describing patients who traveled abroad for treatment and subsequently returned home requiring emergency care, revision surgery, and other forms of postoperative treatment.[18,19] These cases prompt questions about health risks associated with receiving treatment at particular destination clinics and hospitals.

There are significant international variations in the training, qualifications, and capabilities of health care providers, standards for licensure of health care professionals, standards for hospital and clinic accreditation, infection control in operating rooms and patient wards, quality of blood supply, quality of testing and screening for tissues and organs, quality of medical devices and surgical equipment, and quality of medications.[20] For example, India, a leading destination for medical travelers, is known for its inadequate regulation of private medical colleges, selling of places in medical schools on the basis of ability to pay rather than academic qualifications of students, and corrupt national medical council.[21,22] Prevalence rates of infectious disease also vary across countries.[23] Some medical travelers presumably travel to hospitals and clinics providing high-quality professional care that meets or exceeds standards in patients' local communities. In contrast, other medical travelers are at increased risk of acquiring infections or receiving poor-quality care when they travel abroad for treatment. At present, medical travelers do not have access to reliable information that can help protect them from international medical facilities offering low-quality health care. Hospital "report cards," improved accreditation standards, and other initiatives might, in time, improve quality of information available to medical travelers and enable them to distinguish superior international medical centers from facilities providing lower-quality care. Until such information becomes accessible, medical travelers will continue to have much greater access to marketing material than credible information about the quality of care at international hospitals and clinics.

LONG-DISTANCE TRAVEL, SURGERY, AND RISK OF VENOUS THROMBOEMBOLISM

Long-distance air travel in confined spaces is a risk factor for venous thromboembolism, or blood clots. Health researchers use the phrase "economy-class syndrome" to describe the increased risk of thrombosis associated with long journeys undertaken in cramped, confined spaces.[24,25] Surgery shortly before or after long-distance air travel increases risk of venous thromboembolism. Blood clots can cause pulmonary embolisms, potentially life-threatening artery blockages in the lungs. Proper use of prophylactic measures such as compression stockings and anticoagulants can reduce risk of thrombosis. Nonetheless, given the increased risk associated with combining surgery and long-distance travel, coupled with episodes in which medical travelers have not been adequately prepared for travel before or after surgery, there is reason to question the wisdom of promoting a form of health care in which long-distance air travel is a routine component. Case reports reveal that some medical travelers have surgery too soon after flying to distant destinations, and other patients fly home too soon following surgery. One case report documents the case of a Swiss woman who had breast implants surgically inserted in the Dominican Republic and then flew home three days after surgery.[26] Caregivers in Bern diagnosed and treated her for a pulmonary embolism. Another report describes the case of a man who flew from Europe to the United States, underwent surgery at the Mayo Clinic, and died shortly after from a pulmonary embolism believed to be linked to long-haul air travel.[27] Such reports suggest that medical travelers should be encouraged to arrive at destination medical facilities well before surgery and not return home immediately after undergoing invasive medical procedures.

No studies address whether medical tourism facilitators and international patient representatives at destination hospitals tell medical travelers about the risks of combining surgery and air travel. One recent publication examines whether websites of Canadian medical tourism companies disclose the risk of deep vein thrombosis to prospective clients.[28] The researchers found that of 17 Canadian medical tourism company websites, just 2 of them mentioned this risk. Interestingly, the 2 sites noting the risk of deep vein thrombosis indicated that this risk was not relevant to their clients because of the short duration of the flights they organized. Since medical travelers start their journeys from different destinations, fly to different locations around the world, travel for different kinds of procedures, and begin their journeys with different risk profiles, it will be difficult for researchers to conduct systematic studies examining the risks medical travelers assume when they combine surgery with long-haul air travel. However, given that long-distance air travel is a known risk factor for thrombosis, and this risk increases if surgery occurs shortly before or after travel, there is reason to consider the possibility that increased risk to patients is built into the very structure of long-distance travel for medical care.[29] Prospective medical travelers ought to be informed of the risk of combining long-distance travel with surgery. In addition, international medical facilities should routinely use prophylactic measures to reduce risks associated with medical travel.[30]

FRAGMENTATION OF CONTINUITY OF CARE

Continuity of care is a key component of competent, professional, patient-oriented health care. Fragmentation of the continuum of care across institutions, health care providers, and geographic settings is an additional risk factor associated with medical travel. Medical tourism companies and destination hospitals emphasize prompt access to desired medical procedures. Competent and safe health care, however, requires far more than expedited access to surgical interventions. The full continuum of care typically includes visits with health care providers before tests or procedures are performed; access to preventive care; physiotherapy and other low-risk, noninvasive forms of treatment before considering more interventionist approaches; discussion of risks and benefits of medical procedures; provision of information about rehabilitation following surgery or other interventions; treatment; immediate postoperative treatment; and long-term care. Postoperative care and long-term monitoring of patients are vital parts of treating patients who have undergone surgery.[31] In most settings, surgeons are responsible for seeing and treating their patients following surgery or making arrangements to transfer care of patients to suitably qualified health care providers. Treating physicians are accountable for coordinating care and ensuring that postoperative infections and other complications are addressed in a professional manner.

Numerous case reports reveal that some medical travelers return home with no plans for postoperative monitoring and treatment.[32,33] Some patients return to their local communities and require emergency care to treat postoperative complications.[34,35] Other medical travelers do not require admission to emergency care but must be treated and followed by local health care providers. Emergence of symptoms associated with postoperative infections is a common reason why medical travelers seek treatment following their return home. Continuity of care is at risk when patients leave their local communities and travel across vast geographic distances. Continuity of care is also compromised by some physicians' reluctance to treat patients who have gone abroad for care and then returned home requiring wound management, revision surgery, treatment of infections, or other forms of care.[36] Whether justified or not, some physicians are concerned that they will become vulnerable to lawsuits if they treat complications resulting from care provided by other medical professionals.

Many technological developments enable provision of health care across geographic distances.[37] Email, videoconferencing, instant messaging, teleradiology, and other modes of telecommunication provide tools for helping patients and health care providers remain connected across geographic distances. Despite the development of these technologies, disruption of the continuum of care is a significant risk associated with medical travel. Coordinated, continuous care is an integral component of treating illnesses and injuries. The fragmentation of care in medical travel raises troubling questions about risks associated with encouraging significant numbers of patients to enter the global health services marketplace and seek care far from local caregivers. Better coordination of health care providers in both domestic and international settings and ensuring that they communicate with one another could improve continuity of care. In practice, however, such communication often does not occur, and not all physicians are willing to provide postoperative care when a physician based in another country has provided treatment.

RISK OF SIGNING WAIVER OF LIABILITY DOCUMENTS

Legal protections for medical travelers are as varied as the countries to which patients travel for treatment. Depending upon where they go for care, some medical travelers risk having limited prospects for legal redress if they are harmed while receiving care at international medical facilities.[38,39]

Medical tourism companies typically require that their clients sign "waiver of liability" documents. The purpose of these waivers is to have customers sign their agreement that in the event they are harmed while obtaining medical care at international medical facilities, they will not attempt to sue the medical tourism company in the country where it is situated. Medical tourism companies presumably regard waiver of liability documents as legal shields. They are designed to make it difficult for clients to bring lawsuits against medical tourism agencies.

Use of waiver of liability documents by medical tourism companies matters because many destination hospitals and clinics are located in countries where there are multiple obstacles to successfully suing for medical malpractice or personal injury.[40] To launch such lawsuits, medical travelers must find legal representation in the country where they received medical care. Initiating legal action requires finding a court willing to consider the claim. Pursuing a successful lawsuit is challenging in countries where it is difficult to demonstrate that the traveler was the victim of medical negligence, personal injury, or other harm. Financial payouts are highly variable across jurisdictions. Medical travelers who require costly long-term care as a result of personal injury or negligence can find that even if their lawsuit is successful, payouts are miniscule compared to settlements in their local communities. In short, medical travelers can find that they have waived liability of medical tourism companies based in their country of origin and have few realistic legal options in the setting where they received care.

Medical travel is multidirectional; destination health care facilities are located all over the world. It therefore is misleading to claim that all medical travelers are without legal recourse if they receive negligent treatment at international medical facilities. As chapter 9 discusses in detail, many factors are relevant, including the legal systems in the countries medical travelers visit, legal systems in countries of origin, and the effectiveness of waiver of liability documents as a legal shield when medical travelers arrange medical care through medical tourism companies. Recognizing the numerous factors that shape the extent to which medical travelers have legal protections when they travel for care, it is clear that at least some individuals who are harmed while seeking medical care abroad will have little prospect of obtaining legal redress.

RISK OF FRAUD

Fraud is often overlooked as a risk associated with medical travel. However, when prospective medical travelers visit websites that advertise health services provided in distant settings and insist upon receipt of payment before treatment, patients are exposed to risk of fraud. How often fraud occurs in the context of medical travel is unknown. Nonetheless, fraud sometimes occurs, and the effects can be devastating. For example, in one case, Jerome Feldman was arrested in the Philippines and convicted in a U.S. Federal Court of five counts of wire fraud in connection with payment for organ transplant procedures advertised by his website.[41,42] Feldman, a former U.S. psychiatrist who fled the United States as a fugitive after being indicted for Medicare and Medicaid fraud in Florida, relocated to the Philippines. There, he created a website that he used to defraud individuals searching the Internet for kidney and liver transplants. Using multiple aliases, Feldman convinced his victims that if they came to the Philippines, he would arrange kidney and liver transplants for them. Clients would wire money to Feldman's bank account in New York State, and Feldman would then fail to arrange the promised transplants. Feldman's activities attracted the attention of law enforcement authorities after a Canadian patient was defrauded of $75,000 and died in a Manila hospital after being promised and failing to receive a liver transplant.

In another case, the two owners of EcuMedical Resources International, a Canadian medical tourism company, were each charged with eight counts of fraud after accepting payments from clients and then failing to pay U.S. hospitals for the treatments provided to their customers.[43] Clients paid EcuMedical for arranging medical procedures and were then served with debt collection notices sent by the hospitals that did not receive payment from EcuMedical. The company closed following these allegations of fraud.

When researchers address risks related to medical travel, they commonly focus upon threats to health of medical travelers. They fail to acknowledge that financial harm needs to be included in analysis of risks related to medical travel. Of course, fraud can have direct effects upon the health of victims in addition to causing financial losses. Depending upon the condition of medical travelers, fraud can have life-threatening implications if a seriously ill person travels to a distant country with the expectation of prompt access to treatment and then is not provided the treatment he or she has paid to receive.

In addition to being victims of fraudulent activities, medical travelers and international medical facilities have themselves engaged in activities intended to defraud health insurance companies. Proponents of developing an expanded global health services marketplace argue in favor of making health insurance portable across national borders.[44] They propose letting health insurance plans incorporate international health care providers meeting Joint Commission International standards. They claim that the costs of health care will be lowered, and health insurance premiums will drop if health insurance plans are developed in a manner that encourages individuals to travel to countries where medical procedures are available at lower rates than in domestic facilities. While cross-border health insurance might generate cost savings in settings with sufficiently robust regulatory standards and law enforcement capabilities, it is important to understand that increased risk of cross-border health insurance fraud is likely to accompany efforts to globalize health insurance plans.

Since the 1990s, U.S. Federal Bureau of Investigation offices in California, Arizona, and Nevada have pursued several major investigations of fraudulent health insurance claims involving U.S. patients obtaining health care at medical facilities in Mexico.[45,46] These schemes to defraud health insurance companies typically operated in two distinct ways.[47,48] In some instances, health care facilities in Mexico treated U.S. patients suffering from minor medical problems and then inflated bills by submitting insurance claims for "emergency" medical interventions that had not been provided. Fraud was perpetrated by the medical facilities in Mexico and did not involve active participation by U.S. citizens. The second type of health insurance fraud involved U.S. patients colluding with health care providers in Mexico. In these schemes, U.S. citizens traveled to health care facilities in Mexico and underwent cosmetic surgery procedures that were not covered by their private health insurance plans. The hospitals and clinics then submitted bills for emergency medical procedures covered under the terms of the patients' health insurance coverage. The scheme enabled participating patients to receive "free" cosmetic surgery procedures while the medical facilities were paid by insurers for "emergency treatments" that were not provided.

Future efforts to promote portable health insurance plans need to better address the risk of increased cross-border health insurance fraud. Investigating cross-border health insurance fraud is time consuming, labor intensive, and requires appropriate claims-monitoring mechanisms. Some cases raise complicated questions about legal jurisdiction and authority to investigate allegations of fraud. Cross-border health insurance fraud poses significant challenges to law enforcement agencies and the investigative units of health insurance companies facing suspicious claims for out-of-country emergency medical care. Efforts to promote medical travel and make health insurance portable across national boundaries are likely to be accompanied by an increase in health insurance fraud. Just as it is important to protect medical travelers from risk of fraud, it is important to appreciate that health insurers are at risk of being defrauded if adequate transnational regulatory structures are not established to govern the global health services marketplace.

RISKS TO PRIVACY AND CONFIDENTIALITY OF PATIENT INFORMATION

Most countries have national legislation governing privacy and confidentiality of medical records. This legislation typically applies to hospitals and clinics, other health care institutions, and health care professionals. Respect for patients' privacy is an important component of the relationship between patients and health care professionals. Patients need to be able to speak freely about their health and know that this information will not enter the public domain. Laws governing privacy and confidentiality of patient information and medical records do not directly address the role medical tourism companies and destination hospitals play in recording information and transmitting across national boundaries details about patients and their health problems. Rather, legislation governing privacy and confidentiality of medical records typically assumes that health care will be obtained in domestic facilities.

The extent to which medical tourism companies and international hospitals conform to either legislation governing privacy and confidentiality of patient information in the countries where they are located or laws in countries from which their customers travel is unclear. Medical tourism companies are neither hospitals nor clinics; they are not subject to accreditation, inspection, certification or other forms of regulatory oversight. While medical tourism companies must comply with domestic criminal and civil law, it is unclear whether most medical tourism companies have the legal knowledge, training programs, and information technology infrastructure needed to conform to national legislation concerning privacy of patient information and confidentiality of medical records. Health care providers sometimes work for medical tourism companies or serve as consultants to them, but many medical tourism companies are not staffed by licensed health care professionals. With destination health care facilities and medical tourism companies located in different legal contexts and spread over the globe, there is considerable variation in how medical tourism companies and destination medical facilities store, utilize, transmit, and disclose patient information.

Though no studies address how medical tourism companies and destination hospitals store client-related data and transmit patient information, there are grounds to question the adequacy of standards governing privacy and confidentiality of information in transnational medical travel. Many medical tourism companies post to their websites photos, videos, and additional information concerning their clients. Some medical tourism companies and destination hospitals provide information about the procedures their clients underwent and reveal patient identifiers. It is conceivable that some medical travelers consent to disclosure of such detailed personal information. It is also possible that standards for protecting and promoting privacy and confidentiality of patient information vary across cultural and national contexts. At present, insufficient attention is being given to various risks associated with divulging patient information that in domestic contexts is considered confidential. The expansion of medical travel has not been accompanied by legislative developments addressing privacy of patient information and confidentiality of medical records in a transnational context. As a result, many of the standards governing privacy and confidentiality of patient information within national contexts fail to protect patients when health care becomes global in scale.

FINANCIAL RISKS TO PUBLICLY FUNDED HEALTH SYSTEMS

Individual decisions to arrange health care at international facilities can have collective costs when patients return to their local communities and require costly follow-up treatment provided by publicly funded health systems. A report from Australia describes a case in which an Australian man traveled to India and had a total knee arthroplasty even though the patient's local physician had recommended nonsurgical treatment and monitoring for his osteoarthritic knee.[49] The patient experienced multiple complications following surgery in India and required four subsequent operations and an extensive course of antimicrobial therapy following his return to the Australian health care system. While the medical traveler paid just $8,600 in Australian dollars for his surgery in India, the total cost to the publicly funded Australian health care system for postoperative care came to over $AUS140,000. Health care professionals in England and Canada likewise describe cases in which they provided publicly funded health care to treat surgical complications and infections in medical travelers who went abroad for surgery and returned home requiring postoperative medical care.[50,51]

Decisions to seek medical care abroad have collective consequences whenever publicly funded health systems must absorb cost of care required to address surgical complications and infections acquired at international medical facilities. One reason that it is possible for international hospitals and clinics to advertise inexpensive medical procedures is that these facilities know there is little chance that they will be held financially accountable if medical travelers experience postoperative complications and require costly follow-up care. By the time such problems become apparent, medical travelers often have already returned home. Some medical tourism companies and destination hospitals are explicit about this arrangement. They inform medical travelers that if they require follow-up care, they should plan to visit hospitals and clinics in their local communities.

When follow-up care entails trivial expenditures, provision of publicly funded health care to medical travelers who return home with postoperative complications does not raise major ethical concerns. However, when treating complications of medical travelers generates significant costs for publicly funded health systems, it is reasonable to ask whether drawing health care resources from other citizens transforms individual decisions to seek care abroad into collective concerns about fair, equitable use of health resources.

When travel abroad leads to infections and other complications requiring postoperative treatment, publicly funded health care systems are forced to subsidize the decisions of medical travelers going abroad to access health care. Medical travel insurance could address this problem by ensuring that medical travelers are insured when they travel abroad and experience treatment-related complications. However, it is unclear how many medical travelers have such insurance, whether travelers are adequately covered when they make claims on these policies, and what notions of "standard of care," "substandard care," and "medical negligence" mean in contexts where standards of medical professionalism vary across professional and legal jurisdictions. Travel for medical care is often characterized as a personal choice and an "individual right." It is important to understand that these personal choices can have collective consequences and impose financial burdens on public health systems providing care to medical travelers requiring treatment after they return home.

PUBLIC HEALTH AND RISKS ASSOCIATED WITH SPREAD OF INFECTIOUS DISEASES

When medical travelers return home with infections acquired from organ or tissue transplants, blood transfusions, surgical interventions, or hospitals stays, they are at risk of spreading communicable diseases within their home communities.[52,53] Reports of disease outbreaks involving medical travelers are rare. Nonetheless, individuals who travel abroad for medical care and then return home with infectious diseases are at risk of transmitting those diseases to family members, neighbors, and workplace colleagues as well as other patients and health care providers if they are hospitalized for care upon their return home. Some infectious diseases are endemic in leading medical travel destinations and extremely rare in the communities to which medical travelers return. Medical travelers can play a role in increasing risk of transmission of infectious diseases to settings where they are not commonly found. In addition, some medical travelers return home with multidrug-resistant infections. Recent research on New Delhi metallo-beta-lactamase-1 (NDM-1), an enzyme that confers drug resistance to bacteria, suggests that medical travel played a role in the global spread of multidrug-resistant organisms carrying NDM-1 from India and Pakistan to countries around the world.[54,55] Caring for such individuals as well as isolating them from other patients and preventing further spread of antibiotic resistant organisms is costly, labor intensive, and burdensome to health systems treating returned medical travelers.[56]

The role medical travel plays in contributing to the global spread of infectious diseases and antibiotic resistant organisms is a subject of growing interest to public health specialists and infectious disease researchers.[57] The subject is explored at length in chapter 6. Individual choices to travel for health care, because they can result in patients traveling to settings where medical travelers are at increased risk of exposure to infectious diseases and multidrug-resistant organisms, can pose significant risks to public health in the communities to which medical travelers return after receiving treatment.

RISKS TO HEALTH EQUITY IN
MEDICAL TRAVEL DESTINATIONS

India, Singapore, the Philippines, and many other countries promote medical tourism as a national economic development strategy. Developing a medical tourism industry is supposed to attract tourism dollars and boost foreign direct investment. Constructing hospitals, clinics, and "medi-cities" is intended to contribute to health care infrastructure development and improve local access to health care. Though national medical tourism initiatives are typically promoted as generating social and economic benefits, as chapters 4 and 5 note, in some countries the emergence of private, for-profit medical facilities catering to international patients poses risks to health equity.[58,59]

First, efforts to promote medical tourism can have effects upon health human resources and distribution of health care providers. Private hospitals and clinics need to be staffed with trained health care professionals. Doctors, nurses, and other health care providers must be located and recruited in a global marketplace where health care providers are in great demand. Most researchers examining the "brain drain" of health care providers address the international movement of doctors and nurses from such countries as India, Pakistan, South Africa, and the Philippines to such nations as Australia, Canada, England, and the United States. However, migration of health human resources also occurs within nations as health care providers relocate from underfunded and understaffed public health care facilities to private, for-profit hospitals catering to medical travelers and wealthy local elites.[60] In both India and Thailand, construction of private, for-profit "five star" hospitals combined with an influx of international patients has resulted in clinicians, particularly specialists, relocating from overburdened and underfinanced publicly funded facilities providing health care to local populations to health care facilities offering higher salaries and better working conditions.[61,62] Migration of health care personnel from public hospitals to private, for-profit facilities leaves already struggling public health systems even further understaffed.

Second, in India and other countries promoting national medical tourism initiatives, significant expenditures of public funds are used to support construction of private, for-profit health care facilities built for the purpose of treating wealthy local citizens and international patients. Governments pay for road construction, upgrade airports, bridges, and other public infrastructure, and donate inexpensive public land to private corporations. Government support for private health care facilities is typically provided with the understanding that these institutions will reserve a specified number of beds for the care of low-income local citizens. However, numerous studies and legal decisions reveal that private, for-profit hospitals often do not provide such care to local individuals.[63] Instead, public funds are absorbed by business enterprises without a return benefit to local communities. When this occurs, public funds subsidize inexpensive health care for international patients instead of being used to improve local health equity.

Third, promotion of medical travel does not necessarily realize the theoretical economic "trickle down" effect. An increase in the number of medical travelers is supposed to generate economic benefits for hotel employees, hospital employees, taxi drivers, and other individuals. However, there is little evidence that economic benefits from medical travel are broadly distributed and benefit local communities.

Fourth, treating medical travelers and developing medical tourism as an industry promotes a particular kind of biomedicine that may not benefit the general population. Hospitals trying to attract international patients purchase expensive diagnostic imaging suites and advanced biomedical technologies.[64] In many countries promoting medical tourism, most local citizens cannot afford access to these technologies. The practical result is that in some medical tourism destinations, local citizens cannot obtain even basic medical care, while international patients benefit from access to advanced biomedical technologies. A technology-oriented form of medicine is given precedence over preventive medicine, primary care, and public health.[65]

Medical travel risks increasing health inequities rather than improving health equity in countries attracting international patients. Rather than investing in community medicine and basic public health infrastructure, countries promoting medical tourism build health care industries intended to serve local elites and international patients. International patients obtain access to sophisticated technologies and a high ratio of doctors and nurses to patients, while local citizens remain vulnerable to malnutrition and infectious diseases that could be eradicated with increased investments in public health. It might be possible to use a portion of fees paid by international medical travelers, or a tax on treatments provided international patients, to improve health equity in low-income nations. In practice, however, attracting medical travelers often seems to harm rather than promote health equity.

ORGAN TRANSPLANTS AND RISKS
TO VULNERABLE POPULATIONS

Medical travel for commercial organ transplants poses serious risks not just to transplant recipients but also to the impoverished individuals who sell kidneys to international patients. When individuals sell a kidney in India, Egypt, Pakistan, the Philippines, and other countries where buying and selling human organs occurs, they rarely understand the long-term consequences of this choice. Numerous reports indicate that the health and overall quality of life of kidney sellers deteriorates following nephrectomy.[66,67] Sellers experience pain, suffer from increased rates of hypertension and other health problems, and often find it difficult to return to physically demanding forms of employment. Many kidney sellers are promised a particular amount for their kidney and then, after surgery, they are paid less than what they were promised. Researchers studying organ sellers in India, Pakistan, and the Philippines report that the money individuals receive after selling a kidney commonly goes to debt collectors.[68] Whatever earnings remain soon disappear and do not provide long-term economic benefits. Kidney selling to international patients, rather than leading to financial gains for sellers, often causes long-term economic harms in addition to a decline in health.

Medical travel involving kidney buying and selling typically occurs in settings where poverty is accompanied by high levels of corruption. Organ trafficking is illegal in Egypt, India, Pakistan, and the Philippines, but enforcement of legislation is lax. Sellers are desperate—their decisions can hardly be described as "voluntary" if their socioeconomic circumstances are acknowledged—and the entire enterprise is based upon the existence of impoverished, vulnerable populations.[69] Medical travel undertaken for the purpose of purchasing kidneys exploits individuals living in poverty and fails to generate the economic improvements that sellers expect when they decide to exchange kidneys for cash. The practice also poses risks to transplant recipients because often commercially acquired kidneys do not undergo proper testing and screening. Failure to screen transplanted tissues leaves organ buyers at risk of complications and death.[70,71] In addition, transplant recipients are sometimes infected with diseases capable of spreading in the communities to which medical travelers return following transplantation.[72] Buying kidneys from impoverished, vulnerable persons poses significant risks to buyers and sellers. Chapter 7 explores these and other considerations of travel for transplants in depth.

CONCLUSION

Medical tourism companies as well as destination hospitals and clinics benefit from the emergence of a global health services marketplace. Governments in India, Singapore, and other countries regard medical travel as a component of larger efforts to build knowledge-based "bioeconomies." These countries see medical travel as having potential as a national economic development strategy. Advocates for international trade in health services regard global competition in health care as a tool for encouraging local health care providers to reduce the costs of treatment and improve the quality of their services.[73] Global competition, according to proponents of international trade, will generate lower prices for health care, improve consumer experiences, and provide faster access to health care as the world's best medical facilities outperform less efficient, capable, and customer-centric health care providers.

Acknowledging that the emergence of a global health services marketplace benefits some patients, there are many risks associated with increasing the number of patients participating in medical travel. Financial interests of medical tourism companies as well as destination hospitals and clinics can lead to inadequate disclosure of risks of treatment and exaggerated accounts of benefits of care. Involvement of sales representatives at destination health care facilities and sales agents at medical tourism companies prompts questions about what informed consent means in conversations where medical information is provided by individuals who are not trained as health care professionals and profit from selling medical procedures. Privacy of patient information and confidentiality of medical records are at risk in a global marketplace where there are no transnational regulatory standards for protecting information that in the local communities of many medical travelers is subject to strict regulation. Patient safety and quality of medical care are at risk in a global marketplace where health care practices and health care standards vary. Standards for medical education and licensure, hospital accreditation, screening and testing of blood, tissues, and organs, infection control, and clinical care differ around the world. International hospital accreditation is supposed to indicate that select international health care facilities have the "gold seal of approval" provided by Joint Commission International (JCI). However, it is unclear whether JCI sets a sufficiently robust standard when evaluating international medical facilities. Payment of international accreditors for the service of accreditation raises disturbing questions about financial conflicts of interest and the integrity of the accreditation process. Financial arrangements in which institutions undergoing accreditation pay accrediting agencies are vulnerable to a form of regulatory capture in which accrediting organizations must satisfy clients if they wish to retain customers.

Continuity of care is at risk when health care occurs across geographically distant settings. Case reports reveal that some medical travelers go abroad, receive care, and return home with serious postoperative complications. They return to their communities with no plans for postoperative care. Medical travelers must then struggle to gain access to needed treatment. Some clinicians are reluctant to treat patients seen in other settings. In settings where medical travelers return home and require publicly funded postoperative health care, administrators and clinicians in these health systems question whether individuals who return from abroad with complications ought to have nonemergency care covered by publicly funded health insurance.

Across jurisdictions, legislation varies concerning personal injury, medical negligence, and professional standards of care. National variations in legal frameworks can leave medical travelers with little recourse if they are harmed while obtaining medical care at international facilities. Waiver of liability forms routinely used by medical tourism companies are intended to make it difficult for medical travelers to initiate lawsuits against these businesses. Some medical travelers find it difficult to obtain legal redress when they are harmed as a result of receiving care at international medical facilities. Though there is now a global marketplace in health services, this marketplace is not governed by global legal norms and regulatory standards.

Medical travel also poses risks to public health and health equity in destination nations. Countries such as India, Indonesia, Malaysia, and the Philippines have poured public resources into developing medical tourism industries. These public funds subsidize the care of international patients seeking care in elite "five star" medical facilities. Limited public resources might have a more significant impact if they were used to fund public health infrastructure and promote health equity in settings with malnutrition, preventable infectious diseases, and high levels of social and economic inequality. Public health in countries to which medical travelers return after receiving care abroad is also at risk as the number of medical travelers increases. Some medical travelers return home with infectious diseases and multi-drug-resistant organisms. Putting medical travelers with communicable diseases in isolation and establishing rigorous infection control measures imposes economic, organizational, and health human resources burdens on health care systems. These costs will escalate if more medical travelers return home with multidrug-resistant infections. The "personal" choices of medical travelers have public consequences when patients return home and contribute to the spread of infectious diseases.

Proponents of trade in health services provide an idealized account of the many benefits presumed to flow from increased medical travel and expansion of the global health services marketplace. According to advocates of expanding global trade in health services, policy measures can mitigate risks and ensure that medical travelers do not receive substandard medical care, return home with serious postoperative complications, or contribute to the spread of infectious diseases. Advocates of a global marketplace in health services offer a vision of high-quality, low-cost, accessible, and "customer-centric" care. This model fails to adequately address the many different risks associated with medical travel and globalization of health care.

Medical travel benefits some patients. High-quality health care is available in countries around the world, and it is important to acknowledge that many individuals cross national borders and obtain the professional care they seek. However, the idealized model of global trade in health services fails to address the many risks accompanying the emergence of a global health services marketplace. These problems suggest that medical travel is far more complicated and, in at least some circumstances, hazardous than idealized models suggest. Globalization of health care has not been accompanied by globalization of regulatory mechanisms, legal norms, and clinical protections for medical travelers. Until basic issues related to information disclosure and informed consent, patient safety and quality of care, confidentiality and privacy of medical records, legal redress in case of personal injury or medical negligence, and postoperative and long-term care are better addressed by all parties involved in the medical travel industry, there is reason to wonder whether most patients might be better served by seeking care from local health care providers rather than exposing themselves to the numerous risks associated with obtaining treatment in the global health services marketplace.

REFERENCES

1. Bagadia N. The Western "seal of approval": Advanced liberalism and technologies of governing in medical travel to India. *International Journal of Behavioural and Healthcare Research.* 2010;2:85–110.

2. Moore JD, Jr. Going global. JCAHO to accredit foreign healthcare organizations. *Mod Healthc.* 1998;28(14):44, 46.

3. Turner L. "First World health care at Third World prices": Globalization, bioethics and medical tourism. *BioSocieties.* 2007;2:303–325.

4. Sobo E, Herlihy E, Bicker M. Selling medical travel to U.S. patient-consumers: The cultural appeal of website marketing messages. *Anthropology & Medicine.* 2011;18:119–136.

5. Turner L. "Medical tourism" and the global marketplace in health services: U.S. patients, international hospitals, and the search for affordable health care. *Int. J. Health Serv.* 2010;40(3):443–467.

6. Crone RK. Flat medicine? Exploring trends in the globalization of health care. *Acad Med.* 2008;83(2):117–121.

7. Lunt N, Hardey M, Mannion R. Nip, tuck and click: Medical tourism and the emergence of web-based health information. *The Open Medical Informatics Journal.* 2010;4:1–11.

8. Connell J. Medical tourism: Sea, sun, sand and . . . surgery. *Tourism Management.* 2006;27:1093–1100.

9. Passmore R. Converting international patient inquiries @10%–Part 2. *Medical Tourism Magazine.* December 17, 2009.

10. Lunt N, Carrera P. Systematic review of web sites for prospective medical tourists. *Tourism Review.* 2011;66:57–67.

11. Penney K, Snyder J, Crooks V, Johnston R. Risk communication and informed consent in the medical tourism industry: A thematic content analysis of Canadian broker websites. *BMC Medical Ethics.* 2011;12:17.

12. Nassab R, Hamnett N, Nelson K, Kaur S, Greensill B, Dhital S, Juma A. Cosmetic tourism: Public opinion and analysis of information and content available on the Internet. *Aesthetic Surgery Journal.* 2010;30(3):465–469.

13. Mason A, Wright K. Framing medical tourism: An examination of appeal, risk, convalescence, accreditation, and interactivity in medical tourism web sites. *Journal of Health Communication.* 2011;1:1–15.

14. Lunt N, Carrera P. Systematic review of web sites for prospective medical tourists. *Tourism Review.* 2011;66:57–67.

15. Turner L. Quality in health care and globalization of health services: Accreditation and regulatory oversight of medical tourism companies. *International Journal for Quality in Health Care.* 2011;23:1–7.

16. Yang Y, Ani S, Bartlett G, Moazzam A. Cosmetic medical tourism: Its true cost. *ANZ Journal of Surgery.* 2009;79(s1):A60.

17. Newman M, Camberos A, Ascherman J. Mycobacteria absessus outbreak in U.S. patients linked to offshore surgicenter. *Annals of Plastic Surgery.* 2005;55(1):107–110.

18. Birch J, Caulfield R, Ramakrishnan V. The complications of "cosmetic tourism"—an avoidable burden on the NHS. *J Plast Reconstr Aesthet Surg.* 2007; 60(9):1075–1077.

19. Jeevan R, Armstrong A. Cosmetic tourism and the burden on the NHS. *J Plast Reconstr Aesthet Surg.* 2008;61(12):1423–1424.

20. Green S. Medical tourism—a potential growth factor in infection medicine and public health. *Journal of Infection.* 2008;57(5):429.

21. Bal A. Medicine, merit, money and caste: The complexity of medical education in India. *Indian Journal of Medical Ethics.* 2010;7:25–28.

22. Chattopadhyay S. Black money in white coats: Whither medical ethics? *Indian Journal of Medical Ethics.* 2008;5:20–21.

23. Coker R, Hunter B, Rudge J, Liverani M, Hanvoravongchai P. Emerging infectious diseases in southeast Asia: Regional challenges to control. *The Lancet.* 2011;377:599–609.

24. Bhatia V, Arora P, Parida AK, Singh G, Kaul U. Air travel and pulmonary embolism: "Economy class syndrome." *Indian Heart J.* 2008;60(6):608–611.

25. Feltracco P, Barbieri S, Bertamini F, Michieletto E, Ori C. Economy class syndrome: Still a recurrent complication of long journeys. *Eur J Emerg Med.* 2007;14(2):100–103.

26. Handschin A, Banic A, Constantinescu M. Pulmonary embolism after plastic surgery tourism. *Clinical and Applied Thrombosis/Hemostasis.* 2007;13(3):340.

27. Gajic O, Sprung J, Hall BA, Lightner DJ. Fatal acute pulmonary embolism in a patient with pelvic lipomatosis after surgery performed after transatlantic airplane travel. *Anesth Analg.* 2004;99(4):1032–1034.

28. Penney K, Snyder J, Crooks V, Johnston R. Risk communication and informed consent in the medical tourism industry: A thematic content analysis of Canadian broker websites. *BMC Medical Ethics.* 2011;12:17.

29. Lapostolle F, Surget V, Borron SW, et al. Severe pulmonary embolism associated with air travel. *N Engl J Med.* 2001;345(11):779–783.

30. Bartholomew J, Schaffer J, McCormick G. Air travel and venous thrombo-embolism: Minimizing the risk. *Cleveland Clinic Journal of Medicine.* 2011;78:111–120.

31. Hanna S, Saksena J, Legge S, Ware H. Sending NHS patients for operations abroad: Is the holiday over? *Annals of the Royal College of Surgeons of England.* 2009;91:128–130.

32. Birch DW, Vu L, Karmali S, Stoklossa CJ, Sharma AM. Medical tourism in bariatric surgery. *Am J Surg.* 2010;199(5):604–608.

33. Furuya EY, Paez A, Srinivasan A, et al. Outbreak of Mycobacterium abscessus wound infections among "lipotourists" from the United States who underwent abdominoplasty in the Dominican Republic. *CID.* 2008;46:1181–1188.

34. Birch J, Caulfield R, Ramakrishnan V. The complications of "cosmetic tourism"—an avoidable burden on the NHS. *J Plast Reconstr Aesthet Surg.* 2007; 60(9):1075–1077.

35. Jeevan R, Armstrong A. Cosmetic tourism and the burden on the NHS. *J Plast Reconstr Aesthet Surg.* 2008;61(12):1423–1424.

36. Jones JW, McCullough LB. What to do when a patient's international medical care goes south. *J Vasc Surg.* 2007;46(5):1077–1079.

37. Wachter RM. The "dis-location" of U.S. medicine—the implications of medical outsourcing. *N Engl J Med.* 2006;354(7):661–665.

38. Cortez N. Patients without borders: The emerging global market for patients and the evolution of modern health care. *Indiana Law Journal.* 2008;83:71–132.

39. Mirrer-Singer P. Medical malpractice overseas: The legal uncertainty surrounding medical tourism. *Law and Contemporary Problems.* 2007;70:211–232.

40. Cortez N. Recalibrating the legal risks of cross-border health care. *Yale Journal of Health Policy, Law, and Ethics.* Winter 2010:1–89.

41. Barrera J. U.S. man to face trial in global organ scam: Victims include Canadians. *Montreal Gazette.* March 26, 2009.

42. O'Brien J. Former doctor imprisoned 16 years for phony organ transplant scam. *Syracuse Post-Standard.* May 27, 2010.

43. Puzic S. Windsor police lay fraud charges against EcuMedical couple. *Windsor Star.* October 28, 2010.

44. Mattoo A, Rathindran R. How health insurance inhibits trade in health care. *Health Aff.* 2006;25(2):358–368.

45. O'Connor A. 21 arraigned in cross-border fraud scheme. *Los Angeles Times.* October 16, 1997:23.

46. Weber T. Fraudulent foreign medical claims plague insurers; crime: Billings for exaggerated or nonexistent care increase from Mexico to Nigeria. *Los Angeles Times.* October 6, 1996.

47. Kranhold K. U.S. arrests 19 in alleged scheme to bilk insurers. *Wall Street Journal.* October 15, 1997:1.

48. Shroder S. Four accused in surgery scheme. *The San Diego Union-Tribune.* April 25, 2009:B3.

49. Cheung IK, Wilson A. Arthroplasty tourism. *Med J Aust.* 2007;187(11–12): 666–667.

50. Birch J, Caulfield R, Ramakrishnan V. The complications of "cosmetic tourism"—an avoidable burden on the NHS. *J Plast Reconstr Aesthet Surg.* 2007; 60(9):1075–1077.

51. Birch DW, Vu L, Karmali S, Stoklossa CJ, Sharma AM. Medical tourism in bariatric surgery. *Am J Surg.* 2010;199(5):604–608.

52. Farrugia A. Globalisation and blood safety. *Blood Rev.* 2009;23(3):123–128.

53. Harling R, Turbitt D, Millar M, et al. Passage from India: An outbreak of hepatitis B linked to a patient who acquired infection from health care overseas. *Public Health.* 2007;121(10):734–741.

54. Kumarasamy KK, Toleman MA, Walsh TR, et al. Emergence of a new antibiotic resistance mechanism in India, Pakistan, and the UK: A molecular, biological, and epidemiological study. *Lancet Infect Dis.* 2010;10(9):597–602.

55. Poirel L, Lagrutta E, Taylor P, Pham J, Nordmann P. Emergence of metallo-ss-lactamase NDM-1-producing multidrug resistant Escherichia coli in Australia. *Antimicrob Agents Chemother.* 2010;54 (11):4914–4916.

56. Muir A, Weinbren MJ. New Delhi metallo-beta-lactamase: A cautionary tale. *J Hosp Infect.* 2010;75(3):239–240.

57. Hall CM, James M. Medical tourism: Emerging biosecurity and nosocomial issues. *Tourism Review.* 2011;66:118–126.

58. Kanchanachitra C, Lindelow M, Johnston T, Hanvoravongchai P, Lorenzo F, Huong N, Wilopo S, dela Rosa J. Human resources for health in southeast Asia: Shortages, distributional challenges, and international trade in health services. *The Lancet.* 2011;377;769–781.

59. Sen Gupta A. Medical tourism in India: Winners and losers. *Indian J. Med Ethics.* 2008;5(1):4–5.

60. Pachanee CA, Wibulpolprasert S. Incoherent policies on universal coverage of health insurance and promotion of international trade in health services in Thailand. *Health Policy Plan.* 2006;21(4):310–318.

61. NaRanong A, NaRanong V. The effects of medical tourism: Thailand's experience. *Bulletin of the World Health Organization.* 2011;89:336–344.

62. Hazarika I. Medical tourism: Its potential impact on the health workforce and health systems in India. *Health Policy Plan.* 2010;25(3):248–251.

63. Thomas G, Krishnan S. Effective public-private partnership in healthcare: Apollo as a cautionary tale. *Indian J. Med. Ethics.* 2010;7(1):2–4.

64. Mahal A, Karan AK. Diffusion of medical technology: Medical devices in India. *Expert Rev. Med. Devices.* 2009;6(2):197–205.

65. Wilson C. Dis-embedding health care: Marketisation and the rising cost of medicine in Kerala, South India. *Journal of South Asian Development.* 2009;4:83–101.

66. Moazam F, Zaman RM, Jafarey AM. Conversations with kidney vendors in Pakistan: An ethnographic study. *Hastings Cent. Rep.* 2009;39(3):29–44.

67. Naqvi SA, Ali B, Mazhar F, Zafar MN, Rizvi SA. A socioeconomic survey of kidney vendors in Pakistan. *Transpl. Int.* 2007;20(11):934–939.

68. Scheper-Hughes N. The global traffic in human organs. *Curr. Anthropol.* 2000;41(2):191–224.

69. Scheper-Hughes N. Keeping an eye on the global traffic in human organs. *Lancet.* 2003;361(9369):1645–1648.

70. Canales MT, Kasiske BL, Rosenberg ME. Transplant tourism: Outcomes of United States residents who undergo kidney transplantation overseas. *Transplantation.* 2006;82(12):1658–1661.

71. Yakupoglu YK, Ozden E, Dilek M, et al. Transplantation tourism: High risk for the recipients. *Clin. Transplant.* 2010;24(6):835–838.

72. Harling R, Turbitt D, Millar M, et al. Passage from India: An outbreak of hepatitis B linked to a patient who acquired infection from health care overseas. *Public Health.* 2007;121(10):734–741.

73. Mattoo A, Rathindran R. How health insurance inhibits trade in health care. *Health Aff.* 2006;25(2):358–368.

Chapter 13

Medical Tourism Facilitators: Ethical Concerns about Roles and Responsibilities

Jeremy Snyder, Valorie A. Crooks, Alexandra Wright, and Rory Johnston

Within the medical tourism industry are a number of key stakeholders—groups and individuals who champion the development of the industry, provide services within the industry, use the services of the industry, or are directly or indirectly impacted by the industry—who contribute to its expansion. One such group is facilitators, private agents who broker medical travel and foreign care arrangements between patients and destination facilities but are not employed by these facilities.[1] Key to this element of the medical tourism industry is the Internet. Facilitation companies in many countries have a strong web presence and rely primarily on websites (and secondarily on word of mouth) to advertise their services.[1-4]

Medical tourism facilitators' responsibilities toward medical tourists can include securing travel and accommodation needs, suggesting and booking facilities and surgeons abroad, contacting destination clinics, overseeing translation of medical records, arranging for tourist activities, and transferring medical records.[5] These facilitators can play an essential role in facilitating communication, providing information, and securing overall quality control by assessing the reputability and reliability of international facilities.[3] It appears, however, that only a fraction of medical tourists actually use the services of facilitators.[1] Facilitators themselves have indicated this, noting that patients wanting to go abroad for care sometimes seek them out as an informational resource even though they never actually intend to book care through them.[3]

There is no single business model for medical tourism facilitators. This is perhaps not surprising given the range of roles and responsibilities they may take on. Some facilitators refer patients to a number of countries, while others refer only to one or two trusted international facilities.[3] Some arrange care for hundreds of medical tourists each year, while others do so for less than 20 clients per year.[3] Some specialize in arranging care abroad for a particular procedure or group of procedures, while others have no stated limitations on procedures for which they are willing to arrange care.[3] These are but a few of the fundamental differences between medical tourism facilitators' business practices. While some facilitators view themselves as patient advocates and change agents, playing an involved role in patient care coordination and putting forth calls for domestic health system reform, others see their roles and responsibilities as much more limited, primarily focusing on the logistics of securing care abroad.[5] In general, medical tourism facilitation remains relatively fluid and undefined as a profession. There is also no overarching professional organization providing mandatory monitoring of facilitators and their practices.[6]

In this chapter, we review ethical concerns that have been raised in the medical tourism literature with regard to the specific roles and responsibilities of medical tourism facilitators, including as they relate to business practices. We also examine the evidence available in the scholarly literature to support or refute these concerns. As we outline below, most of the scholarly literature that offers primary data-based insights on facilitators' roles and practices uses facilitator websites, interviews with facilitators, or legal cases as empirical sources. We compare the ethical concerns raised in the ethical and legal literature to the empirical findings about facilitators' roles and practices in reviews of facilitator websites, interviews, and legal cases to identify which of these concerns have been borne out thus far. Finally, we use the gaps that emerge between these two bodies of scholarly literature to assess proposed regulation (i.e., the creation of an institutional framework, such as laws or operating regulations) of medical tourism facilitators and to identify future research directions. In doing so, we aim to present the current state of knowledge about the ethical issues raised by medical tourism facilitation and guide continued research on this topic.

EXISTING ETHICAL CONCERNS ABOUT MEDICAL TOURISM FACILITATORS

Through our review of the ethical and legal literature about medical tourism, we identified five areas of ethical concern most commonly discussed about the roles and responsibilities of facilitators. These areas are (1) facilitator training and accreditation (i.e., facility- or organizational-level systems for enacting and assessing standards), (2) facilitator conflicts of interest, (3) transparency and patients' consent to risks, (4) problems with continuity of care and follow-up care, and (5) liability for harms. In the remainder of this section of the chapter, we outline the scope of the ethical concerns in each of these areas and then examine the extent to which the empirical medical tourism literature confirms that these problems actually are occurring. Table 13.1 provides an overview of the data available in the empirical sources we discuss.

Table 13.1
Empirical sources reviewed

Source title	Authors	Year	Source(s) of data
The Potential for Bi-lateral Agreements in Medical Tourism: A Qualitative Study of Stakeholder Perspectives from the UK and India	Alvarez, Chanda, Smith	2011	30 medical tourism stakeholder interviews (10 in United Kingdom, 20 in India), including 2 with facilitators
Medical Travel Facilitator Websites: An Exploratory Study of Web Page Contents and Services Offered to the Prospective Medical Tourist	Cormany, Baloglu	2011	website review (reviewed 57 websites of facilitators—24 N. American, 11 Asian, 8 European, 8 Central and S. American, 6 African)
Patients Without Borders: The Emerging Global Market for Patients and the Evolution of Modern Health Care	Cortez	2008	legal review (including consideration of specific facilitator websites)
An Industry Perspective on Canadian Patients' Involvement in Medical Tourism: Implications for Public Health	Johnston, Crooks, Adams, Snyder, Kingsbury	2011	12 interviews with Canadian medical tourism facilitators
Systematic review of web sites for prospective medical tourists	Lunt, Carrera	2011	website review (reviewed 50 English language websites of facilitators)

(continued)

Table 13.1 (continued)

Source title	Authors	Year	Source(s) of data
Framing Medical Tourism: An Examination of Appeal, Risk, Convalescence, Accreditation, and Interactivity in Medical Tourism Web Sites	Mason, Wright	2010	website review (reviewed 66 websites of United States-based facilitators)
International medical travel and the politics of therapeutic place-making in Malaysia	Ormond	2011	49 medical tourism stakeholder interviews in Malaysia, including 7 with facilitators
Risk Communication and Informed Consent in the Medical Tourism Industry: A Thematic Content Analysis of Canadian Broker Websites	Penney, Snyder, Crooks, Johnston	2011	website review (reviewed 17 websites of Canadian facilitators)
The 'Patient's Physician One-Step Removed': The Evolving Roles of Medical Tourism Facilitators	Snyder, Crooks, Adams, Kingsbury, Johnston	2011	12 interviews with Canadian medical tourism facilitators
Selling Medical Travel to US Patient-Consumers: The Cultural Appeal of Website Marketing Messages	Sobo, Herlihy, Bicker	2011	website review (reviewed 27 websites of United States-based facilitators)
Medical Tourism: Protecting Patients from Conflicts of Interest in Broker's Fees Paid by Foreign Providers	Spece	2010	legal review (including consideration of specific facilitator websites)

Note: Most existing studies of medical tourism facilitators rely on interviews with facilitators and reviews of websites and legal cases.

Facilitator Training and Accreditation

The global nature of medical tourism complicates patients' abilities to assess the credentials of the hospitals, physicians, and other health workers they may encounter in distant facilities. Patients often must navigate a bewildering array of regulatory environments, accreditation systems, and facilities in deciding whether and where to seek care. This problem extends to distinguishing the quality of medical tourism facilitators, upon whom patients may depend for help in guiding their medical decision making.[3] So while facilitators might, in principle, help patients to overcome difficulties in assessing the quality of the care they will receive abroad, patients may first find it difficult to assess the quality of facilitators and facilitation companies themselves.

While some facilitators specialize in and have detailed knowledge about specific destinations, there is no limit to the destinations—and thus different regulatory and accreditation environments—to which they may direct their clients.[6] Similarly, while some facilitators have a medical background, such training is not required for entry into the profession. It has been speculated that many facilitators come from a tourism background, with experience booking vacations, flights, and other tourist services, but lack the background to help facilitate medical tourists' medical needs.[7] This lack of training is part of a wider area of ethical concern regarding facilitators' roles and responsibilities—namely, the lack of universal standards of training and accreditation for members of this profession and, more strikingly, a lack of barriers to entering the facilitation industry, including any requirement that facilitators receive training or accreditation.[7] Meanwhile, facilitators can play a substantial role in patient decision making about the care they will receive. Facilitators who see giving medical advice as falling within their roles may suggest certain medical interventions; advise patients on the safety and outcomes of these interventions; and help guide, with substantial advice and influence, patients' health care decisions. Consequently, there is the danger that potential medical tourists will make treatment decisions without the benefit of direct consultation with medical professionals and rely instead on the recommendation of facilitators who may lack medical training or even clear standards for what information they should provide to patients.

There has been little consideration of how aware medical tourists are about facilitators' level of training. If this awareness is minimal, they are unlikely to be in a position to judge the quality of advice that they receive from these individuals. Some facilitators have the word "medical" in their titles, make seemingly informed claims about the success rates of procedures and quality of care in specific facilities and by specific physicians, and take on the role of patient advisor and even advocate.[1,5] These roles may easily confuse patients, thereby leading them to put unjustified weight on facilitators' advice. If patients are not willing to discuss their decisions to seek medical care abroad with their own physicians (or even other members of their social networks), or do not have access to a physician due to financial constraints, then the facilitators' perspectives will not be balanced by other, less financially interested views.

Just as other medical providers, including hospitals, physicians, and private clinics are regulated to instill practices that do not harm the health and safety of patients, it has been argued that medical tourism facilitators should be similarly regulated based on some kind of accreditation standards.[6] The content of these accreditation standards is still a matter of debate; for example, it is not immediately clear whether facilitators should be required to obtain some degree of medical training or whether requiring limits on the advice they give to clients would be sufficient to protect clients' interests. Without accreditation requirements, as is presently the case, there are no restrictions on who can take on the role of facilitator or repercussions for those who violate professional norms.

In a content analysis of Canadian facilitation company websites, Kali Penney and colleagues observed that the websites did not consistently refer to a single facilitator organization that represents a comprehensive monitoring body.[1] This was confirmed in Alicia Mason and Kevin Wright's analysis of facilitator websites, which found that website logos that appeared to signify quality were typically branding devices rather than evidence of facilitator certification.[8] Of the websites that Penney et al. examined, 35.3 percent contained logos or representations of various organization memberships, but only rarely were these evidence of facilitator certification (i.e., individual-level training and credentialing) by any regulatory organization. Although some sites referred to external accreditation bodies, those bodies' reputability and assessment standards are not always clear to medical tourists. This particular analysis also found that the sites generally did not indicate which of the hospitals they recommended were accredited, although 52.9 percent of websites provided information on physicians and their credentials.[1]

Mason and Wright reported that 29.3 percent of the reviewed sites gave evidence of some form of accreditation for preferred destination hospitals, such as indications that the facilities have met the standards of the Joint Commission International (JCI) or the International Organization for Standardization (ISO).[8] JCI accreditation has been used as a marker of quality and safety in the medical tourism industry and is often highly sought by facilities seeking to attract international patients.[6] But the display of hospital accreditation information on facilitator websites may confuse potential clients. Medical tourists may feel confident accepting a facilitator's services based on the mistaken belief that a preferred destination facility's accreditation also applies to the facilitator and/or facilitation company when, in fact, it says nothing about the facilitator's qualifications or knowledge.[1]

Facilitator Conflicts of Interest

Medical tourism is characterized by patients arranging for private medical services that they typically pay for out of pocket.[3] As we explained earlier, facilitators are private operators who are paid in exchange for the services they provide to those seeking this private care. But patients may not be aware of how much or in what manner facilitators are paid, since patients may not pay directly for facilitators' services. These services may be covered by referral fees paid for by the destination hospital or as part of an overall "package deal" that does not include a detailed cost breakdown. Consequently, the financial structures of medical tourism as they relate to facilitators' involvement may be opaque to individual patients.

Because medical tourism facilitators receive fees to arrange for medical services, there is potential for a conflict between the interests of the facilitators and those of patients. While some facilitators receive fees directly from their clients, and so align their interests more directly with them, other facilitators receive fees or other benefits from medical facilities or physicians abroad with whom they book procedures.[9] Thus, in some cases, the facilitator has an incentive to book procedures independent of any benefit to the patient. This conflict of interest can take the form of supplier-induced demand, in which the facilitator encourages the client to purchase specific forms of medical care, introduces the client to new options for care, or even alerts the client to previously unknown medical conditions or perceived medical needs, all while receiving payment from providers for the provision of these services.[10]

The potential for conflict of interest in medical tourism facilitators' business practices extends to facilitators recommending or encouraging clients to obtain procedures that are unavailable or illegal in their home countries. If facilitators receive booking fees, they have an incentive to encourage their clients to receive these procedures regardless of whether they are legal in the client's home country. The international dimension of medical tourism allows facilitators to promote and aid their clients in escaping the legal jurisdiction of their home countries, which undermines the ability of countries to regulate access to medical care at home.[11] While such regulations may exhibit ethically problematic paternalistic attitudes, or state enforcement of public morality on individuals (e.g., in reproductive decisions), states do have a legitimate interest in regulating the medical care provided to citizens to promote patient safety and public health.[12] In some cases, states with high regulatory thresholds for patient safety will make certain treatments unavailable out of concern for efficacy, side effects, or other threats to health. By enabling patients' access to these treatments outside of domestic regulatory frameworks, facilitators can expose clients to risks that they would not have faced in their home health systems.[6] At the same time, access to unavailable, illegal, or experimental treatment such as experimental stem cell therapies can be highly desirable for patients who are well informed about their associated uncertainties and risks; and in some of these cases, facilitators are crucial to enabling such access. (For further discussion of circumvention tourism, see chapter 10.)

Unfortunately, there is little empirical evidence to support or refute claims that medical tourism facilitators face conflicts of interest in enacting their roles and responsibilities. In a legal review, Roy Spece found that information about facilitators' fees is generally not provided up front to clients.[9] As a result, some clients may assume that facilitators are working on a nonprofit basis. The likelihood for misunderstandings regarding facilitators' referral fees received from medical tourism providers and fee structures charged to patients can be heightened by clients' unfamiliarity with medical referral fees, in light of the prohibition of referral fees in some domestic health care contexts. Rory Johnston et al. confirmed this in their study, in which Canadian facilitators speculated that Canadian patients may find the notion of paying a facilitator to assist with booking and coordinating care to be off-putting since Canada's public health care system does not require citizens to pay out of pocket for any aspect of necessary medical care.[3]

Transparency of and Consent to Risks

Medical tourism has been associated with a range of risks to the patient, including deep vein thrombosis (blood clots) due to flying soon after surgery, exposure to infectious disease, poor quality of care, and the creation of a discontinuous medical record.[13] Informed consent requires that patients receive and comprehend information pertaining to treatment options, success rates, and risks of complications prior to undergoing care. Patients may not be aware of the risks associated with medical tourism and therefore may not be able to give fully informed consent to be exposed to these potential complications.[1]

Facilitators' websites are thought to be a key, initial source of information about medical tourism for many patients.[1–4] These websites serve as a means of advertising facilitation services to potential clients, and so there is likely to be a great incentive to inform people of the potential benefits of medical tourism and to assuage any fears associated with traveling abroad for medical care. These positive messages may not be balanced against information about the risks inherent in medical travel, so patients may not receive the information necessary to give informed consent to these risks. Many patients opt for medical tourism based on the lower price of the treatments offered abroad.[13] Since cost savings are often associated with inferior quality,[14] facilitators' websites may feature an abundance of quality assurance messages as an anticipatory strategy to head off potential clients' concerns about whether these lower costs reflect poor quality.[7]

Facilitators' use of branding techniques in advertising their services, including noting that physicians at preferred destination facilities have trained in North America and Europe, and partnering with internationally recognized hospital and university brands, can help to reassure patients about the quality of care abroad. Similarly, use of accrediting agencies like the JCI may signal quality and safety to potential customers. Advertising high staffing levels and excellent customer service abroad also helps to assuage the concerns of potential medical tourists. Facilitators' references in their promotional materials to state-of-the-art medical devices and technologies available in destination hospitals counter concerns that lower levels of economic development in host countries mean lower standards of care and less technologically advanced medical equipment.[7] Again, these messages reflect facilitators' concerns with reassuring medical tourists about the quality of care received abroad and may not accurately represent the risks associated with medical travel.

Since facilitators will be motivated to communicate the potential benefits of medical tourism, it is possible for a medical tourist to book care through a facilitator and never receive a comprehensive list of the risks and dangers associated with this practice. In fact, the patient may only receive an account of the high quality of the care available abroad or at a specific facility. The accuracy of this information may be very difficult for the medical tourist to verify. Because norms and legal requirements for informed consent vary by country, the patient may have expectations for receiving information about risks that are not shared by the facilitator.[7] This problem is exacerbated by the lack of a single set of professional norms about communicating risks in the industry and an overall lack of oversight.

In reviews of facilitator websites, risk information—which is necessary for informed consent—has been found to be limited. For example, Penney et al. found that only 17.6 percent of Canadian medical tourism facilitator websites addressed possible risks and negative outcomes, and those that did most often did so in the "facts" or "disclaimer" pages.[1] Mason and Wright also found that websites rarely addressed risks and concerns on their main pages. Their study found only 4.9 percent of websites addressed postoperative care, 1.1 percent legal recourses, 2.2 percent complications, and 2.2 percent procedural risk.[8] An additional study found 16 percent of reviewed facilitator websites mentioned possible risks, but these risks were again consistently downplayed in favor of positive outcomes and benefits of medical travel.[15] Elisa Sobo et al. observed the theme of a "worry free experience" was particularly evident among medical tourism websites. Prospective clients were depicted as empowered to take control of their own medical care, with the companies' facilitators being available to assist. Risks were often addressed in "Terms and Conditions" pages of websites.[16] These reviews confirm that, "[d]espite great importance of postoperative care, procedural risk and potential medical complications when making informed decisions about undergoing a medical procedure, the issues appear to be discussed in limited ways, if at all, on the websites."[8(p173–174)] They also show that discussion of risk is rarely given "front-page" coverage on these websites.

Facilitators are commonly focused on increasing patient confidence and on the attractiveness of medical tourism destinations in terms of quality, experience, and price.[1] To heighten patient confidence, facilitators usually focus on statements of accreditation, training and experience of physicians, statements of advanced technology used in the hospitals, patient testimonials, and enjoyable environments and tourist activities.[1,16] Facilitators' marketing materials consistently demonstrate an emphasis on the likely benefits of seeking treatment abroad. As such, there is a focus on characterizing positive experiences, benefits, and outcomes of medical tourism. Penney et al. found that any mention of risk in facilitators' websites was carefully worded to emphasize the unlikelihood of negative outcomes in order to maintain a generally positive message. Some websites are careful to remind patients that similar risks occur when seeking medical treatment in their own country, which is another strategy for minimizing risk messages in marketing materials.[1]

Problems with Continuity of Care and Follow-Up Care

Medical tourism can undermine both informational continuity of care (i.e., the maintenance of a continuous and complete medical record) and access to care following treatment.[13] When medical tourism involves international travel, medical records must be transferred between countries. The geographical, cultural, and linguistic distances involved in these transfers may complicate continuity of care. The patient's medical records may become discontinuous; different groups of caregivers may have difficulty communicating with one another; or the patient may be subjected to multiple, potentially conflicting standards of care. Similarly, the self-directed nature of medical tourism means that patients may have difficulty accessing follow-up care, including for unexpected complications. The patient's domestic care providers may be unfamiliar with the care received abroad or reluctant to provide follow-up care out of a concern for legal liability for complications arising from this care—if the patient has access to care at home at all.

Facilitators may not have the capacity or background necessary to help patients arrange for continuity of care and follow-up care. Facilitators may not inform their clients of the need to work with their home country physician to arrange for medical record transfer and follow-up care if needed. They may not be aware of the need to take these steps or might be concerned that emphasizing these care coordination logistics will detract from the appeal of their services.[7] Depending on the facility, there may or may not be international patient coordinators (i.e., staff employed by the destination facility to oversee the off- and on-site logistics of treating international patients) with which the facilitator can work to ensure continuity of the patient's care.[17] In some cases, attempts to facilitate continuity of care are limited to suggestions that patients communicate with their home country doctors before and after receiving care abroad.[17] Patient-initiated conversations of this kind can however be limited if patients are ill-informed about the care they will be receiving abroad or hesitant about speaking with their regular physicians about leaving the country for care because they fear that the physician will disapprove.[3] Moreover, patients may not be aware of the potential expenses associated with receiving follow-up care upon return home, further complicating coordinating aftercare.[17] In short, there is no guarantee that patients seeking care abroad will consult with a physician before or after travel or that facilitators will aid them in doing so.[6]

Empirical studies presenting the findings of interviews with facilitators show that their roles in arranging follow-up care vary greatly.[3,5] Johnston et al. recorded a diverse spectrum of facilitator approaches to follow-up care. Some interviewees reported arranging follow-up care by request of the client only. Other interviewees frequently contacted clients upon return home from medical care abroad to discuss follow-up arrangements.[3] Facilitators who demonstrated the most involvement in follow-up care reported only accepting clients once such care had been secured. Even when facilitators want to take a role in arranging follow-up care, their efforts may be restricted in cases when clients' regular physicians do not support, or even openly disapprove of, the pursuit of care abroad and thus decline to provide the necessary tests or referrals.[3,5]

In a content analysis of 17 websites, Penney et al. found that facilitation companies claimed a wide variety of responsibilities regarding the transfer of medical records and coordination of follow-up care. Some websites clearly stated that the facilitator has no role in monitoring patient care upon arrival home. Others offered a range of services, including "arranging phone calls between the patient and specialist abroad, having report sent to home physician, organizing rehabilitation, telehealth consultations, and answering questions,"[1] However, whether these services would require additional fees or specific requests was typically not made clear. Additional website analyses support the findings of Penney et al. that follow-up care is not consistently addressed. For example, Neil Lunt and Percivil Carrera found that although preoperative consultations were often offered to potential patients, only 10 percent of websites addressed follow-up care.[15] Mason and Wright found only 4.9 percent of websites addressed follow-up care on the main page of their site, with 18.2 percent addressing follow-up care on other pages.[8]

Legal Liability for Harms

When patients seek care abroad, they may be subjected to unfamiliar legal environments. Legal protections for patients and medical liability standards differ greatly from jurisdiction to jurisdiction. Low malpractice insurance costs have been cited as one factor allowing some medical tourism destinations to offer less expensive care,[18] but patients may find it challenging to factor the value of decreased malpractice protection into their decision making. Facilitators can help patients navigate these issues, but they too inhabit a murky international arena complicated both by the relatively unregulated status of medical tourism facilitation and the international dimension of the practice.

Some facilitators try to insulate themselves from the legal risks of medical tourism—including suits for malpractice, poor quality of care, or any complications that might arise from seeking medical care abroad—by distancing themselves from actual medical provision, and instead framing themselves as merely facilitating contact with medical facilities and physicians abroad and arranging for travel to these facilities.[7] Then, if complications arise from the care provided, the responsibility for these problems theoretically would be shifted to the physician and medical facilities abroad instead of the facilitators themselves.[7] In this way, if facilitators simply provide clients with information and contacts, along with a warning to beware of the complications that may arise from receiving medical care abroad, patients take on the responsibilities for the outcomes of their own decisions.[19]

Facilitators' attempts to limit their own liability sometimes take the form of statements warning patients that the facilitator has no legal liability for malpractice or complications arising from treatment received abroad or dissatisfaction with the care received. In other instances, facilitators require clients to sign contracts that waive the facilitator's legal liability in the event of complications.[7] When this occurs, the facilitator not only warns patients that they are on their own when risking medical treatment abroad, but also creates a legal barrier against seeking redress from the facilitator. While facilitators may encourage patients to seek legal redress from their medical providers abroad, doing so is problematic in two respects. First, pursuing a legal course of action abroad may be very expensive and difficult. Doing so requires navigating a foreign legal system, possibly using a language other than the patient's own.[20,21] If the patient is required to return to the country where the care was received in order to pursue damages, this creates additional burdens and costs. Second, adequate legal recourse may not even be available to the patient if the host country has limited medical malpractice protections for patients.[17,21] For a more detailed discussion of the issues surrounding legal liability in medical tourism, see chapter 9.

Interviews with Canadian facilitators show that they emphasize to clients that they are not medical professionals and are instead offering information and referrals that patients have requested.[5] In this sense, facilitators do not view themselves as being responsible for adverse outcomes that occur as a result of patients acting on the information or referrals. Some facilitators do perform certain actions that could help lessen the risk of liability issues and patient complications. For instance, one facilitator reported visiting potential destination facilitates to see, firsthand, if the facilitator would feel comfortable referring patients there.[5] However, since facilitators lack standardized professional training, their capacity to discern quality medical locations from unsafe ones is questionable. In website analyses, very few facilitator sites addressed issues of legal recourse for patients. For example, Mason and Wright found only 6.1 percent of websites that they examined addressed legal concerns,[8] while Lunt and Carerra reported that 3 of the 5 sites they examined stated that it was the surgeon's responsibility to address postoperative complications.[15]

DISCUSSION

Our review of ethical concerns tied to the practice of medical tourism facilitation and the emerging body of empirically based research on facilitators confirms, gives context to, and enhances our understanding of certain of these ethical concerns. At the heart of these concerns is the pressing question that many health systems confront: who holds responsibility for managing patient care across the continuum? As we have emphasized above, in the case of medical tourism, this continuum extends across countries, legal systems, regulatory approaches, and sometimes even languages.

It is clear that potential medical tourists face challenges in their informed decision making. Reviews of facilitator websites consistently show that patients are not made sufficiently aware of the risks associated with medical tourism through these sources alone. As these websites are initial and formative sources of information, this lack of information raises questions about patients' ability to give fully informed consent to face these risks. Other information gaps undermine informed decision making as well. Should decisions be based solely on publicly available information through facilitator websites, potential medical tourists are likely to be confused about facilitators' pay structures, among other factors. Moreover, reviews of facilitator websites give evidence that most do not offer clear guidance on the legal protections afforded to medical tourists if they choose to travel abroad for care. Statements and waivers of facilitator liability vary among websites, and patients are not likely to be in a position to judge the enforceability of these waivers, particularly if they have not yet been tested in court. Moreover, these websites lack information on the variability of malpractice protections in host countries, further compromising patients' ability to make informed decisions.

The lack of a requirement for accreditation reinforces ethical concerns around the roles and responsibilities of medical tourism facilitators. For example, our review demonstrated a lack of clear protocols for providing follow-up care and ensuring informational continuity of care, a problem due in part to a lack of standardization among facilitators. While some facilitators oversee follow-up care for their clients and facilitate continuity of care, the treatment of these issues on facilitators' websites suggests the quality and scope of these services is uneven. The lack of accreditation undermines patients' ability to assess facilitators' training and qualifications. While symbols of accrediting agencies and other signifiers of quality were common on facilitator websites, they generally did not pertain to accreditation of the facilitators themselves. This can be misleading or confusing for medical tourists attempting to evaluate facilitators.

However, our review of the literature on medical tourism facilitators shows that a number of commonly cited ethical concerns have yet to be evidenced in practice. For example, while concerns have been raised that payments from destination facilities to facilitators for referrals creates a potential conflict of interest and may negatively impact patient care or motivate unnecessary or overly expensive treatments, we do not yet have evidence of whether or how this conflict of interest has influenced facilitators' recommendations for care. While the financial incentive referrals create may work against patients' interests, facilitators also have an interest in developing and maintaining a reputation for quality service and satisfied customers that may outweigh those incentives. Furthermore, it is difficult to assess the legal vulnerability of patients given the lack of case law around facilitator liability waivers. While the findings of website review studies make us suspect that the content of these waivers is variable, we do not have access to the content of these statements since they are generally not made public. We also do not know how common signed waivers are in the industry. Finally, evidence of the negative health impacts of engaging in medical tourism and of gaps in continuity of and follow-up care is lacking. While anecdotes of complications emerging from medical tourism are common and alarming, as are examples of problems with continuity of and follow-up care, more data are needed in order to identify and assess trends. Importantly, complications and risks created by medical tourism are likely to vary by procedure and location, making it difficult to issue blanket statements about the safety of this practice.

The ethical concerns associated with medical tourism facilitation highlight the need for greater regulation and transparency.[6,22] The emerging literature on facilitators clearly supports the need for greater transparency to help patients understand the risks medical tourism entails, as well as facilitators' potential for conflicts of interest.[4] Facilitators could promote transparency by fully disclosing the source and amount of their fees and by providing more information about the risks of medical tourism on their websites.[9] Requiring facilitators to receive training and accreditation could help ensure that facilitators provide this information about risks and funding sources to potential patients.[5,6] An accreditation process could also help to establish uniform procedures for providing medical tourists with better continuity and follow-up care. Other proposed regulations, including restrictions on facilitators' contracts, requirements for travel insurance, patient compensation for malpractice, and restrictions on the procedures that facilitators can advertise[6] are less directly supported by the existing empirically based literature. Additional research into the impacts of medical tourism on patient health and the adequacy of patient information on the risks entailed by medical tourism might support these additional regulatory interventions and is thus needed.

In interviews, facilitators stated a desire for standardization and regulation as a way to professionalize their practice.[5] However, it is not clear what organization or group should assume this responsibility. Norms and standards of facilitator services have not yet developed, no regulatory body has formed to oversee facilitator practices, and a code of practice has not been adopted. Medical tourism facilitation companies work in a wide variety of legal and regulatory contexts, and without the oversight of one professional accrediting body. The international nature of medical tourism, where patients, providers, and facilitators may each be based in different countries, makes regulation difficult to impose, especially given the significant financial incentives to limit regulatory policies in medical tourism destinations. Voluntary participation in an accreditation system akin to JCI accreditation for health providers would be a first, feasible step toward greater regulation of the industry. While such a system would be voluntary and thus limited in force, JCI accreditation is increasingly seen as a de facto requirement for medical tourism providers targeting patients in North America.

CONCLUSION: RESEARCH DIRECTIONS

Our review suggests several areas of research that are needed in order to expand our understanding of the ethical dimensions of medical tourism facilitation. Most pressing is an understanding of patient–facilitator interactions beyond what is known from public facilitator websites. This information will help to bridge several gaps in our understanding of medical tourism and of facilitators' roles and responsibilities. These gaps include the limited understanding of the degree to which facilitators convey information on the risks of medical tourism, the content and presentation of liability waivers, and discussions of follow-up and continuity of care. While ethical concerns about all of these areas are well founded, a better understanding of the full range of patient–facilitator interactions will help to add detail to these concerns, illuminate differences in how facilitators interact with their clients, and suggest interventions for overcoming or mitigating these concerns.

More data are needed on the numbers of medical tourists using facilitators to plan their travel abroad for care, medical tourists choosing not to use facilitators, and patients who interacted with facilitators but chose not to engage in medical tourism. This data will help to better understand patients' decision-making processes around medical tourism and facilitators' roles and responsibilities in this process. More data also are needed on patient outcomes following travel abroad for medical care. This data could help differentiate outcomes for those patients using facilitators and help to uncover facilitators' roles in improving or worsening health outcomes for medical tourists. It is possible that these outcomes will differ by destination and procedure, but ideally such data would help to determine whether facilitators who are accredited and have a medical background have better outcomes than other facilitators.

Information is greatly needed on how patients, facilitators, and other industry stakeholders, including physicians, perceive the facilitators' roles and responsibilities. While this information is starting to appear through facilitator interviews, facilitator self-perception may vary by location, thus creating the need for comparative insights. Moreover, our understanding of patient and other stakeholders' views of facilitators' roles is limited at this time. A better understanding of facilitators' roles will help shape regulatory responses and inform procedures for facilitator accreditation.

Given the dynamic nature of medical tourism and relative newness of facilitation as an entrepreneurial venture within this global health services industry, the literature on ethical concerns about this practice has been quick to develop. The expanding body of empirically based research on facilitation is helping to define our understanding of the ethical dimensions of facilitation. Continued research along existing pathways and in the areas described here, while logistically difficult and time and money intensive, will help to shape policy responses to medical tourism generally and facilitation specifically. Medical tourism facilitation is a business that is likely to continue playing a role in securing (or perhaps worsening) patient health, thus making it clear that a better understanding of the practice of facilitation and diversity of facilitators' roles and responsibilities toward medical tourists and the industry is needed.

REFERENCES

1. Penney K, Snyder J, Crooks VA, Johnston R. Risk communication and informed consent in the medical tourism Industry: A thematic content analysis of Canadian broker websites. *BMC Medical Ethics.* 2011;12:17.

2. Cormany D, Baloglu S. Medical travel facilitator websites: An exploratory study of web page contents and services offered to the prospective medical tourist. *Tourism Management.* 2011;32(4):709–716.

3. Johnston R, Crooks VA, Adams K, Snyder J, Kingsbury P. An industry perspective on Canadian patients' involvement in medical tourism: Implications for public health. *BMC Public Health.* 2011;11:416.

4. Lunt N, Hardey M, Mannion R. Nip, tuck and click: Medical tourism and the emergence of web-based health information. *The Open Medical Informatics Journal.* 2010;4:1–11.

5. Snyder J, Crooks VA, Adams K, Kingsbury P, Johnston R. The "patient's physician one-step removed": The evolving roles of medical tourism facilitators. *Journal of Medical Ethics.* 2011;37(9):530–534.

6. Turner L. Quality in health care and globalization of health services: Accreditation and regulatory oversight of medical tourism companies. *International Journal for Quality in Health Care.* 2011;23(1):1–7.

7. Turner L. "First world health care at third world prices": Globalization, bioethics and medical tourism. *Biosocieties.* 2007;2(3):303–325.

8. Mason A, Wright K. Framing medical tourism: An examination of appeal, risk, convalescence, accreditation, and interactivity in medical tourism web sites. *Journal of Health Communication.* 2011;16(2):163–177.

9. Spece RG. Medical tourism: Protecting patients from conflicts of interest in broker's fees paid by foreign providers. *Journal of Health and Biomedical Law.* 2010;6:1–36.

10. Lunt N, Machin L, Green S, Mannion R. Are there implications for quality of care for patients who participate in international medical tourism? *Expert Review of Pharmacoeconomics & Outcomes Research.* 2011;11(2):133–136.

11. Hunter D, Oultram S. The ethical and policy implications of rogue medical tourism. *Global Social Policy.* 2010;10(3):297–299.

12. Cohen I. Medical tourism: The view from ten thousand feet. *The Hastings Center Report.* 2010;40(2):11–12.

13. Crooks VA, Kingsbury P, Snyder J, Johnston R. What is known about the patient's experience of medical tourism? A scoping review. *BMC Health Services Research.* 2010;10:266–277.

14. Crooks VA, Turner L, Snyder J, Johnston R, Kingsbury P. Promoting medical tourism to India: Messages, images, and the marketing of international patient travel. *Social Science & Medicine.* 2011;72(5):726–732.

15. Lunt N, Carrera P. Systematic review of web sites for prospective medical tourists. *Tourism Review.* 2011;66(1/2):57–67.

16. Sobo E, Herlihy E, Bicker M. Selling medical travel to U.S. patient-consumers: The cultural appeal of website marketing messages. *Anthropology & Medicine.* 2011;18(1):119–136.

17. Kirkner R. Liability concern balances medical tourism's cost appeal. *Managed Care.* 2009;18(6):34.

18. Johnston R, Crooks VA, Snyder J, Kingsbury P. What is known about the effects of medical tourism in destination and departure countries? A scoping review. *International Journal for Equity In Health.* 2010;9:24.

19. Klaus M. Outsourcing vital operations: What if U.S. health care costs drive patients overseas for surgery? *Quinnipiac Health Law Journal.* 2005;9:219–247.

20. Álvarez MM, Chanda R, Smith R. The potential for bi-lateral agreements in medical tourism: A qualitative study of stakeholder perspectives from the UK and India. *Globalization and Health.* 2011;7:11.

21. Cortez N. Patients without borders: The emerging global market for patients and the evolution of modern health care. *Indiana Law Journal.* 2008;83:71–132.

22. Crooks VA, Snyder J. Regulating medical tourism. *The Lancet.* 2010; 376:1465–1466.

Chapter 14

Conclusion: High Stakes Market

Ann Marie Kimball and Jill R. Hodges

HEALTH CARE FOR SALE

The analyses in the preceding chapters describe an expanding, global market for health services that in some senses resembles many other markets but in other, critical respects is quite different. In the global market for health services, suppliers leverage comparative advantages such as cost, capacity, technology, and customer service to capitalize on international demand. Purchasers seek the best quality for the lowest possible cost. But of course, in this global market, the good on offer is health services—or ultimately health—arguably the most universally valued commodity of all. And customers may undertake their purchases during particularly vulnerable times, when they are facing chronic or life threatening illnesses. The product, health services, is complex in nature, intertwining cultural and social values, technological interventions, and the particular features of each individual's health. In essence, although, as we have seen, health services can certainly be sold and delivered internationally via market mechanisms, these services are not widgets that can easily be assessed, processed, tracked, and consumed in a standardized manner.

The size and value of the medical tourism market is unknown; there are, in fact, stunning disparities among attempts to quantify this trade. What is known is that the market has expanded in recent decades. Medical travel, once primarily the domain of wealthy individuals who traveled in search of advanced medical interventions, now extends to members of the middle class, who travel chiefly for relief from high costs and long waiting lists. These individuals travel for essential as well as elective services, from transplants to tummy tucks. The entry of the middle class, kindled by the growing ease and affordability of global travel and Internet marketing, has along with diminishing trade barriers spurred industry growth. The volume of travelers, distances traveled, and range of health services sold and purchased make up a complex, global, multibillion-dollar market that has outpaced any regulatory infrastructure.

The distinct features of the product for sale and the dynamic and unregulated nature of this market both complicate and heighten the importance of critically examining medical tourism and the global market for health services. By drawing together contributions from leading researchers in this field, we have sought to contextualize and interpret recent developments in this market from a variety of perspectives. The chapters in this collection show a market that poses risks not only for individuals and domestic health systems but also for global public health. While medical tourism enables patients who have sufficient resources to access health services that may otherwise be out of reach, individuals often make their "purchases" without adequate information about the potential risks to themselves or to other individuals who may be involved in the transaction, such as those who provide organs or surrogacy services. In other words, as with any market, consumers may be sold products that they do not need, that are of poor quality, or that were obtained in a manner that harmed others; what's notable in the medical tourism industry is that the potential risks and harms involve individuals' health. Similarly, while medical tourism may provide a revenue source for national economies, it also may disrupt domestic public health systems by redirecting scarce resources to the private sector, an issue that chapters 4 and 5 explore in the context of Southeast Asia and Costa Rica. Globally, this trade promises to support the exchange of opportunities and resources but also perhaps to disseminate problems, most notably infectious disease, as the scenarios in chapter 6 demonstrate. Inadequate oversight and regulation of this market make it more difficult to identify and address such problems. Documentation of medical travel is haphazard and fragmentary. Patients are not batched or tracked in their journeys abroad—there is no register to identify or "recall" medical errors or patients carrying infectious disease.

Two central themes weave through this multidisciplinary examination of medical tourism. First, it is an industry that recasts patients as consumers and underscores the commercial aspects of health care as a product to be marketed and sold. And second, these exchanges occur in a market that is largely undocumented, unstructured, and unregulated—or, as Nathan Cortez puts it in chapter 9, the industry has evolved in a regulatory void. In this concluding chapter, we discuss how these characteristics contribute to the central risks and controversies surrounding medical tourism, and examine what mechanisms exist to address these concerns. We offer potential approaches for consideration by consumers; the medical tourism trade; and national, regional, and international policy makers. Finally, we consider the future of this rapidly evolving global market and highlight key issues that warrant further attention if this market is to develop in a manner that realizes the greatest possible benefits and minimizes potential harms.

CALCULATING RISK

The commercial nature of the medical tourism industry presents risks for patients who undertake medical tourism, individuals who supply services or biological materials to medical tourists, and the public health systems that send and receive medical tourists. Complicating and potentially elevating these risks are two central and related problems with the global medical tourism market—a lack of reliable data on the market; and a lack of common infrastructures, standards, or regulations.

Risks for Patients

In the United States and increasingly in other developed countries, patients are electing and being encouraged to take a more active role in selecting their health care services; to consider themselves as savvy, engaged consumers instead of passive recipients of services to which they're entitled under private or government health plans. The global market in health services in some respects supports this trend—it enables individuals with adequate resources to decide what services they want, when and where they want to have them, and how much they'll pay for them. They can shop around to avoid queues, find the best prices, and access experimental therapies or limited resources, such as organs. The unfettered nature of the market encourages providers to offer whatever services consumers seek—in some cases, regardless of whether the services are effective or not.

At the same time, two features of the medical tourism industry compromise patients' ability to safely act as discriminating consumers. First, as Leigh Turner discusses in chapter 12, many providers in this market are paid for selling health services and procedures, and not necessarily for improving health. This profit-oriented, private health care model is the same fee-for-service model that predominates in the U.S. health care system. But in the medical tourism market, health care providers aren't the only ones selling medical services. Also promoting these services to consumers are the facilitators that arrange health care travel, and national tourism boards and even health ministries. Since most medical travelers pay out of pocket, the insurance providers and health ministries that might play a quality control role or gatekeeper function typically are not part of the transaction. In some cases, patients, or consumers, have only biased or insufficient information to make potentially complicated and consequential health care decisions on their own. Even in cases in which it is reasonably easy for patients to determine what services they need, they must select health care providers largely without the benefit of any reliable data on service quality or infection rates from one facility to the next. In the global health care bazaar, instead of hanging out a shingle on Main Street, providers advertise their services on the Internet. And rather than walking through a nearby clinic or making inquiries in the neighborhood, patients select providers from afar with little to go on other than the recommendation of a facilitator who may be paid for referrals. As the discussion in chapter 9 demonstrates, should problems arise, there may be few if any legal remedies to address them.

Risks for Donors and Surrogates

Prospective patients are not the only vulnerable individuals in the global market for health services. A small but significant part of the medical tourism industry involves travel to acquire organs and commercial surrogacy services. While exploitation is a possibility in any market that facilitates interactions between individuals in high- and low-resource settings, the potential consequences are particularly grave when the commodities being exchanged are body parts or services that may compromise individuals' health or well-being. As we saw in the discussion of commercial transplant and stem cell procedures by Dominique Martin in chapter 7 and reproductive services by Andrea Whittaker in chapter 8, the prospect of compensation may induce organ sellers or commercial surrogates to consider procedures that result in health problems that far outweigh any potential payments.

Risks for Health Systems

Southeast Asia, one of the major centers of medical tourism, provides vivid examples of the opportunities and dilemmas that arise in nations with thriving medical tourism industries. Malaysia, the Philippines, Singapore, and Thailand are among the countries that embraced medical tourism as a strategy to fill private hospital beds and generate export revenues in the wake of the Asian economic crisis in the late 1990s. Governments in these countries have partnered with private industry and adopted a variety of tactics, from tax breaks and other incentives to ambitious promotional campaigns, to nurture their medical tourism industries. As Churnrurtai Kanchanachitra, Cha-aim Pachanee et al. detail in chapter 4, while each of these Southeast Asian countries has fostered its own brand of medical tourism, emphasizing its distinctive selling points, all struggle to balance the benefits of building this high-end market with the potential costs to their public health systems, including the loss of specialists and other health care providers who are lured to the more lucrative private sector that caters to medical travelers. Theoretically, the benefits of medical tourism extend to the public sector in the form of additional resources in tax coffers, but there are few mechanisms in place to ensure that redistribution.[1] Proponents of the industry suggest that medical tourism and the jobs it generates enable countries to retain health workers who might otherwise seek work abroad. But even if this claim is true, it is of limited benefit if these workers are employed in the private sector, which many patients cannot afford. India, which is one of the more popular medical tourism destinations, remains among the countries that WHO classifies as having a critical shortage in health workers.[2] In addition to workforce shortages, medical tourism can lead to price increases in both the public and private sectors as well as an emphasis on services that target medical tourists instead of the local population. Like these Southeast Asian countries, Latin American medical tourism destinations also confront the implications of the incursion of a private industry into their public health systems. Courtney Lee's ethnographic profile of medical tourism in Costa Rica in chapter 5 reveals health care providers who are at once drawn by the prospect of increased wages in the growing private sector and troubled by the challenges these opportunities pose to the country's highly successful socialized health system. Medical tourism can exacerbate inequities in sending countries as well since it is an option that is only available to those who can afford to travel for health care.

As we elucidate in chapter 6, cross-border disease transmission can also take a toll on public health resources in the countries where medical tourists both originate and travel. The geographic expansion of bacteria carrying the gene that makes the highly drug resistant enzyme NDM-1, for instance, has been linked to patients who traveled to India and Pakistan for care.[3] While it is not possible to definitively attribute this rapid spread to medical tourism, it is equally difficult to imagine its occurrence without the infected patients moving postoperatively across continents. Receiving countries face similar risks—Singapore's first case of extensively drug resistant tuberculosis (XDR-TB), which requires lengthy and costly isolation, arrived with a patient from Indonesia.[4]

Weighing Risks

Reliable estimates of the full costs and benefits of medical tourism to individual economies are elusive. The absence of precise data concerning the scope of the medical tourism industry is a repeated theme throughout this book. For a variety of reasons, researchers have had limited success to date quantifying with certainty the extent and specifics of medical travel. First, as the preceding chapters note, there is no general agreement about which patients and procedures to count, not to mention who might do the counting—candidates include everyone from individual providers to national or global travel bodies. Second, health services are not an ordinary commodity that can be readily tracked and monitored, particularly when most patients pay out of pocket for a variety of services, some of which they may be pursuing against the recommendations of their physicians, or even the laws of their countries, and therefore may be reluctant to disclose. Third, any figures reported by providers, governments, or business consulting firms could be inflated. To the extent that the definitions and categories of medical tourism remain in flux, those who hope to foster the industry may well adopt the most generous terms to enhance counts. Finally, the medical tourism volumes and revenues that national ministries and others report do not consistently factor in funds foregone in tax breaks, or expended to promote the industry, provide additional infrastructure, or address resulting problems such as workforce shifts to the private sector. It is also not always clear whether these figures include hospitality revenues, which may well account for a significant portion of medical travelers' benefit to the domestic economy, and whether they reflect trips that may have been taken anyway, regardless of the need for health services. A calculus that articulated and incorporated all these elements would more accurately represent the net value of medical tourism to individual nations.

Who Are You Going to Call?

Closely related to the inadequate documentation of the medical tourism industry is its lack of global standards, regulations, and overall infrastructure. There are no overarching health quality, legal, business, or information technology standards governing this industry. While frameworks are beginning to emerge to meet these needs, such as accreditation schemes and various guiding principles, all of these approaches are voluntary. For the most part, the only regulations governing health care providers are those of their respective countries. Similarly, there are no legal remedies, health information systems, disease surveillance mechanisms, or advertising standards that effectively span all borders. In reality, most national health systems have not managed to construct interconnected systems for patient records and disease surveillance within their own borders. These inconsistencies and disconnects, like the lack of reliable data, can make it difficult to identify and address the problems in the global market for health services.

ADDRESSING RISKS

The evidence set forth in this book highlights four major areas of risk associated with medical tourism: (1) patient safety, (2) cross-border spread of disease, (3) donor and surrogate safety, and (4) threats to public health systems. A broad variety of measures, mechanisms, and initiatives are necessary to effectively address these concerns, from more comprehensive and reliable standards and regulations to improved data collection. The challenges of realizing these improvements are significant. Increased global trade in health services at once demands and defies greater documentation, standardization, and regulation. Patients' and corporations' privacy rights complicate potential solutions for better data collection and interoperable patient records that would support continuity of care. Cultural and economic differences and the complexities of medical care make it difficult to devise and impose common standards and regulations. Table 14.1 details some of the major challenges and supports in addressing the risks of medical tourism.

Table 14.1

Addressing risks

Goal	Supports	Challenges
Increase patient safety	—Accreditation —Oversight by third-party payers —Collaboration with/counsel from home doctors —Reliable information and resources for patients —Interoperable electronic medical records —Competition for patients on the basis of quality of care	—High cost of accreditation —Commercial nature of medical tourism (potential for "sales" and low-cost orientation to overshadow effectiveness and quality) —Internet marketing and claims that are difficult to verify —Lack of regulation and legal protections —Lack of common standards —Patients' and providers' desire for privacy/autonomy
Improve infectious disease surveillance and control	—Cross border disease surveillance networks —Shared laboratory and surveillance expertise and resources —WHO International Health Regulations —Desire to reduce disease-related costs —Desire to attract medical tourists with reputation as "safe" health care destination/facility	—Uncontrolled/undocumented nature of travel —Emerging diseases that are difficult to detect and identify —Diverse systems for detecting disease —Facilities and regions with different rates of disease and resources for detecting and controlling outbreaks —Patients with compromised immunity —Potential for lost business after reporting infectious disease outbreaks

(continued)

Table 14.1 (continued)

Goal	Supports	Challenges
Promote ethical practices (e.g. avoid exploitation in organ sales)	—Public image —Commitment to treat people equitably —Pressure from interest and professional groups —Interest in avoiding expenses due to poor health outcomes for donors and recipients	—Income potential for activities such as organ sales —Income disparities that promote exploitation —Power differentials —Lack of awareness of potential risks to donors and recipients
Protect domestic public health systems	—Government interest in promoting public health —Potential to use medical tourism revenues to capitalize on economies of scale or enhance pubic health systems —Growing recognition of interconnected nature of health of all people	—Comparatively high wages in private practice —Political power of private interests —Lack of mechanisms/will to enforce commitments to use medical tourism revenues to bolster public services —National economic strategies focused on attracting revenues via medical tourism —Lack of data illustrating problems
Develop more comprehensive and accurate data	—Increasing interest in developing reliable data to guide policy —Participation of third-party payers —OECD guidelines —Electronic medical records	—Patients' and providers' desire for privacy/autonomy —Lack of common classification system —No requirements for data collection —Private providers' reluctance to share data

Note: A variety of existing forces support and pose challenges to efforts to address the potential risks that arise from medical tourism.

There is need for leadership in these efforts. As various authors have pointed out, the World Health Organization (WHO), through its World Health Assembly, is well positioned to work with member nations to create partnerships and alliances to address health matters of global concern.[5] Indeed, in 2009, WHO convened experts for an initial exploration of the health, economic, legal, and ethical implications of cross-border travel for health services. Ideally, next steps would involve collaborating with relevant organizations such as the World Trade Organization (WTO) and World Tourism Organization to establish a common agenda for addressing risks and concerns. To be effective, deliberations would need to include representatives from a variety of disciplines and extend beyond aspirational guidelines to debate and development of specific goals and mechanisms for achieving those goals. The WHO Commission on Macroeconomics and Health (2000) demonstrated that such transdisciplinary consultation is both feasible and essential for progress. Many individuals consider the current global campaign for the Millennium Development Goals—targets for reducing poverty and hunger, improving health and education, empowering women, and ensuring environmental sustainability—to be a direct result of such leadership by WHO and other UN agencies. The commission's work led to the establishment of regional and national commissions to tailor the recommendations to accommodate the diverse circumstances and resources of individual economies.

However, it is unrealistic to look to WHO or any single international body to "fix" all of the potential problems or govern all aspects of medical tourism, an industry that spans health, travel, and trade and involves an array of public and private interests. The development of a safe, effective, and equitable market relies on a variety of approaches and on the combined efforts of international nongovernmental organizations, supranational organizations, national governments, scientific communities, private industry, payers, providers, and patients. The preceding chapters have highlighted examples of efforts from all these sectors that offer promise in addressing the risks that accompany medical tourism.

International Nongovernmental Organizations—Although WHO has not pursued any major initiatives specifically focused on medical tourism, it has led important efforts to address related issues of global concern, such as patient safety and health worker shortages. Chapter 6 describes several WHO initiatives to reduce infections and curb cross-border spread of disease, including the revised International Health Regulations (IHRs), which contain some strong potential control points for the industry. The IHRs compel WHO's 194 member countries to report outbreaks occurring within their borders that rise to the level of "international concern." In addition, they include recommended practices for airlines to avoid transporting infectious passengers. Of course, these measures rely upon tracking and detecting infections in the first place, a challenge for even the most well-resourced countries, especially in the case of emerging infections.

Supranational Organizations—The European Union's recently adopted Directive on the Application of Patients' Rights in Cross Border Health Care, described by Richard Smith and Helena Legido-Quigley et al. in chapter 3, addresses some of the legal questions, ambiguities, and issues inherent in medical travel by articulating common processes and patients' rights. While the supranational structure of the European Union facilitated the enactment of common structures and processes, the Directive might serve as a model that could be modified and incorporated into bilateral or multilateral trade agreements governing trade in health services.

National Governments—Concerns regarding whether investments in the private health sector will drain resources from publicly funded health systems are largely the domain of national governments. As chapter 4 describes, this topic has been debated at Thailand's National Health Assembly, where participants developed a proposal that private hospitals receiving tax breaks provide care for public health enrollees in exchange. Similarly, the Philippines requires private hospitals to allocate at least 10 percent of their authorized bed capacity for "charity beds."

The potential toll on the public health system is also a topic for national governments to consider as they develop bilateral and multilateral agreements for trade in health services. Among other things, these agreements can help regulate the migration of health workers, the degree of foreign investment in health facilities, and the cross-border movement of patients.

National governments also must determine how much to invest in their public health systems to reduce the health conditions that contribute to illness that may ultimately prompt medical tourism. And, as Dominique Martin suggests in chapter 7, governments must consider how to devise systems such as national organ donor banks to avoid unhealthy interdependencies with other nations in the global market for health services.

Scientific Communities—Chapter 7 also provides examples of international groups of experts that have convened to address concerns related to markets for commercial organ transplantation and unproven stem cell treatments, areas in which both patients and potential donors may be especially desperate and vulnerable. In both cases, professional and scientific societies have played an important role in attempting to limit instances of exploitation and other problems, drafting the Declaration of Istanbul on Organ Trafficking and Transplant Tourism (at the suggestion of WHO) and the Guidelines for the Clinical Translation of Stem Cells. These agreements serve as guidelines rather than regulations, and participation is voluntary. Nonetheless, they provide models for attempting to combat organ trafficking and marketing of stem cell therapies that have not been approved for use in humans.

Private Industry—Numerous efforts are underway to improve the quality and safety of care provided at health care facilities that attract international patients. The International Standards Organization (ISO) provides a source of standards for health care facilities, and the Joint Commission International (JCI) and other schemes offer accreditation through inspection. But as Stephen T. Green and Hannah King point out in chapter 11, there is no one organization that is overseeing these various groups or devising a common set of standards that would enable patients to compare quality across borders and medical facilities. Furthermore, it remains unclear whether current accreditation systems ultimately result in improved quality of care. Facilities serving international patients also have the responsibility and capacity to address health care quality concerns on an individual level by attending to areas such as infection control, translation services, and interoperable electronic medical records.

Private enterprises that profit from medical tourism also can help by devoting a portion of those profits to help subsidize care for local populations. There already are some very limited instances of this happening on both mandatory and voluntary bases, but if medical tourism is to live up to its billing of benefiting the larger economy and population, it will need to happen more. An example of a successful model for this is the Aravind Eye Care System in Southern India. Aravind uses revenues from patients paying market rates to cover surgeries for those who cannot pay. Roughly half of the 300,000 surgeries performed annually at Aravind's seven hospitals are free.[6] Dr. G. Venkataswamy founded Aravind in 1976, well before the medical tourism wave, to reduce unnecessary blindness, not to attract medical tourists; and it is a charitable organization, not a for-profit entity. Nonetheless, its model of dedicating operating surpluses to cover services for those who cannot afford them could apply equally to those facilities catering to international patients.

Payers—If participation by private and public health insurers increases in the medical tourism market, these insurers might serve as quality control agents by carefully reviewing the providers they will reimburse for services. They can also negotiate better rates for their members, which may serve to make potential medical tourists less alluring prospects for providers focused primarily on attracting lucrative customers.

Patients and Providers—Patients and providers have roles to play on both individual and organizational levels. While patients currently are typically not sufficiently informed to assess the quality of care provided by health care facilities, they can at least attempt to protect themselves from harm when deciding whether or where to travel abroad for health care. Patients undertaking medical travel should strive to access whatever reliable information is available to assess the risks of the procedures, facilities, and destinations they are considering for any health services. They should also speak with their local physicians before going abroad for treatment regarding access to postoperative care following their return home, and obtain and provide to their local physicians any documentation of the services they receive. Patient representatives also play key roles in initiatives such as WHO's Patient Safety program, which promotes access to standards and information around patient safety concerns.

Likewise, health care providers in sending countries can help patients understand and assess safety risks as they consider medical travel. Treating providers in destination facilities can help by providing comprehensive information to patients and their home providers about treatments received and potential complications, as well as detailed and easy-to-understand discharge instructions. Physician groups can develop medical tourism guidelines and standards such as those provided by the American Medical Association.[7]

The points above represent just a few of the strategies, possibilities, and work underway to address the potential problems that might arise in a global market for health services. Gaps remain, most notably in regulation of medical tourism facilitators and other parties that organize medical travel, and in data collection.

UNCERTAIN OUTCOMES

There is still much to be understood about the benefits and risks of medical tourism and the emergence of a globe-spanning market for health care. Similarly, the manner in which the industry may grow and change is uncertain. Various unpredictable forces will influence how medical tourism develops. Just as the Asian economic crisis in the 1990s propelled the development of medical tourism in that region, the economic troubles confronting the United States and many European nations in recent years may drive more medical travelers into the market in search of more affordable care. Conversely, it is also possible that individuals will refrain from cosmetic surgery and other elective services that constitute a significant segment of medical travel, or lack the funds to travel for more essential health care services. As chapters 2 and 9 discuss, health reform in the United States also could reduce or increase the flow of patients abroad. The rise of multidrug resistant infections like NDM-1 also could ultimately cause medical travelers to avoid certain regions or to seek services close to home. The stalled negotiations in the WTO Doha Round may cause national economies to steer clear of multinational trade agreements and focus more on bilateral and regional trade agreements, which in turn could influence the volume and direction of patient flows and provider migrations.

In addition to these dynamic factors, there are the particularities and complexities of health care that might ultimately limit growth, including the cultural aspects of care; the desirability of accessing care close to home where a support network is nearby; and the growing emphasis on integrated, holistic care that runs contrary to the fragmented care processes that are inherent in medical travel. There are also larger ethical questions to consider in relation to this global market that relies upon inequities in resources and access to care. As Courtney A. Lee notes in chapter 5, medical tourism exists because not all individuals can afford or access the health care services that they need or want at home, and because of the huge cost differentials from one region or country to the next. As a number of our contributors have highlighted, nations and health care providers that foster medical tourism must balance the rights of individuals to access the care they want against the well-being of individuals who are at risk of being harmed by these transactions.

CONCLUSION

Although it remains to be seen how the medical tourism industry will evolve, it is clear that it is a phenomenon of increasing importance to global health. Medical tourism's potential impacts on public services, infection risks, and the commodification of health services all have ripple effects well beyond the providers and recipients of care who are immediately involved. The internal migration of health providers from the public to private sector and the marginalization of the state in the provision of health services could have potentially profound impacts, particularly in countries where the public sector has traditionally been the major provider of care. The social, legal, and ethical issues raised in the preceding chapters are critical to the health of the global population, and they require serious consideration. Areas of particular importance for future research and deliberation include the following:

- **Health care outcomes and quality of care**—More systematic studies are needed to determine how outcomes and quality of care vary by procedures, destinations, and ideally individual facilities that target medical tourists. It is also important to explore the extent to which receiving care within the context of one's local community may influence health care outcomes.

- **Infectious disease surveillance and control**—International efforts to develop global systems for identifying and tracking infectious disease become ever more critical as new drug resistant agents continue to emerge and spread via medical tourists and other international travelers.

- **Legal and regulatory systems**—The legal and regulatory ambiguities that surround medical tourism create an accountability void and increase the vulnerability of patients and others who are affected by medical tourism. It is important to explore whether agreements such as the EU's Directive on the Application of Patients' Rights in Cross Border Health Care might be applied in other contexts to better protect patients, donors, and others.

- **Facilitators' roles**—As Jeremy Snyder, Valerie A. Crooks, and colleagues demonstrate in chapter 13, there is a need for greater transparency around the practices and payment systems of the facilitation companies that arrange medical travel.

- **Data collection**—Underlying all of these concerns is the need for a better understanding of medical tourists' travel patterns and motivations for travel. The work by the OECD to standardize definitions and data collection methods (see chapter 1) could help in moving this effort forward. This understanding, and ultimately a transnational system tracking patient flows, could inform and facilitate infection detection and control, outcomes research, and the development of effective systems to protect both individual patients and national and global public health.

While health care services have been traded in most cultures for centuries, the current unregulated global market poses unprecedented risks. As medical tourism continues to develop, the extent to which these risks remain undefined and unresolved will influence public health on local, regional, national, and global levels.

ACKNOWLEDGMENTS

The authors would like to thank the contributors to this volume for their research and insights that are reflected in this chapter. Special thanks to Nathan Cortez, Dominique Martin, Richard D. Smith, Leigh Turner, and Andrea Whittaker for their perspectives and comments.

REFERENCES

1. Blouin C. Trade in health services: Can it improve access to health care for poor people? *Global Social Policy.* 2010;10(3):293–295.

2. O'Brien P, Gostin LO. *Health worker shortages and global justice.* Milbank Memorial Fund. 2011. http://www.milbank.org/publications/milbank-reports/158-reports-health-worker-shortages-and-global-justice-2. Accessed April 13, 2012.

3. Kumarasamy KK, Toleman MA, Walsh TR, et al. Emergence of a new antibiotic resistance mechanism in India, Pakistan, and the UK: A molecular, biological, and epidemiological study. *Lancet Infect Dis.* 2010;10(9):597–602.

4. Phua CK, Chee CBE, Chua APG, et al. Managing a case of extensively drug-resistant (XDR) pulmonary tuberculosis in Singapore. *Ann. Acad. Med. Singap.* 2011;40(3):132–135.

5. Buse K, Hein W, Drager N. *Making sense of global health governance: A policy perspective.* Basingstoke, England: Palgrave Macmillan. 2009.

6. Ydstie, J, India eye care center finds middle way to capitalism. NPR, November 29, 2011. http://m.npr.org/news/Health/142526263. Accessed January 23, 2012.

7. American Medical Association. Setting the standards for medical tourism. 2008. http://www.ama-assn.org/amednews/2008/08/04/edsa0804.htm. Accessed January 15, 2012.

About the Editors and Contributors

EDITORS

Jill R. Hodges, MPH, MSL, is a Seattle-based writer and editor who explores how globalization affects individuals' lives. She has worked in public health and journalism, including as a health analyst at the U.S. Government Accountability Office; senior producer at ABCNEWS.com; and staff writer at the *Star Tribune* in Minneapolis, MN. She holds an MPH from the University of Washington School of Public Health and an MSL from Yale Law School.

Leigh Turner, PhD, is an Associate Professor in the University of Minnesota's Center for Bioethics, School of Public Health, and College of Pharmacy. His research examines ethical and social issues related to transnational medical travel and globalization of health care. He is coeditor of *The View From Here: Bioethics and the Social Sciences.*

Ann Marie Kimball, MD, MPH, FACPM, is a Senior Program Officer, Epidemiology and Surveillance, Infectious Diseases, Global Health at the Gates Foundation. Dr. Kimball founded and directs the Asia Pacific Economic Cooperation Emerging Infections Network and has published widely on global trade and infectious diseases, international health regulations, and disease surveillance. An emerita Professor of Epidemiology in the Schools of Public Health and Medicine, University of Washington, she published *Risky Trade: Infectious Diseases in an Era of Global Trade* (2006, Ashgate Ltd.), which has been highly acclaimed in technical reviews in the *Lancet, NEJM,* and *Emerging Infections.*

CONTRIBUTORS

Molly Allen, MS-HSM, is the Project Coordinator for University Health-System Consortium in Chicago's Market Development Cooperator Program award from the U.S. Department of Commerce, which seeks to expand the medical exports market in the United States. Mrs. Allen oversees the three-year award, which is a collaborative effort between the International Trade Administration, UHC, and Rush University. Allen's previous experience includes work at Rush University Medical Center, Health Care Services Corporation, and local government administration. She holds a Master of Science in Health Systems Management degree from Rush University, a Master of Public Administration degree from Northern Illinois University, and a Bachelor of Arts degree from the University of Notre Dame.

I. Glenn Cohen, JD, is an Assistant Professor at Harvard Law School and Co-Director of the Petrie-Flom Center for Health Law Policy, Biotechnology, and Bioethics at Harvard Law School. Professor Cohen is one of the world's leading experts on the intersection of bioethics, health, and the law. He has spoken at legal, medical, and industry conferences around the world; and his work has been covered on ABC, CBS, FOX, NBC, PBS, NPR, in *Mother Jones,* the *Economist,* the *Boston Globe,* the *New York Times,* and several other media venues. His award-winning academic work has appeared in leading journals such as the *New England Journal of Medicine;* the *American Journal of Public Health;* the *Stanford, Southern California, Georgetown, Cornell, Minnesota, Iowa,* and *Hastings Law Reviews;* the *Virginia Journal of International Law;* the *Food and Drug Law Journal;* the *Journal of Law, Medicine, and Ethics;* and the *Hastings Center Report.*

Nathan Cortez, JD, is an Assistant Professor at Southern Methodist University, Dedman School of Law, where he teaches and writes about health care regulation, administrative law, and the legislative process. He has written a number of articles and book chapters on medical tourism and cross-border health care, and has given commentary to NPR, CNN, the Associated Press, and the *Chicago Tribune,* among others, on these topics. Previously, he was a health care regulatory attorney at Arnold & Porter in Washington, DC.

Valorie A. Crooks, PhD, is Associate Professor in the Department of Geography at Simon Fraser University (British Columbia, Canada). She is a health geographer whose research focuses mainly on health services. Her research is primarily funded from grants awarded by the Canadian Institutes of Health Research. She established the SFU Medical Tourism Research Group (www.sfu.ca/medicaltourism).

Manuel M. Dayrit, MD, MSc, is Director of the Department of Human Resources for Health at the headquarters of the World Health Organization in Geneva. He was Secretary of Health (Minister) of the Department of Health of the Republic of the Philippines from 2001–2005. He has worked in government and the private for-profit and nonprofit sectors as well as in academia. In these various capacities, his work has focused on improving the health care of populations through improving the delivery of health services to individuals and communities.

Andrew Garman, PsyD, is a faculty member and practitioner at Rush University Medical Center and chief executive officer of the National Center for Healthcare Leadership in Chicago. Over the past several years, he has led several projects investigating patterns in international travel for medical care, including an industry studies project funded by the Alfred P. Sloan Foundation. With support from the U.S. Department of Commerce and in collaboration with UHC, this work has expanded into an evaluation of trends in the health services trade. Additionally, Dr. Garman is a recognized authority in evidence-based leadership assessment and development. He received his BS in psychology/mathematics from Penn State, an MS in personnel and human resource development from Illinois Institute of Technology, and a PsyD in clinical psychology from the College of William and Mary/Virginia Consortium. Dr. Garman is also an Illinois-licensed clinical psychologist and a senior fellow with the Health Research and Educational Trust.

Stephen T. Green, MD, MBChB, BSc, MRCP(UK), FRCP(Lond &Glas), FFTM(RCPSGlas), DTM&H, FSLCV, is Director of QHA Trent Accreditation UK. He is also Consultant Physician in Infectious Diseases and Tropical Medicine in Sheffield, UK; Honorary Professor of International Health at Sheffield Hallam University; and Honorary Senior Clinical Lecturer at Sheffield University Medical School. Dr. Green qualified for his MBChB at Dundee University Medical School in Scotland, UK. He holds Fellowships of the Royal College of Physicians of London, the Royal College of Physicians and Surgeons of Glasgow, and the Faculty of Travel Medicine of the Royal College of Physicians and Surgeons of Glasgow, as well as the Diploma in Tropical Medicine and Hygiene of the Royal College of Physicians of London. He also holds the degree of BSc (First Class Honours in Physiology) and the postgraduate degree of MD (with Commendation), both from Dundee University.

Samuel F. Hohmann, PhD, MS-HSM, is Principal Consultant—Research for the Comparative Data and Informatics group at University HealthSystem Consortium in Chicago. There he facilitates member engagement in data resources provided by the Clinical Data and Informatics enterprise. His focus is on encouraging the use of UHC data for medical and health services research. Dr. Hohmann also provides advice on development of UHC's integrated data environment, serves as an end user in testing new software performance, conducts audits of internal data bases, and contributes to UHC's drive for internal data quality. In addition to his responsibilities at UHC, Dr. Hohmann is an Assistant Professor of Health Systems Management at Rush University.

Daniel Horsfall, PhD, is a member of the academic staff at the University of York. He teaches comparative social policy and has published in this field. He is currently a member of a team undertaking a research project geared toward understanding the impact of medical tourism.

Tricia J. Johnson, PhD, is Associate Professor and health economist in the Department of Health Systems Management and Director of the Center for Health Management and Policy Research at Rush University in Chicago. Dr. Johnson is a leader in forecasting trends in health care innovation and globalization and predicting the ways in which innovations in quality, safety, and efficiency will shape the future of health care. This work includes a collaboration with UHC and the U.S. Department of Commerce to evaluate health services trade for the United States. Dr. Johnson was a 2008–2009 Fulbright Scholar in Austria, where she worked with faculty in the Institute for Social Policy at the Vienna University of Economics and Business. Dr. Johnson earned her BA in economics and business administration from Coe College, an MA in hospital and health administration from the University of Iowa, and MS and PhD in economics from Arizona State University.

Rory Johnston is a graduate student in the Geography Department at Simon Fraser University in Vancouver, Canada. His research interests are broadly concerned with global health equity and international trade in health services, most specifically with regard to medical tourism.

Churnrurtai Kanchanachitra, PhD, is an Associate Professor and Vice President for Collaboration and Networking, Mahidol University, Thailand. She has more than 30 years of experience in health policy development at the country level both as a researcher and a policy actor. She is an expert in health policy, gender and health, and poverty and equity in health. She has participated in the development of the National Health Assembly since 2001. She is a Chair of the National Health Assembly Organizing Committee and was a President of National Health Assembly in 2010 and 2011. In addition, she serves as Member of the Reform Assembly Organizing Committee (RAOC) and Chair of the Technical Subcommittee under the RAOC. At the international level, she is actively involved in global health issues. She is a member of the steering committee of the

Global Health Diplomacy Network. She also represents the South East Asia (SEA) constituency in the Policy and Strategy Committee of the Global Fund to Fight AIDS, TB, and Malaria; and represents Thailand in the board meetings.

Hannah King, PhD, is a member of the teaching staff in the Department of Social Policy and Social Work at the University of York, UK. A former Local Government Senior Policy Officer, she has published in the field of youth studies and on the subject of medical tourism.

Courtney A. Lee is a PhD candidate in the Health and Behavioral Sciences Department at the University of Colorado Denver and holds a masters degree in anthropology from the University of Colorado at Boulder. She has studied medical tourism in various contexts, including Costa Rica, where she conducted her dissertation research, and in Austria at the Institute for Applied Systems Analysis in the Health and Global Change Program.

Helena Legido-Quigley, BSc, MSc, PhD, is a research fellow at the London School of Hygiene and Tropical Medicine. She is currently working on an EU-funded project on cross-border health care that seeks to contribute to a process whereby a patient in one member state can make an informed choice about whether to seek health care in another member state. In this project, she is exploring how specialists work in different member states, how regulatory bodies function across Europe, how policies affecting these groups are developed and implemented, and the possibilities and barriers of telemedicine across borders.

Neil Lunt, PhD, is Senior Lecturer in the Department of Social Policy and Social Work, University of York, UK. He has published widely in the areas of medical tourism, global social policy, and welfare reform, including reports supported by the OECD, World Health Organization, and International Labour Organization. He was Principal Investigator on a project funded by the National Institute for Health Research, "Implications for the NHS of Inward and Outward Medical Tourism."

Dominique Martin, MBBS/BA, PhD, recently graduated from the Centre for Applied Philosophy and Public Ethics at the University of Melbourne. Her thesis examined the ethical procurement of human biological materials, in particular the issue of selling such materials. She is a member of the Declaration of Istanbul Custodian Group and works part time in emergency medicine.

Steven Meurer, MBA/MHS, PhD, is University HealthSystem's Senior Vice President for Comparative Data and Informatics, a position he has held since April of 2007. Dr. Meurer's background includes 15 years of health care administration experience, including the Chief Quality & Information Officer at the DeKalb Regional Healthcare System in Atlanta, and the Vice President of Operations and Performance Improvement at St. Mary's Medical Center in Langhorne, PA. Dr. Meurer has spent time in increasing roles of responsibility at a number of organizations, including the Orlando Regional Healthcare System, University Pittsburgh Healthcare System, and BJC Healthcare. Dr. Meurer's passion is in understanding and promoting improvement and the role of data in those efforts. He has published a number of articles and speaks regularly on this topic. In addition, Dr. Meurer has taught quality to masters students at Loyola (Chicago), Rush, Georgia Tech, and Georgia State.

Cha-aim Pachanee, PhD, has been working at the Bureau of Policy and strategy and International Health Policy Program (IHPP), Ministry of Public Health, Thailand, for 10 years. She has her PhD in Epidemiology and Population Health at the National Centre for Epidemiology and Population Health, the Australian National University, Australia. Her main interests are in international health, international trade in health services, human resources for health, health systems, and health policies.

Richard D. Smith, PhD, is Professor of Health System Economics and Head of the Faculty of Public Health and Policy at the London School of Hygiene and Tropical Medicine. He is also an Honorary Professor of Health Economics at the Universities of Hong Kong and East Anglia; an Associate Fellow at the Royal Institute of International Affairs, Chatham House; Associate Editor of *Health Economics*; and Member of the editorial boards for the *Journal of Public Health* and *Globalization and Health*. Richard has worked in a number of areas of health economics, most recently concerning the application of macroeconomics to health; the economics of globalization and health; and aspects of trade in health goods, services, people, and ideas. Richard has received over £25 million in grant income, published 5 books, and more than 100 journal papers.

Jeremy Snyder, PhD, is an Assistant Professor in the Faculty of Health Sciences at Simon Fraser University, BC. His research focuses on applied ethics, including medical tourism, theories of exploitation, and human subject research.

Viroj Tangcharoensathien, MD, PhD, is the Senior Advisor to the International Health Policy Program of the Ministry of Public Health of Thailand. He has more than 25 years of research experience in health systems and health policy, and in policy process and translating research into policy at the national and regional levels. His areas of expertise are health care financing, health economics, and health policy. He earned his medical degree from Mahidol University and obtained a PhD in health care financing from the London School of Hygiene and Tropical Medicine. He is the Edwin Chadwick medalist granted by the London School of Hygiene and Tropical Medicine in 2011. He has published more than 100 articles in international peer-reviewed journals.

Andrea Whittaker, PhD, is an Australian Research Council Future Fellow at the School of Psychology and Psychiatry at Monash University in Melbourne. Prior to that, she was an Associate Professor in Medical Anthropology at the School of Population Health, University of Queensland. She received her PhD in Medical Anthropology and BA (Hons) in Anthropology from the University of Queensland. Her research interests include reproductive health in Thailand, the consequences of unplanned pregnancy in Thailand, medical travel and HIV, and social isolation in Australia. She is also involved in research on autism in Vietnam, postpartum complications and abortion in PNG, and has previously worked on reproductive morbidity in Timor Leste. Her major publications include *Intimate Knowledge: Women and Their Health in Northeast Thailand* (2000), *Women's Health in Mainland Southeast Asia* (2002), *Abortion, Sin and the State in Thailand* (2004), and *Abortion in Asia: Local Dilemmas, Global Politics* (2010).

Alexandra Wright, BA, received her undergraduate degree in Health Sciences at Simon Fraser University. During that time, she was a Research Assistant for the SFU Medical Tourism Research Group. She is currently reading for an MSc in Comparative Social Policy at the University of Oxford.

Index

Lightning Source UK Ltd.
Milton Keynes UK
UKHW02n2021110518
322491UK00008B/51/P